CRC Desk Reference
for NUTRITION

CRC Desk Reference Series

Series Editor
Gerald Kerkut
University of Southampton
Southampton, England

Published Titles

CRC Desk Reference for Nutrition
Carolyn Berdanier, University of Georgia, Athens, Georgia

CRC Desk Reference of Clinical Pharmacology
Manuchair Ebadi, University of Nebraska, Omaha, Nebraska

Forthcoming Titles

CRC Desk Reference for Hematology
N. K. Shinton, University of Warwick, Coventry, United Kingdom

CRC Desk Reference *for* NUTRITION

Carolyn D. Berdanier

With Contributions by
Anne Dattilo
and
Wilhelmine P.H.G. Verboeket-van de Venne

Illustrations by
Toni Kathryn Adkins White

CRC Press

Boca Raton Boston London New York Washington, D.C.

QP
141
.B523
1998

Acquiring Editor:	Marsha Baker
Project Editor:	Andrea Demby
Marketing Manager:	Becky McEldowney
Cover design:	Denise Craig
PrePress:	Kevin Luong
Manufacturing:	Carol Royal

Catalogue record is available from the Library of Congress

DESK REFERENCE BOOKS

This series of volumes will form a set of concise medical science encyclopedias.

Very few people read a medical or science book right through from cover to cover. They tend to dip into the book, reading a few pages here and a few pages there. More often they look up subjects in the Index at the back of the book and with a finger in the index page, they look up the different page references, often having difficulty in finding the reference subject on the given page. This is partly because the index usually gives the page references in numerical order (though the more important references are often printed in bold) and partly because the indexer likes to give every possible reference — major, minor, and miniscule.

The present book is in effect an annotated index. The topics are arranged in alphabetical order so that they are easy to find. The intention is that each topic should be concise so that after having read it, the reader will be able to remember the important information in that topic. There is a "take away message." Too often in larger encyclopedias, the item has to be read several times to get the key information, i.e., they are discursive instead of being didactic. The intention in the present book is to give the time-pressed reader the necessary data quickly and concisely.

On the other hand some subjects have to be given in more detail to provide the background information necessary to have a fuller understanding of the subject.

In addition the book contains "orientation" subjects that give the background and bring the reader up to date. Medicine and Science advance very quickly these days and although recent graduates can be assumed to have the modern information, even those graduating five years ago can sometimes find themselves unsure about new facts, ideas, and terminology that are now currently mentioned in the news and have come into vogue.

It is difficult to get a correct balance between being sufficiently informative so as to be useful, being too concise so that the required information is not present, and being so long that the reader can't find the time to read the item.

It is hoped that these Desk References get near the correct balance and will be a useful source of information for the reader.

Gerald Kerkut
Supervising Editor of the Series

Preface

This is a book of terms together with their definitions that should answer many of the questions that arise with respect to nutrition as it relates to human health and well being. The book includes many common medical terms as well as descriptions of biochemical pathways and physiological processes. Some short descriptions of nutrition-related genetic diseases are included as well.

The reader might well wonder why such a diverse list of terms have been collected together in one text. The answer to this question relates to the nature of the science we call nutrition. Nutrition science is a hybrid science with origins in what is now known as biochemistry and molecular biology. The early discoveries of vitamin deficiency diseases and their cures were published in the *Journal of Biochemistry* and in *Medical Annals*. Journals of Physiology and Pathology also published reports of research concerning the importance of specific nutrients or a nutrient class on normal cell and organ function as well as normal growth and development. This work is ongoing and becoming evermore specialized as the tools of biotechnology are used to test hypotheses about the roles of specific nutrients in the control of gene expression.

As nutrition science has evolved and become more sophisticated, the application of the results of this scientific endeavor has become more difficult. Those who specialize in high technology science have significantly departed from those who help people make appropriate food choices to optimize their health and well being. Many people need this help for a variety of reasons. They need someone who can interpret their physician's instructions with respect to food choices. This individual, a dietitian, has the skills and training to make these interpretations. As well, the dietitian has localized knowledge about the cost of food, its variety, the cultural practices of the local population and may be in a good position to guide and advise less knowledgeable persons in their food choice. While the dietitian may not be a skilled nutrition scientist or a physician, he/she is a vital component of the health care team. It is hoped that this book will have information of value not only to the physician, nurse, dietitian, physical therapist, and pharmacist but also to the student who has one of these careers as an objective.

ACKNOWLEDGMENTS

The authors would like to express their appreciation to Dr. Gerald Kerkut who proposed that such a book be prepared and to Mr. David Grist who agreed to publish it. Without the encouragement of these two the book never would have been written. Our appreciation is also extended to Toni Kathryn Adkins White who prepared both the illustrations and the initial draft. Lastly, Tonya Whitfield, my wonderfully competent secretary, should be thanked and thanked again for her patience and endurance throughout this project. Thanks Tonya!

HOW TO USE THIS BOOK

Terms of nutritional importance are listed in alphabetical order. Cross referencing is used when more than one term is used for the same definition. An appendix containing general considerations for food selection can be found at the end of the text. Because this is an alphabetical list of terms, there is no index.

CONTENTS

LIST OF LONGER ARTICLES

LIST OF TABLES

LIST OF FIGURES

A

ABETALIPOPROTEINEMIA

A mutation in the gene for apolipoprotein b. The human intestinal cell has two lipid carrying proteins called ApoA-I and b. Apolipoprotein b is essential for chylomicron release by the intestinal cell. ApoA-I is the lipoprotein of the gut VLDL. Should apolipoprotein b be aberrant in function as happens in the genetic disorder called A-b-lipoproteinemia, there will be a total or partial (depending on the mutation) absence of lipoproteins in the blood. The prefix A is used for the disorder name and refers to a lack of the ApoA-I transport protein. Patients with A-b-lipoproteinemia are characterized by very low blood lipids and lipid malabsorption (steatorrhea). The feces contain an abnormally large amount of fat and have a characteristic peculiar odor. In this disorder, not only is the triglyceride absorption affected but so too are the fat soluble vitamins. Without the ability to absorb these energy rich food components and the vital fat soluble vitamins, the patient does not thrive and survive. The disorder is inherited as an autosomal recessive trait.

ABCESS

A circumscribed collection of pus.

ABSORPTION

Nutrients in the diet are absorbed by cells lining the gastrointestinal tract (the enterocytes) by one of three mechanisms: active transport, facilitated diffusion, and passive diffusion. The absorption of both micro- and macronutrients is described below as separate entries.

1. **Active Transport**. A process which moves essential nutrients against a concentration gradient and which requires energy (usually from ATP) and a nutrient carrier. Most carriers are specific for specific nutrients. Almost all required nutrients are actively transported. The exceptions are the minerals. These nutrients are absorbed by processes that involve both passive diffusion and carrier mediated transport.
2. **Passive Diffusion**. Movement of compounds across the cell membrane so as to equalize the concentration of the substrate on both sides of the membrane. This process only applies to small molecules such as electrolytes, water, small sugars and amino acids. It does not apply to large molecules such as starch or large proteins.
3. **Facilitated Diffusion**. Movement of nutrients against a concentration gradient; usually does not require energy but does require a carrier.

Carbohydrate Absorption

Once the monosaccharides are released through the action of the digestive enzymes they are absorbed by one of several mechanisms. Glucose and galactose are absorbed by an energy-dependent, sodium-dependent, carrier-mediated mechanism. This mechanism is termed active transport because glucose is transported against a concentration gradient. Because the transport is against a concentration gradient, energy is required to "push" the movement of glucose into the enterocyte. Glucose and galactose appear to compete for the same active transport system. They also compete for a secondary transporter, a sodium-independent transporter found in the contraluminal membrane. The two transporters differ in molecular weight. The sodium-dependent transporter has a weight of 75 kDa while the sodium-independent transporter weighs 57 kDa. This sodium-independent transporter is a member of a family of transporters called GLUT 1, 2, 3, 4, or 5. Each of these transporters is specific to certain tissues (See mobile glucose transporters). Fructose is not absorbed via an active transport system but by facilitated diffusion. This process is independent of the sodium ion and is specific for fructose. In the enterocyte much of the absorbed fructose is metabolized such that little fructose can be found in the portal blood even if the animal is given an intraluminal infusion of this sugar. Of the other monosaccharides present in the lumen, passive diffusion is the means for their entry into the enterocyte. Pentoses such as those found in plums or cherries, and other minor carbohydrates will find their way into the system only to be passed out of the body via the urine if the carbohydrate cannot be used.

Amino acid absorption

Most amino acids are actively transported and require a carrier for this transport. These are listed in Table 1.

TABLE 1
Carriers for Amino Acids

Carrier	Amino Acids Carried
1	Serine, Threonine, Alanine
2[a]	Phenylalanine, tyrosine, methionine, valine, leucine, isoleucine
3	Proline, hydroxyproline
4	Taurine, β alanine
5	Lysine, arginine, cysteine-cysteine
6	Aspartic and glutamic acid

[a] When a mutation in the gene that codes for this carrier occurs, the individual is unable to absorb these amino acids from the gut contents or reabsorb these amino acids through the renal tubule. Patients with this disorder will manifest symptoms of protein malnutrition. These people can absorb these amino acids as partners in a dipeptide or tripeptide. However, because of the defect in the renal tubule they cannot conserve their supply. This genetic disease is called Hartnup's disease or neutral amino aciduria.

Fat absorption

After the dietary lipids are hydrolyzed, fat absorption occurs by passive diffusion. Only 30–40% of the dietary cholesterol is absorbed. The percent cholesterol absorbed depends on a number of factors including the fiber content of the diet, the gut passage time, and the total amount of cholesterol present for absorption. At higher intake levels, less is absorbed and vice versa at lower intake levels. Compared to fatty acids and the acylglycerides, the rate of cholesterol absorption is very slow. It is estimated that the half-life of cholesterol in the enterocyte is 12 hours. With high fiber intakes, less cholesterol is absorbed because the fiber acts as an adsorbent, reducing cholesterol availability. Celluloses and lignens are good adsorbents of cholesterol, and they also decrease transit time. Pectins and gums lower serum cholesterol levels by creating a gel-like consistency of the chyme rendering the cholesterol in the chyme less available. High fiber diets reduce gut passage time which in turn results in less time for cholesterol absorption. The fate of the absorbed fatty acids depends on chain length. Those fatty acids having 10 or fewer carbons are quickly passed into the portal blood stream without further modification. They are carried to the liver bound to albumin. Those fatty acids remaining are bound to a fatty acid binding protein and transported through the cytosol to the endoplasmic reticulum whereupon they are converted to their CoA derivatives and re-esterified to glycerol to reform the triacylglyceride. These reformed triacylglycerides adhere to phospholipids and a fat transporting protein called apolipoprotein b. This relatively large lipid-protein complex migrates to the Golgi complex in the basolateral basement membrane of the enterocyte. The lipid rich vesicles fuse with the Golgi surface membrane whereupon the lipid-protein complex is exocytosed and secreted into the intercellular space which, in turn, drains into the lymphatic system. The lymphatic system contributes these lipids to the circulation as the thoracic duct enters the jugular vein prior to its entry into the heart.

After gastric resection
When the stomach is fully or partly removed, the individual loses (depending on the part removed) storage capacity and/or HCl production and/or the churning and mixing action of this organ. Food digestibility is reduced.

After intestinal resection
Depending on what section and how much of the intestine is removed, digestion is impaired as is absorption.

In lactose intolerance
Lactose must be hydrolyzed to glucose and galactose which are then actively transported from the gut. In the absence of normal lactase activity, lactose accumulates and exerts an osmotic effect on the gut. Water diffuses into the gut and stimulates peristalsis. Diarrhea results. Some of the lactose is fermented by gut flora producing gas and discomfort.

In gluten-induced enteropathy
Diarrhea, flatulence, and discomfort are the results of an inability to digest the wheat protein, gluten. If diarrhea persists, the gut cells are abraided and absorption of other nutrients is impaired. Gluten accumulates in the gut with resultant osmotic effects as described above for lactose intolerance.

Mineral absorption
Of all the minerals needed by animals, few enter the absorptive cell by passive diffusion. Several are carried into the body by proteins to which the minerals are loosely attached. Iron, zinc, and copper are imported via these transporters. Sodium and potassium enter (or are exchanged) by an ATPase specific for these ions. Chloride, iodide, and fluoride enter by way of an anion-cation exchange mechanism. The uptake of calcium and phosphorus (as phosphate) occurs by a protein-mediated process. It is known that optimal absorption occurs when the calcium:phosphorus ratio is between 1:2 and 2:1 and that an adequate vitamin D supply is essential. Intestinal calcium uptake is mediated by a vitamin D-dependent, calcium binding protein (calbindin). It is suspected that the uptake is also dependent on a phosphorylation/dephosphorylation process; hence, the importance of the calcium:phosphorus ratio that should be between 1:2 and 2:1.

Although all of these mechanisms of uptake are operative for the minerals, few of the minerals are 100% absorbable. The exceptions are sodium, potassium, chloride, selenium, and magnesium. For the others, the absorption process is dependent on a number of factors: the binding capacity of the transport protein (if needed), solubility, the composition of the diet, the mixture of the elements present in the gut contents, the presence of materials such as phytate and EDTA which bind specific minerals thus changing the mineral mixture presented to the enterocyte, and the actual amount of the mineral to be absorbed. All of these factors contribute to the bioavailability of the anion and cations that are essential micronutrients. In addition, there are physiological factors (age, hormonal status, and health status) that also influence absorption and subsequent use. Those minerals that are variable in terms of their absorption are those that are either divalent ions or multivalent, that is, an ion that has more than one charged state. Iron and chromium fit into this category while calcium, magnesium, selenium, manganese, zinc, copper, and molybdenum fit into the former category.

Vitamin absorption

All three mechanisms of absorption are used for the uptake of the vitamins. The fat soluble vitamins A, D, E, and K are absorbed along with the dietary fat and combined with proteins in the chylomicrons. Vitamin A requires a specific retinol-binding carrier protein, while vitamins D, E, and K do not have such a requirement. The water-soluble vitamins are largely absorbed by facilitated diffusion. The exception is ascorbic acid. This vitamin is actively absorbed via an energy- and sodium-dependent transport mechanism.

ACANTHOCYTOSIS

A rare blood condition characterized by deformed red blood cells having irregular cell surfaces and pseudopod-like projections. These cells are very fragile.

ACARBOSE

A drug which interferes with starch digestion.

ACAT

Acyl coenzyme A: cholesterol acyl transferase. An enzyme that catalyzes the formation of an ester linkage between a fatty acid and cholesterol.

ACCEPTABLE DAILY INTAKE (ADI)

Estimation of the maximum allowable level of a food component or contaminant. These values serve as guides in health policy. For noncarcinogenic components, the ADI is derived from the No-Observed-Adverse Effect Level (NOAEL) determined in experimental animals. NOAEL is divided by safety factors (e.g., 10 for taking into account the extrapolation from animals to humans and 10 for taking into account a susceptible human subpopulation, such as infants), resulting in an integral safety factor of 100. Factors considered in establishing the ADI are:

1. biochemical studies, including absorption kinetics, tissue distribution, excretion route, excretion rate, metabolic conversion, biological half-life, effect on enzymes, and other critical targets;
2. toxicological studies such as carcinogenicity, mutagenicity, neurotoxicity, potentiation, and antagonism among different factors; reproductive effects: teratogenicity, acute and chronic toxic effects; on either progeny or mother involving several species and multigeneration studies;
3. epidemiological studies, including observations on occupational or accidental exposure;
4. human volunteer studies.

ACETALDEHYDE

An aldehyde formed from the oxidation of ethanol; can be converted to acetate and thence to acetyl CoA.

ACETALDEHYDE DEHYDROGENASE

An enzyme that metabolizes ethyl alcohol.

ACETOACETATE

A four carbon ketone found in large amounts in the uncontrolled insulin-dependent diabetic; acetoacetate is a normal end product of fatty acid oxidation which is usually oxidized further to CO_2 and water.

$$CH_3-\overset{\overset{\displaystyle O}{\|}}{C}CH_2COOH$$

ACETONE

One of the common ketones found in blood and tissues. Its structure is

$$CH_3-\overset{\overset{\displaystyle O}{\|}}{C}-CH_3.$$

It can accumulate if the citric acid cycle is not working fully. Levels of acetone can become toxic; high levels of acetone are a typical sign of uncontrolled insulin dependent diabetes mellitus.

ACETONEMIA

Higher than normal (3–20 mg/l) levels of acetone in the blood.

ACETONURIA

Higher than normal (1 mg/l/24 hr) levels of acetone in the urine.

ACETYL CoA

A two carbon metabolic intermediate that is the starting substrate for fatty acid synthesis or the product of fatty acid oxidation. When joined to oxalacetate it enters the citric acid cycle as citrate and the CoA portion of the molecule removed and reused.

$$CH_3-\overset{\overset{\displaystyle O}{\|}}{C}\sim S-CoA$$

ACETYLCHOLINE

A neurotransmitter released by a calcium-dependent process in response to the arrival of an action potential. Acetylcholine initiates changes in ion permeability that occur at the neuro-muscular junction. Acetylcholine is hydrolyzed by acetylcholine esterase. The choline is then recycled.

ACETYLCHOLINESTERASE INHIBITORS

Natural toxins with alkaloids as active components. They have been detected in several edible fruits and vegetables, such as potato, eggplant, and tomato. The most potent inhibitors are found in potatoes, and, of these, the most active component is the glycoalkaloid solanine. The solanine concentration of potato tubers varies with the degree of maturity at harvest, rate of nitrogen fertilization, storage conditions, greening by exposure to light, and variety. Commercial potatoes contain 2–15 mg of solanine per 100 g fresh weight. Greening of potatoes may increase the solanine content to 80–100 mg/100 g. Most of the alkaloid is concentrated in the skin, whereas sprouts may contain lethal amounts of solanine. It is generally accepted that 20 mg solanine per 100 g fresh weight is the upper safe limit. Since potatoes also contain other glycoalkaloids (chaconine and tomatine), with biological properties similar to solanine, the symptoms seen in potato poisoning may be due to combined actions of the alkaloids. Potato poisoning is a very rare event.

ACHALASIA

Constriction or malfunction of muscles controlling peristalsis by the esophagus. Because the muscles do not readily relax and because there is a loss in the synchrony of constriction and relaxation, ingested food does not readily pass into the stomach.

ACHLORHYDRIA

Absence of HCl in stomach either through gastric cell malfunction or through the surgical removal of the acid secreting cells of the stomach. Iron absorption is impaired in achlorhydria.

ACID-BASE BALANCE

Minute to minute regulation of the hydrogen ion concentration (pH) in the body; accomplished through the action of the bicarbonate buffering system, the phosphate buffering system, and the action of proteins as buffers.

ACIDIC AMINO ACIDS

Amino acids having two carboxyl groups in their structure. These amino acids are aspartic acid and glutamic acid. See Table 5 (page 25) for structure.

ACIDOSIS

When the blood pH falls below 7.4 acidosis develops. Metabolic acidosis refers to changes in the bicarbonate concentration in blood; respiratory acidosis refers to changes in carbon dioxide pressure. Dehydration, uncontrolled diabetes, low carbohydrate diets, cardiac failure, and pulmonary insufficiency can result in acidosis.

ACNE

Skin disease characterized by eruptions of infected sebaceous cells.

ACP

Acyl carrier protein. A pantothenic acid-protein-thio-ethanolamine structure which is an essential component of fatty acid biosynthesis.

ACRODERMA ENTEROPATICA

A genetic disease characterized by an inability to normally absorb zinc.

ACROLEIN

Excessively oxidized fats due to excessive heat.

ACROMEGALY

Disease that results from excess growth hormone production and release from the anterior pituitary; characterized by coarsening of facial features through growth of facial bones. Excess fatty acid mobilization and glucose intolerance is observed. Whereas excess growth is characteristic of excess growth hormone in the young, acromegaly occurs in adults whose long bones are closed making further growth impossible. In adults, this condition is characterized by a coarsening of facial features. Treatment consists of removing the source of the excess growth hormone.

ACTIVE SITE

A three-dimensional region of a catalyst or receptor or carrier where the substrate binds prior to catalysis or binding or carriage.

ACTIVE TRANSPORT

See absorption.

ACTIVITY INCREMENT

Energy needed to sustain body activities. Typical energy costs are shown in Table 2.

ACTH

A polypeptide hormone synthesized and released by the pituitary. ACTH stimulates the adrenal cortex to release the glucocorticoids (cortisol, corticosterone, and hydrocortisone) and the mineralocorticoid, aldosterone.

ACTUARIAL DATA

Information used to create mortality tables and life expectancy numbers.

ACUTE RENAL FAILURE

Sudden cessation of renal function.

ACUTE TOXICITY

A potentially lethal condition caused by a very large intake of a substance that the body cannot metabolize or excrete.

ACUTE TUBULAR NECROSIS

Most common form of acute renal failure that results when an ischemic or nephrotoxin damages the renal tubules.

ACYLATION

The addition of an acyl group (carbon chain) to a substrate.

ACYL CARRIER PROTEIN

A protein that has pantothenic acid as its prosthetic group. It is active in fatty acid synthesis as it carries the acyl groups that are bound to the CoA molecule in the multienzyme complex of fatty acid synthase.

AD LIBITUM

A latin term meaning unrestricted access to food; to eat freely.

ADDISON'S DISEASE

Adrenocortical insufficiency resulting from inadequate production of one or more hormones by the adrenal cortex.

ADDITIVES

Substances added to food to enhance its flavor, texture, or appearance or to retard spoilage or augment its nutritional value.

GRAS

Abbreviation for the U.S. Food and Drug Agency term meaning Generally Recognized As Safe. A list of additives approved by U.S. Food and Drug Agency. The substances so listed are generally regarded as safe. Table 3 lists the various types of food additives and their functions. Table 4 lists some of the more common additives.

TABLE 2
Energy Cost of Activities Exclusive of Basal Metabolism and Influence of Food

Activity	kcal/kg/hr	Activity	kcal/kg/hr
Bedmaking	3.0	Paring potatoes	0.6
Bicycling (century run)	7.6	Playing cards	0.5
Bicycling (moderate speed)	2.5	Playing Ping Pong	4.4
Boxing	11.4	Piano playing	
Carpentry (heavy)	2.3	Mendelssohn's Song Without Words	0.8
Cello playing	1.3	Beethoven's Appassionata	1.4
Cleaning windows	2.6	Liszt's Tarantella	2.0
Crocheting	0.4	Reading aloud	0.4
Dancing		Rowing	9.8
Moderately active	3.8	Rowing in a race	16.0
Rhumba	5.0	Running	7.0
Waltz	3.0	Sawing wood	5.7
Dishwashing	1.0	Sewing	
Dressing and undressing	0.7	Hand	0.4
Driving car	0.9	Foot-driven machine	0.6
Eating	0.4	Electric machine	0.4
Exercise		Singing in loud voice	0.8
Very light	0.9	Sitting quietly	0.4
Light	1.4	Skating	3.5
Moderate	3.1	Skiing (moderate speed)	10.3
Severe	5.4	Standing at attention	0.6
Very severe	7.6	Standing relaxed	0.5
Fencing	7.3	Sweeping with broom, bare floor	1.4
Football	6.8	Sweeping with carpet sweeper	1.6
Gardening, weeding	3.9	Sweeping with vacuum sweeper	2.7
Golf	1.5	Swimming (2 mi/hr)	7.9
Horseback riding		Tailoring	0.9
Walk	1.4	Tennis	5.0
Trot	4.3	Typing	
Gallop	6.7	Rapidly	1.0
Ironing (5-lb iron)	1.0	Electric typewriter	0.5
Knitting sweater	0.7	Violin playing	0.6
Laboratory work	2.1	Walking (3 mi/hr)	2.0
Laundry, light	1.3	Walking rapidly (4 mi/hr)	3.4
Lying still, awake	0.1	Walking at high speed (5.3 mi/hr)	8.3
Office work, standing	0.6	Washing floors	1.2
Organ playing (1/3 handwork)	1.5	Writing	0.4
Painting furniture	1.5		

Adapted from *Rose's Laboratory Handbook for Dietetics*, 5th ed., Macmillan, New York, 1949.

TABLE 3
Terms Used to Describe the Functions of Food Additives

Term	Function
Anticaking agents and free-flow agents	Substances added to finely powdered or crystalline food products to prevent caking.
Antimicrobial agents	Substances used to preserve food by preventing growth of microorganisms and subsequent spoilage, including fungicides, mold and yeast inhibitors, and bacteriocides.
Antioxidants	Substances used to preserve food by retarding deterioration, rancidity, or discoloration due to oxidation.
Colors and coloring adjuncts	Substances used to impart, preserve, or enhance the color or shading of a food, including color stabilizers, color fixatives, and color-retention agents.
Curing and pickling agents	Substances imparting a unique flavor and/or color to a food, usually producing an increase in shelf-life stability.
Dough strengtheners	Substances used to modify starch and gluten, thereby producing a more stable dough.
Drying agents	Substances with moisture-absorbing ability, used to maintain an environment of low moisture.
Emulsifiers and emulsifier salts	Substances which modify surface tension of two (or more) immiscible solutions to establish a uniform dispersion of components. This is called an emulsion.
Enzymes	Substances used to improve food processing and the quality of the finished food.
Firming agents	Substances added to precipitate residual pectin, thus strengthening the supporting tissue and preventing its collapse during processing.
Flavor enhancers	Substances added to supplement, enhance, or modify the original taste and/or aroma of a food, without imparting a characteristic taste or aroma of its own.
Flavoring agents and adjuvants	Substances added to impart or help impart a taste or aroma in food.
Flour treating agents	Substances added to milled flour, at the mill, to improve its color and/or baking qualities, including bleaching and maturing agents.
Formulation aids	Substances used to promote or produce a desired physical state or texture in food, including carriers, binders, fillers, plasticizers, film-formers, and tableting aids.
Fumigants	Volatile substances used for controlling insects or pests.
Humectants	Hygroscopic substances incorporated in food to promote retention of moisture, including moisture-retention agents and antidusting agents.
Leavening agents	Substances used to produce or stimulate production of carbon dioxide in baked goods to impart a light texture, including yeast, yeast foods, and calcium salts.
Lubricants and release agents	Substances added to food contact surfaces to prevent ingredients and finished products from sticking to them.
Non-nutritive sweeteners	Substances having less than 2% of the energy value of sucrose per equivalent unit of sweetening capacity.
Nutrient supplements	Substances which are necessary for the body's nutritional and metabolic processes.
Nutritive sweeteners	Substances having greater than 2% equivalent unit of sweetening capacity.

TABLE 3 (CONTINUED)
Terms Used to Describe the Functions of Food Additives

Term	Function
Oxidizing and reducing agents	Substances which chemically oxidize or reduce another food ingredient, thereby producing a more stable product.
pH control agents	Substances added to change or maintain active acidity or alkalinity, including buffers, acids, alkalis, and neutralizing agents.
Processing aids	Substances used as manufacturing aids to enhance the appeal or utility of a food or food component, including clarifying agents, clouding agents, catalysts, flocculents, filter aids, and crystallization inhibitors.
Propellants, aerating agents, and gases	Gases used to supply force to expel a product or used to reduce the amount of oxygen in contact with the food in packaging.
Sequestrants	Substances which combine with polyvalent metal ions to form a soluble metal complex to improve the quality and stability of products.
Solvents and vehicles	Substances used to extract or dissolve another substance.
Stabilizers and thickeners	Substances used to produce viscous solutions or dispersions, to impart body, improve consistency, or stabilize emulsions, including suspending and bodying agents, setting agents, gelling agents, and bulking agents.
Surface-active agents	Substances used to modify surface properties of liquid food components for a variety of effects, other than emulsifiers but including solubilizing agents, dispersants, detergents, wetting agents, rehydration enhancers, whipping agents, foaming agents, and defoaming agents.
Surface-finishing agents	Substances used to increase palatability, preserve gloss, and inhibit discoloration of foods, including glazes, polishes, waxes, and protective coatings.
Synergists	Substances used to act or react with another food ingredient to produce a total effect different or greater than the sum of the effects produced by the individual ingredients.
Texturizers	Substances which affect the appearance or feel of the food.

Source: From Ensminger et al., *Foods and Nutrition Encyclopedia*, 2nd ed., CRC Press, Boca Raton, FL, 1994, 11.

TABLE 4
Common Food Additives

Name	Function[a]	Food Use and Comments
Acetic acid	pH control; preservative	Acid of vinegar is acetic acid. Miscellaneous and/or general purposes; many food uses; GRAS additive.
Adipic acid	pH control	Buffer and neutralizing agent; use in confectionery; GRAS additive.
Ammonium alginate	Stabilizer and thickener; texturizer	Extracted from seaweed. Widespread food use; GRAS additive.
Annatto	Color	Extracted from seeds of *Bixa crellana*. Butter, cheese, margarine, shortening, and sausage casings; coloring foods in general.

TABLE 4 (CONTINUED)
Common Food Additives

Name	Function[a]	Food Use and Comments
Arabinogalactan	Stabilizer and thickener; texturizer	Extracted from Western larch. Widespread food use; bodying agent in essential oils, non-nutritive sweeteners, flavor bases, nonstandardized dressings and pudding mixes.
Ascorbic acid (Vitamin C)	Nutrient; antioxidant; preservative	Widespread use in foods to prevent rancidity, browning; used in meat curing; GRAS additive.
Aspartame	Sweetener; sugar substitute	Soft drinks, chewing gum, powdered beverages, whipped toppings, puddings, gelatin, and tabletop sweetener.
Azodicarbonamide	Flour treating agent	Aging and bleaching ingredient in cereal flour.
Benzoic acid	Preservative	Occurs in nature in free and combined forms. Widespread food use; GRAS additive.
Benzoyl peroxide	Flour treating agent	Bleaching agent in flour; may be used in some cheeses.
Beta-apo-8' carotenal	Color	Natural food color. General use not to exceed 30 mg/lb or pt of food.
BHA (butylated hydroxyanisole)	Antioxidant; preservative	Fats, oils, dry yeast, beverages, breakfast cereals, dry mixes, shortening, potato flakes, chewing gum, and sausage; often used in combination with BHT; GRAS additive.
BHT (butylated hydroxytoluene)	Antioxidant; preservative	Rice, fats, oils, potato granules, breakfast cereals, potato flakes, shortening, chewing gum, and sausage; often used in combination with BHA; GRAS additive.
Biotin	Nutrient	Rich natural sources are liver, kidney, pancreas, yeast, and milk; vitamin supplement; GRAS additive.
Calcium alginate	Stabilizer and thickener; texturizer	Extracted from seaweed. Widespread food use; GRAS additive.
Calcium carbonate	Nutrient	Mineral supplement; general purpose additive; GRAS additive.
Calcium lactate	Preservative	General purpose and/or miscellaneous use; GRAS additive.
Calcium phosphate	Leavening agent; sequestrant; nutrient	General purpose and/or miscellaneous use; mineral supplement; GRAS additive.
Calcium propionate	Preservative	Bakery products, alone or with sodium propionate; inhibits mold and other micro-organisms; GRAS additive.
Calcium silicate	Anticaking agent	Used in baking powder and salt. GRAS additive.
Canthaxanthin	Color	Widely distributed in nature. Color for foods; more red than carotene.
Caramel	Color	Miscellaneous and/or general purpose use in foods for color; GRAS additive.
Carob bean gum	Stabilizer and thickener	Extracted from bean of carob tree (Locust bean). Numerous foods like confections, syrups, cheese spreads, frozen desserts, and salad dressings; GRAS additive.
Carrageenan	Emulsifier; stabilizer and thickener	Extracted from seaweed. A variety of foods, primarily those with a water or milk base.
Cellulose	Emulsifier; stabilizer and thickener	Component of all plants. Inert bulking agent in foods; may be used to reduce energy content of food; used in foods which are liquid and foam systems.

TABLE 4 (CONTINUED)
Common Food Additives

Name	Function[a]	Food Use and Comments
Citric acid	Preservative; antioxidant; pH control agent; sequestrant	Widely distributed in nature in both plants and animals. Miscellaneous and/or general purpose food use; used in lard, shortening, sausage, margarine, chili con carne, cured meats, and freeze-dried meats; GRAS additive.
Citrus Red No. 2	Color	Coloring skins of oranges.
Cochineal	Color	Derived from the dried female insect, *Coccus cacti*; raised in West Indies, Canary Islands, southern Spain, and Algiers; 70,000 insects to 1 lb. Provides red color for such foods as meat products and beverages.
Corn endosperm oil	Color	Source of xanthophyll for yellow color. Used in chicken feed to color yolks of eggs and chicken skin.
Cornstarch	Anticaking agent; drying agent; formulation aid; processing aid; surface-finishing agent	Digestible polysaccharide used in many foods often in a modified form; these include baking powder, baby foods, soups, sauces, pie fillings, imitation jellies, custards, and candies.
Corn syrup	Flavoring agent; humectant; nutritive sweetener; preservative	Derived from hydrolysis of cornstarch. Employed in numerous foods, e.g., baby foods, bakery products, toppings, meat products, beverages, condiments, and confections; GRAS additive.
Dextrose (glucose)	Flavoring agent; humectant; nutritive sweetener; synergist	Derived from cornstarch. Major uses of dextrose are confections, wine, and canned products; used to flavor meat products; used in production of caramel; variety of other uses.
Diglycerides	Emulsifiers	Uses include frozen desserts, lard, shortening, and margarine; GRAS additive.
Dioctyl sodium sulfosuccinate	Emulsifier; processing aid; surface active agent	Employed in gelatin dessert, dry beverages, fruit juice drinks, and noncarbonated beverages with cocoa fat; used in production of cane sugar and in canning.
Disodium guanylate	Flavor enhancer	Derived from dried fish or seaweed.
Disodium inosinate	Flavor adjuvant	Derived from seaweed or dried fish; sodium guanylate is a by-product.
EDTA (ethylenediamine-tetraacetic acid)	Antioxidant; sequestrant	Calcium disodium and disodium salt of EDTA employed in a variety of foods including soft drinks, alcoholic beverages, dressings, canned vegetables, margarine, pickles, sandwich spreads, and sausage.
FD&C colors: Blue No. 1 Red No. 40 Yellow No. 5	Color	Coloring foods in general including dietary supplements.
Gelatin	Stabilizer and thickener; texturizer	Derived from collagen by boiling skin, tendons, ligaments, bones, etc. with water. Employed in many foods including: confectionery, jellies, and ice cream; GRAS additive.
Glycerine (glycerol)	Humectant	Miscellaneous and general purpose additive; GRAS additive.
Grape skin extract	Color	Colorings for carbonated drinks, beverage bases, and alcoholic beverages.
Guar gum	Stabilizer and thickener; texturizer	Extracted from seeds of the guar plant of India and Pakistan. Employed in such foods as cheese, salad dressings, ice cream, and soups.

TABLE 4 (CONTINUED)
Common Food Additives

Name	Function[a]	Food Use and Comments
Gum arabic	Stabilizer and thickener; texturizer	Gummy exudate of Acacia plants. Used in variety of foods; GRAS additive.
Gum ghatti	Stabilizer and thickener; texturizer	Gummy exudate of plant growing in India and Ceylon. A variety of food uses; GRAS additive.
Hydrogen peroxide	Bleaching agent	Modification of starch and bleaching tripe; GRAS bleaching agent.
Hydrolyzed vegetable (plant) protein	Flavor enhancer	To flavor various meat products.
Invert sugar	Humectant; nutritive sweetener	Main use in confectionery and brewing industry.
Iron	Nutrient	Dietary supplements and food; GRAS additive.
Iron-Ammonium citrate	Anticaking agent	Used in salt.
Karraya gum	Stabilizer and thickener	Derived from dried extract of *Sterculia urens* found primarily in India. Variety of food uses; a substitute for tragacanth gum; GRAS additive.
Lactic acid	Preservative; pH control	Normal product of human metabolism. Numerous uses in foods and beverages; a miscellaneous general purpose additive; GRAS additive.
Lecithin (phosphatidyl-choline)	Emulsifier; surface active agent	Normal tissue component of the body; edible and digestible additive naturally occurring in eggs; commercially derived from soybeans. Margarine, chocolate, and wide variety of other food uses; GRAS additive.
Mannitol	Anticaking; nutritive sweetener; stabilizer and thickener; texturizer	Special dietary foods; GRAS additive; supplies 1/2 the energy of glucose; classified as a sugar alcohol or polyol.
Methylparaben	Preservative	Food and beverages; GRAS additive.
Modified food starch	Drying agent; formulation aid; processing aid; surface finishing agent	Digestible polysaccharide used in many foods and stages of food processing; examples include baking powder, puddings, pie fillings, baby foods, soups, sauces, candies, etc.
Monoglycerides	Emulsifiers	Widely used in foods such as frozen desserts, lard, shortening, and margarine; GRAS additive.
MSG (monosodium glutamate)	Flavor enhancer	Enhances the flavor of a variety of foods including various meat products; possible association with the Chinese restaurant syndrome.
Papain	Texturizer	Miscellaneous and/or general purpose additive; GRAS additive; achieves results through enzymatic action; used as meat tenderizer. Heat inactivated.
Paprika	Color; flavoring agent	To provide coloring and/or flavor to foods; GRAS additive.
Pectin	Stabilizer and thickener; texturizer	Richest source of pectin is lemon and orange rind; present in cell walls of all plant tissues. Used to prepare jellies and jams. GRAS additive.
Phosphoric acid	pH control	Miscellaneous and/or general purpose additive; used to increase effectiveness of antioxidants in lard and shortening. GRAS additive.

TABLE 4 (CONTINUED)
Common Food Additives

Name	Function[a]	Food Use and Comments
Polyphosphates	Nutrient; flavor improver; sequestrant; pH control	Numerous food uses; most polyphosphates and their sodium, calcium, potassium, and ammonium salts. GRAS additive.
Polysorbates	Emulsifiers; surface active agent	Polysorbates designated by numbers such as 60, 65, and 80; variety of food uses including baking mixes, frozen custards, pickles, sherbets, ice creams, and shortenings.
Potassium alginate	Stabilizer and thickener; texturizer	Extracted from seaweed. Wide usage; GRAS additive.
Potassium bromate	Flour treating agent	Employed in flour, whole wheat flour, fermented malt beverages, and to treat malt.
Potassium iodide	Nutrient	Added to table salt or used in mineral preparations as a source of dietary iodine.
Potassium nitrite	Curing and pickling agent	To fix color in cured products such as meats.
Potassium sorbate	Preservative	Inhibits mold and yeast growth in foods such as wines, sausage casings, and margarine; GRAS additive.
Propionic acid	Preservative	Mold inhibitor in breads and general fungicide; GRAS additive; used in manufacture of fruit flavors.
Propyl gallate	Antioxidant; preservative	Used in products containing oil or fat; employed in chewing gum; used to retard rancidity in frozen fresh pork sausage.
Propylene glycol	Emulsifier, humectant; stabilizer and thickener; texturizer	Miscellaneous and/or general purpose additive; uses include salad dressings, ice cream, ice milk, custards, and a variety of other foods; GRAS additive.
Propylparaben	Preservative	Fungicide; controls mold in sausage casings; GRAS additive.
Saccharin	Non-nutritive sweetener	Special dietary foods and a variety of beverages; baked products; tabletop sweeteners.
Saffron	Color; flavoring agent	Derived from plant of western Asia and southern Europe. All foods except those where standards forbid; to color sausage casings, margarine, or product branding inks.
Silicon dioxide	Anticaking agent	Used in feed or feed components, beer production, production of special dietary foods, and ink diluent for marking fruits and vegetables.
Sodium acetate	pH control; preservative	Miscellaneous and/or general purpose use; meat preservation; GRAS additive.
Sodium alginate	Stabilizer and thickener; texturizer	Extracted from seaweed. Widespread food use; GRAS additive.
Sodium aluminum sulfate	Leavening agent	Baking powders, confectionery, and sugar refining.
Sodium benzoate	Preservative	Variety of food products; margarine to retard flavor reversion; GRAS additive.
Sodium bicarbonate	Leavening agent; pH control	Miscellaneous and/or general purpose uses; separation of fatty acids and glycerol in rendered fats; neutralize excess and clean vegetables in rendered fats, soups and curing pickles; GRAS additive.
Sodium chloride (salt)	Flavor enhancer; formulation acid; preservation	Used widely in many foods; GRAS additive.
Sodium citrate	pH control; curing and pickling agent; sequestrant	Evaporated milk; miscellaneous and/or general purpose food use; accelerate color fixing in cured meats; GRAS additive.

TABLE 4 (CONTINUED)
Common Food Additives

Name	Function[a]	Food Use and Comments
Sodium diacetate	Preservative; sequestrant	An inhibitor of molds and rope forming bacteria in baked products; GRAS additive.
Sodium nitrate (Chile saltpeter)	Curing and pickling agent; preservative	Used with or without sodium nitrite in smoked or cured fish, and cured meat products.
Sodium nitrite	Curing and pickling agent; preservative	May be used with sodium nitrate in smoked or cured fish, cured meat products, and pet foods.
Sodium propionate	Preservative	A fungicide and mold preventative in bakery products; GRAS additive.
Sorbic acid	Preservative	Fungistatic agent for foods, especially cheeses; other uses include baked goods, beverages, dried fruits, fish, jams, jellies, meats, pickled products, and wines; GRAS additive.
Sorbitan monostearate	Emulsifier; stabilizer and thickener	Widespread food usage such as whipped toppings, cakes, cake mixes, confectionery, icings, and shortenings.
Sorbitol	Humectant; nutritive sweetener; stabilizer and thickener; sequestrant	A sugar alcohol or polyol. Used in chewing gum, meat products, icings, dairy products, beverages, and pet foods. Provides less energy than sucrose.
Sucrose	Nutritive sweetener; preservative	The most widely used additive; used in beverages, baked goods, candies, jams and jellies, and other processed foods.
Tagetes (Aztec marigold)	Color	Source is flower petals of Aztec marigold. To enhance yellow color of chicken skin and eggs, incorporated in chicken feed.
Tartaric acid	pH control	Occurs free in many fruits; free or combined with calcium, magnesium, or potassium. Used in soft drinks industry, confectionery products, bakery products, and gelatin desserts.
Titanium dioxide	Color	For coloring foods generally, except standardized foods; used for coloring ingested and applied drugs.
Tocopherols (Vitamin E)	Antioxidant; nutrient	To retard rancidity in foods containing fat; used in dietary supplements; GRAS additive.
Tragacanth gum	Stabilizer and thickener; texturizer	Derived from the plant *Astragalus gummifier* or other Asiatic species of *Astragalus*. General purpose additive.
Turmeric	Color	Derived from rhizome of *Curcuma longa*. Used to color sausage casings, margarine, or shortening and ink for branding or marking products.
Vanilla	Flavoring agent	Used in various bakery products, confectionery and beverages; natural flavoring extracted from cured, full grown unripe fruit of Vanilla panifolia; GRAS additive.
Vanillin	Flavoring agent and adjuvant	Widespread confectionery, beverage, and food use; synthetic form of vanilla; GRAS additive.
Yellow prussiate of soda	Anticaking agent	Employed in salt.

[a] Function refers to those defined in Table 3.

Source: Adapted from Ensminger et al., *Foods and Nutrition Encyclopedia*, 2nd ed., CRC Press, Boca Raton, FL, 1994, 13–18.

Legal definition

The U.S. Food and Drug Administration (FDA) defines food additives as follows:

> The intended use of which results or may reasonably be expected to result, directly or indirectly, either in their becoming a component of food or otherwise affecting the characteristics of food. A material used in the production of containers and packages is subject to the definition if it may reasonably be expected to become a component, or to affect the characteristics, directly or indirectly, of food packaged in the container. "Affecting the characteristics of food" does not include such physical effects as protecting contents of packages, preserving shape, and preventing moisture loss. If there is no migration of a packaging component from the package to the food, it does not become a component of the food and thus is not a food additive. A substance that does not become a component of food, but that is used, for example, in preparing an ingredient of the food to give a different flavor, texture, or other characteristic in the food, may be a food additive.
>
> (Code of Federal Regulations, Title 21, Section 170.3; revised 4/1/78.)

ADENINE

A purine base that is an essential component of the genetic material, DNA; when joined to ribose via a phosphate bond, it becomes adenylnucleotide or forms adenosine.

ADENOSINE

When phosphorylated, adenosine becomes AMP (one phosphate group), ADP (two phosphate groups), and ATP (three phosphate groups).

ADENYL CYCLASE

The enzyme responsible for the conversion of ATP to cyclic AMP, an important 2nd messenger for hormones that stimulate catabolic processes.

ADENYLATE

See AMP (adenosine monophosphate).

ADH

Antidiuretic hormone; also called vasopressin. Acts to conserve body water by increasing water resorption by the renal distal tubule.

ADHESIONS

Fibrous bands of material that connect two surfaces which are normally separate.

ADIPOCYTES, ADIPOSE TISSUE

Cells that store fat.

ADIPSIA

Lack of thirst sensation.

ADOLESCENCE

That period of growth in which the transition between childhood and adulthood occurs.

ADP

Adenosine diphosphate. Metabolite of ATP. Energy is released when ATP is split to ADP and Pi.

ADRENAL GLAND

Bean- or pea-shaped gland composed of an outer cortex and an inner medulla attached to the superior surface of each kidney.

ADRENOCORTICAL HORMONES

A group of steroid hormones synthesized and released by the cortex of the adrenal gland. These hormones include cortisol, corticosterone, hydrocortisone, and aldosterone.

ADSORB

To attract and retain substances on the surface.

ADULT RESPIRATORY DISTRESS SYNDROME (ARDS)

Condition characterized by increased capillary permeability in the lung circulation resulting in noncardiogenic pulmonary edema.

ADVANCED CARDIAC LIFE SUPPORT (ACLS)

Advanced resuscitation techniques including airway management, arrhythmia detection, drug therapy, and defibrillation.

AEROBIC METABOLISM

Metabolic reactions that require the presence of oxygen.

AEROPHAGIA

The habit of swallowing air.

AFLATOXINS

Contaminants of food produced by molds. The most important mycotoxins, the aflatoxins, are very toxic and carcinogenic substances formed by *A. flavus* and *A. parasiticus*. They are derivatives of coumarin fused to either a cyclopentanone (B group) or to a six-membered lactone (G group). Different types of aflatoxins include aflatoxin B_1, B_2 (dihydroderivative of B_1), G_1, G_2 (dihydroderivative of G_1), M_1 (metabolic product of B_1), and M_2 (metabolic product of B_2). In view of occurrence and toxicity, aflatoxin B_1 is the most important, followed by aflatoxin G_1, B_2, and G_2. Aflatoxins are heat-stable and hard to transform to nontoxic products. They are produced both pre- and post-harvest, at relatively high moisture contents and temperatures. The toxicity of aflatoxins has been demonstrated in many domestic and experimental animals. A common feature is its potent hepatotoxicity. Factors affecting aflatoxin toxicity and carcinogenicity are:

1. species (very susceptible — dog, duckling, guinea pig, neonatal rat, rabbit, turkey poult, rainbow trout; moderately susceptible — chicken, cow, ferret, hamster, mink, monkey, pheasant, pig, rat; very resistant — mouse, sheep);
2. sex (male rats appear more susceptible to the effect of aflatoxin than females);
3. age (young animals appear more susceptible than adults);

4. nutritional factors (protein, methionine, choline, Vitamin A);
5. other factors (cocarcinogenic compounds — ethionine, cyclopenoid fatty acids, malvalic acid, sterculic acid; anticarcinogenic compounds — urethane, diethylstilbestrol, phenobarbitone).

Foodstuffs most likely to become contaminated by aflatoxins are peanuts, various other nuts (e.g., pistachios, almonds, walnuts, filberts), cottonseed, corn, figs, and certain grasses. Human exposure can also occur from intake of aflatoxins from tissues and milk (in particular aflatoxin M1) from animals that have eaten contaminated hay or feeds. Prevention of aflatoxin contamination is achieved by discouraging fungal growth, particularly by adequate post-harvest crop-drying. Aflatoxin consumption has been associated with an inability to respond to oxytocin (dystocia), an inability to lactate, and certain forms of cancer.

AGAR

Food additive that is extracted from seaweed; acts as a gelling agent (see food additives, Table 4).

AGARITINE

A member of a series of hydrazine derivatives, occurring in mushrooms, including the common edible mushroom A. *bisporus.*

AGE ADJUSTED DEATH RATE

The number of deaths in a specific age group for a given calendar year divided by the population of that same age group and multiplied by 1000.

AGRANULOCYTOSIS

Considerable decrease in leukocytes resulting from depression of granulocytes formed in the bone marrow.

AIDS

Acquired immune deficiency syndrome. A disease which results when a specific virus (HIV) attacks elements of the immune system rendering it unable to respond to incoming antigens.

ALANINE

A nonessential amino acid (see Table 5) which can be synthesized from pyruvate and an amino group donated by glutamate.

ALANINE CYCLE

A cycle that plays an important role in maintaining blood glucose levels in the normal range (80–120 mg/dl or 4–6 mmol/l). The cycle uses alanine released by the muscle and deaminated by the liver to produce glucose via gluconeogenesis. This glucose is transported to the muscle where it is oxidized to produce pyruvate which is aminated to form alanine. This cycle is an important defense against hypoglycemia during starvation. Figure 1 illustrates the alanine cycle.

ALAR

Plant growth regulator; chemical name; daminozide.

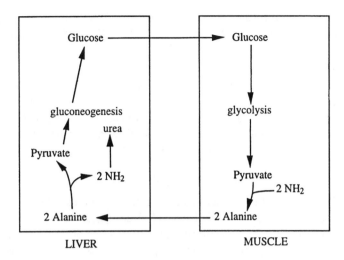

FIGURE 1 Alanine cycle.

ALBINISM

A genetic disease characterized by a failure of melanocytes to synthesize melanin, the pigment responsible for skin color. The gene for tyrosine hydroxylase is mutated in this disorder producing an inactive gene product.

ALBUMIN

Small molecular weight protein found in blood and sometimes in urine. It is a single chain globular protein consisting of 610 amino acids. It assists in the maintenance of the osmotic pressure of the intravascular spaces. It is also a major carrier for free fatty acids in the blood. Albumin found in the urine is considered an early warning sign of renal disease. Normally, it does not cross the renal cell membrane but is conserved by the glomerular cell.

ALBUMINURIA

Condition where albumin is found in the urine.

ALCAPTONURIA

A rare hereditary disease in which homogentisic acid (a metabolite of phenylalanine and tyrosine) accumulates because of a mutation in the gene for homogentisic acid oxidase.

ALCOHOL

A hydrocarbon containing a hydroxyl (–OH) group attached to one of the carbons. The most common alcohol in the diet is ethanol.

ALCOHOL ABUSE AND CARDIOMYOPATHY

Although the precise cause of cardiomyopathy (see below) is unknown, alcohol abuse is the major cause of dilated cardiomyopathy which leads to intractable congestive heart failure.

ALCOHOL ABUSE AND DIABETES MELLITUS

Significant alcohol consumption (>2 ounces daily) in diabetics has been associated with hypoglycemia. Alcohol decreases gluconeogenesis in the liver and, as a result, hypoglycemia can readily develop several hours after alcohol ingestion. If light to moderate quantities of alcohol (1–2 drinks) are consumed with a mixed meal, blood glucose levels can be maintained.

ALCOHOL ABUSE AND GOUT

Hyperuricemia is positively correlated to alcohol intake in adult males. When significant quantities of alcohol (>2 ounces daily) are ingested, the lactic acid accumulation that results inhibits renal secretion of urates potentially resulting in an acute gout attack. Light to moderate quantities of alcohol (1–2 drinks) consumed with a mixed meal appear to have little effect on accumulation of uric acid and gout (see below).

ALCOHOL ABUSE AND HYPERLIPIDEMIA

Significant intakes of alcohol (>2 ounces daily) are positively associated with hypertriglyceridemia. Light to moderate intakes of alcohol (1–2 drinks) are associated with increased high density lipoprotein (HDL) levels. However, the subfraction of HDL that is elevated does not appear to be the one most protective with respect to the risk for heart disease.

ALCOHOL ABUSE AND HYPERTENSION

Significant alcohol consumption (>2 ounces daily) is positively associated with hypertension. However, no effect is consistently reported for alcohol intakes <2 ounces daily. During withdrawal in alcoholic individuals, hypertension is frequently noted, but returns to normal once abstinence is maintained.

ALCOHOL ABUSE AND HYPOMAGNESEMIA

Alcoholism increases the need for magnesium at a time when the intake is low due to the substitution of alcohol for magnesium containing foods.

ALCOHOL ABUSE AND HYPONATREMIA

Alcoholism may be characterized by low levels of sodium in the blood.

ALCOHOL ABUSE AND HYPOPHOSPHATEMIA

Alcoholism is characterized by a low level of phosphate groups in the blood. This impairs the regulation of pH.

ALCOHOL ABUSE AND METABOLIC ACIDOSIS

Metabolic pH falls when excessive alcohol intake occurs.

ALCOHOL ABUSE AND NIACIN DEFICIENCY

Niacin as part of NADH and NADPH is needed for alcohol metabolism. This excess need in the face of deficient intake can result in pellagra.

ALCOHOL ABUSE AND SEPTIC SHOCK

Due to a decreased immune response, alcoholics are at high risk for developing the end result of a process initiated by sepsis known as septic shock.

ALCOHOL WITHDRAWAL

Abstinence of alcohol in an alcoholic individual associated with neurologic symptoms, cardiovascular symptoms, and fluid volume deficit.

ALCOHOLISM

An addictive disease with strong genetic factors. It has been estimated that upwards to 90 million Americans consume alcoholic beverages every day and that about 10% of these people are addicted to its consumption. This affliction is called alcoholism which has a strong genetic linkage. Although the gene(s) is unidentified, there is ample evidence in the literature that supports the concept that the tendency toward alcoholism is inherited. An alcoholic is more likely than a nonalcoholic to have an alcoholic relative. At least 33% of alcoholics have an alcoholic parent. Monozygotic (identical) and dizygotic (fraternal) twins have a high degree of concordance for alcoholism. If one twin becomes an alcoholic, the other twin also becomes one if that twin chooses to consume alcohol. The concordance is greater in identical twins than in fraternal twins. Ethanol consumption increases the need for thiamin, niacin, pyridoxine, and pantothenic acid. Alcoholism may be accompanied by nutritional anemia, beriberi, pellegra, pantothenic acid, and pyridoxine deficiency (see ethanol metabolism).

ALDEHYDE

A carbon compound containing a

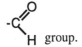 group.

ALDOLASE DEFICIENCY

A mutation in the gene for aldolase which results in accumulation of fructose 1,6 bisphosphate. Aldolase catalyzes the cleavage of fructose 1,6 bisphosphate to glyceraldehyde 3 phosphate and dihydroxyacetone phosphate (see glycolysis, Figure 40, page 148). Muscular dystrophy is characterized by a decrease in aldolase activity in addition to decreases in phosphorylase activity, phosphoglucomutase activity, and total glycolytic activity.

ALDOSTERONE

A steroid hormone released by the adrenal cortex and which acts on the cells bordering the distal tubules of the kidney stimulating them to reabsorb sodium. When sodium is resorbed, water is retained. Thus, aldosterone has an important role in sodium and water conservation.

ALIMENTARY CANAL

See Gastrointestinal tract.

ALIMENTARY TOXIC ALEUKIA (ATA)

See mycotoxins, trichothecenes.

ALIPHATIC

A chain of carbon atoms.

ALIPHATIC AMINO ACIDS

Amino acids which consist of a chain of carbons. These include alanine, cysteine, glycine, isoleucine, leucine, methionine, serine, threonine, and valine.

ALKALOSIS

A condition where the blood pH rises above 7.4. Metabolic alkalosis may be caused by a loss in body acid or chloride ion as happens in excessive vomiting or an excess of antacid intake or depletion of potassium ion as happens with excessive diarrhea.

ALLELE

Any one of a series of different genes that may occupy the same location (locus) on a specific chromosome.

ALLERGENS

Substances capable of eliciting an immunologic response. Allergens in food are either proteins, glycoproteins, or polypeptides. Allergens can also be airborne or can be transmitted through the skin. The allergenicity is associated with the type of structure of the proteins and the peptides: primary, secondary, or tertiary. In the case of tertiary structures, allergenicity often disappears on denaturation, whereas in the case of an allergic response to a primary structure, allergenicity remains. Furthermore, the protein has to be large enough to be recognized by the immune system as a foreign compound. In general, allergenic substances with molecular weights of <5000 elicit little immunologic response, unless they are bound to endogenous proteins. On the other hand, dietary substances with a molecular weight >70,000 are not absorbed and thus do not elicit an immune response. Food proteins that are not digested and absorbed elicit an enteric response, i.e., diarrhea and/or flatulence, which is different from the allergic response.

ALLERGY

A condition whereby body tissues of sensitive persons react to allergens which have no effect on nonsensitive persons similarly exposed. It is essentially an antigen-antibody reaction triggering the release of histamine or similar compounds from injured cells. An allergic reaction differs from other toxic reactions in that the reaction is highly subjective, manifesting only in sensitive individuals. It can be a toxic reaction, producing toxic symptoms, including urticaria, eczema, rash, asthma, hay fever, headache (including migraine), hemorrhage, and gastrointestinal disturbances. Other signs of an allergic reaction can include conjunctivitis, nausea, vomiting, and in rare cases, circulatory collapse, shock, and death. These symptoms indicate that the organs frequently involved are the skin, respiratory tract, vascular system, and the gastrointestinal tract. In general, four different types of immunological hypersensitivity reactions are recognized: types I, II, III, and IV hypersensitivity.

Type I Hypersensitivity. After contact with an allergen certain white blood cells (B lymphocytes) are triggered to produce antibodies of a special type, the immunoglobulin E (IgE) antibodies. These antibodies bind to cells (mainly mast cells and basophils). When there is a subsequent exposure to the same allergen, the allergen becomes bound to two adjacent IgE molecules resulting in degranulation of the cell to which the IgE is bound. Several types of (pre-existing or newly formed) mediators are released, which result in a complex reaction — muscle contraction, dilatation and increase of permeability of blood vessels, chemotaxis (a mediator-triggered process by which other cells are attracted to the site of reaction), and release of other immune mediators. The reaction occurs mostly within one hour, and is sometimes followed by a so-called late reaction which starts hours later.

Type II Hypersensitivity. Antibodies of the immunoglobulin G (IgG) or immunoglobulin M (IgM) class are generated against a cell surface antigen or an antigen bound to a cell surface. This leads to an inflammatory reaction by which the cells are destroyed. Transfusion reactions due to blood incompatibility work according to this mechanism. There is no evidence that this type of allergic reaction plays a role in food allergy.

Type III Hypersensitivity. Antibodies of the types IgG and IgM are formed against antigens that circulate in the blood. This results in the formation of antigen-antibody complexes which activate the complement system, followed by the release of different mediators from mast cells and basophils. When there is an optimal ratio of antibody to antigen, the complexes may precipitate at different sites in the body, e.g., the joints, the kidneys, and the skin. This type of reaction may play a role in some types of food allergic reactions. Type III hypersensitivity reactions also include a number of drug reactions and a few types of vasculitis.

Type IV Hypersensitivity. In contrast to types I, II, and III hypersensitivity, no antibodies are involved in this type of reaction. After contact with an antigen, T-lymphocytes are sensitized. These T-lymphocytes then produce cytokines which activate other cells. An example is contact allergy of the skin due to cosmetics. In food allergy, this type of reaction is sometimes seen when food comes into contact with the skin in a person allergic to that specific food.

ALLICIN

The primary active component of garlic giving it its characteristic aroma.

ALLOGENIC

Referring to the use of tissue or organs from other humans that have a different genetic composition.

ALLOSTERISM

The binding of an inhibitor or activator to an enzyme at a site removed from the active site but which inhibits or activates the enzyme.

ALLOTRIOPHAGY-PICA

Consumption of nonfood items; deranged appetite.

ALOPECIA

Loss of hair.

α-AMINOPROPIONIC ACID DERIVATIVES

Non-nutritive natural food components of important toxicological relevance. They occur in peas of certain Lathyrus-species. These substances are known to cause skeletal malformations (osteolathyrism) and neurotoxic effects (neurolathyrism). The peas are easily grown on poor soil and are often used as feed. Both diseases have occurred in northern India in years with a poor harvest. At present, osteolathyrism has largely disappeared, whereas neurolathyrism still poses a serious health problem. Neurolathyrism is associated with the long-term intake of the peas of *Lathyrus sativus*. The disease is characterized by muscular weakness, degeneration of spinal motor nerves, and paralysis. The peas have been found to contain a neurotoxin — N-oxalyl-diaminopropionic acid (ODAP). In addition, the peas may be contaminated with a vetch species (*Vicia sativa*), also containing a neurotoxic α-aminopropionic derivative, β-cyano-L-alanine. The neurotoxicity of the amino acids is attributed to their structural relationship with the neurotransmitter glutamic acid. ODAP and β-cyano-L-alanine are believed to bind irreversibly to the glutamate receptors on specific nerve cells. Long occupation of the glutaminergic receptors has been reported to result in neurological damage.

ALUMINUM HYDROXIDE

Common antacid; chronic use is associated with lowering serum phosphorus and excess urinary calcium loss.

ALVEOLI

Cells in the lung responsible for O_2/CO_2 exchange.

ALZHEIMER'S DISEASE

Progressive disease characterized by deterioration of memory and other cognitive function; the major cause of dementia in the elderly.

AMENORRHEA

Cessation of menses. May be due to cessation of ovulation as happens in pregnancy or at the end of the female reproductive period (menopause). Can also be due to inadequate food intake as in anorexia nervosa or starvation.

AMIDE BOND

A bond involving an amino group. The peptide bond is the most common amide bond and is formed when two amino acids are joined together. Figure 2 illustrates this reaction.

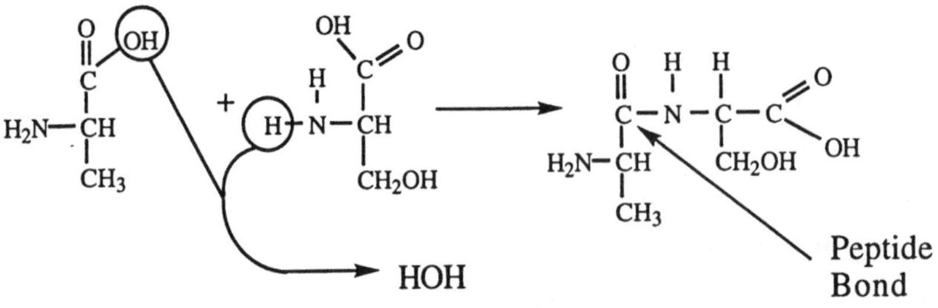

FIGURE 2   Formation of a dipeptide from two amino acids.

AMINO ACIDS

Simple organic nitrogenous compounds that are the building blocks of proteins. They also serve as precursors of several nonprotein compounds, e.g., thyroxine, epinephrine, serotonin, creatine, creatinine, ethanolamine, and others. Amino acids have two reactive groups on their carbon skeletons — the carboxyl (–COOH) and the amino ($–NH_3^+$) groups. They may also have –SH groups or additional hydroxyl, carboxyl, or amino groups. Table 5 gives the names and structures of the 20 amino acids of importance to mammals. These amino acid structures are shown in their nonionized form. In physiological solutions they occur in ionized forms with a positively charged amino group ($–NH_3^+$) and/or a negatively charged carboxyl group (–COO–). Metabolism is shown in Figures 4–8. Typical reactions are listed in Table 6 (page 33). Recommended Dietary Allowances for protein are provided in Table 7.

AMINO ACID METABOLISM

Amino acids are subject to three general reactions as shown in Figure 3. The metabolism for the biologically important amino acids is shown in Figures 4–8.

TABLE 5
Amino Acid Structures

Name	Abbreviation	Structure
Glycine	Gly	$H-\underset{NH_2}{\overset{H}{C}}-COOH$
Alanine	Ala	$CH_3-\underset{NH_2}{CH}-COOH$
Valine	Val	$\overset{CH_3}{\underset{H_3C}{>}}CH-\underset{NH_2}{CH}-COOH$
Leucine	Leu	$\overset{CH_3}{\underset{H_3C}{>}}CH-CH_2-\underset{NH_2}{CH}-COOH$
Isoleucine	Ile	$\overset{CH_3}{\underset{}{CH_2}}$ $\underset{H_3C}{>}CH-\underset{NH_2}{CH}-COOH$
Serine	Ser	$\underset{OH}{CH_2}-\underset{NH_2}{CH}-COOH$
Threonine	Thr	$CH_3-\underset{OH}{CH}-\underset{NH_2}{CH}-COOH$
Cysteine (Cystein)	Cys	$\underset{SH}{CH_2}-\underset{NH_2}{CH}-COOH$
Methionine	Met	$\underset{S-CH_3}{CH_2}-CH_2-\underset{NH_2}{CH}-COOH$
Aspartic Acid	Asp	$HOOC-CH_2-\underset{NH_2}{CH}-COOH$
Asparagine	Asn	$H_2N-\underset{O}{\overset{}{C}}-CH_2-\underset{NH_2}{CH}-COOH$

TABLE 5 (CONTINUED)
Amino Acid Structures

Name	Abbreviation	Structure
Glutamic Acid	Glu	$HOOC-CH_2-CH_2-CH-COOH$, NH_2
Glutamine	Gln	$H_2N-C-CH_2-CH_2-CH-COOH$, O, NH_2
Arginine	Arg	$H_2N-C-N-CH_2-CH_2-CH_2-CH-COOH$, NH H, NH_2
Lysine	Lys	$CH_2-CH_2-CH_2-CH_2-CH-COOH$, NH_2, NH_2
Hydroxylysine	Hyl	$CH_2-CH-CH_2-CH_2-CH-COOH$, NH_2 OH, NH_2
Histidine	His	$CH_2-CH-COOH$, $HN\!\!=\!\!N$, NH_2
Phenylalanine	Phe	$CH_2-CH-COOH$, NH_2
Tyrosine	Tyr	$HO-$⟨ring⟩$-CH_2-CH-COOH$, NH_2
Tryptophan	Trp	$CH_2-CH-COOH$, NH_2
Proline	Pro	$-COOH$
Hydroxyproline	Hyp	HO, $-COOH$

1. Transamination

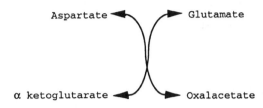

Aspartate can donate its
amino group to α ketoglutarate
which becomes glutamate while
aspartate becomes oxalacetate.
The reverse can also occur.

2. Oxidative deamination

$$Glutamate + NAD(P)^+ + HOH \longrightarrow \alpha \text{ ketoglutarate} + NAD(P)H^{++}$$

$$+ NH_3$$

3. Amino acid oxidase

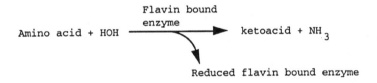

FIGURE 3   General reactions of amino acids that result in the removal or transfer of an amino group.

AMINO ACID REACTIONS

Typical reactions are shown in Table 6 (page 33).

AMINO ACID REQUIREMENTS

The recommended daily intake for amino acids as protein is given in Table 7 (page 33). It is approximately twice that absolutely required for survival. These figures allow for individual variation in need.

AMINO ACID POOL

The free amino acids present in the cytosol of every cell and in the fluids around the cell.

AMINOACIDOPATHY

Inborn error of metabolism resulting from inadequate utilization of one or more amino acids. Common examples include phenylketonuria which results from inadequate activity of the enzyme, phenylalanine hydroxylase, or tyrosinemia and maple syrup urine disease in which an enzyme necessary for metabolism of branch chain amino acids is missing.

AMINOTRANSFERASES (TRANSAMINASES)

Enzymes that catalyze the transfer of an amino group from one carbon chain to another.

AMNIOTIC FLUID

The fluid which surrounds the unborn child.

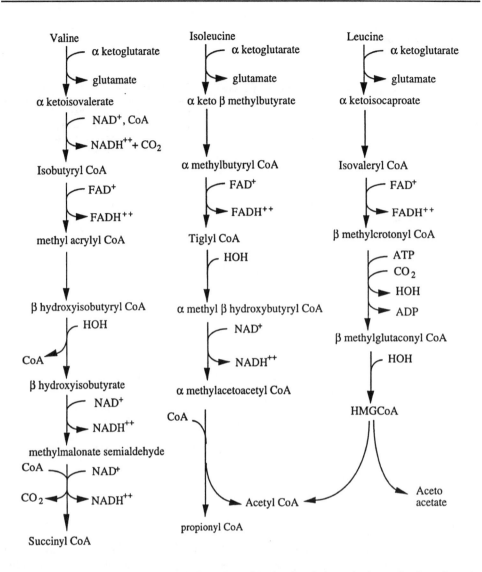

FIGURE 4 Catabolism of branched chain amino acids showing their use in the production of metabolites that are either lipid precursors or that can be oxidized via the Krebs cycle.

AMP

Adenosine monophosphate. Metabolite of ADP. Energy is released when ADP is split to AMP and Pi.

AMPHIPATHIC

The characteristic of a compound containing both polar and nonpolar groups. This allows it to be soluble in polar and nonpolar solvents. Water is a polar solvent while acetone, ether, methanol, and chloroform are nonpolar solvents.

AMPHOTERIC

The characteristic of a compound which allows it to have either an acidic or a basic function, depending on the pH of the solution.

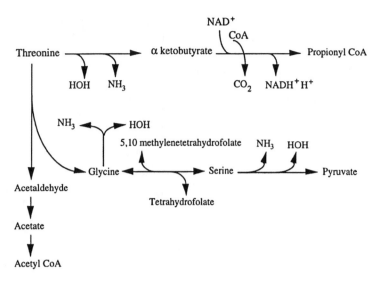

FIGURE 5   Catabolism of threonine showing its relationship to that of serine and glycine.

AMYLASE
An enzyme that catalyzes the cleavage of glucose molecules from amylose (starch).

AMYLOPECTIN
A branched chain polymer of glucose found in plants.

AMYLOSE
A straight chain polymer of glucose found in starch; the storage carbohydrate in plants.

ANABOLISM
The totality of reactions that account for the synthesis of the body's macromolecules.

ANAEROBIC METABOLISM
Metabolic reactions that occur in the relative absence of oxygen.

ANAPHYLACTIC RESPONSE
A systemic allergic reaction to a food or food additive or to an exogenous chemical such as bee venom (see anaphylaxis).

ANAPHYLAXIS
Severe allergic response which, if untreated, leads to coma and death. The response is due to a massive release of histamine that causes blood vessels to dilate and blood pressure to fall.

ANASTOMOSIS
Joining of two normally separate structures by a surgical procedure.

ANDERSON'S DISEASE
One of the glycogen storage diseases (Type IV). A genetic disease where the mutation occurs in the gene for the glycogen branching enzyme.

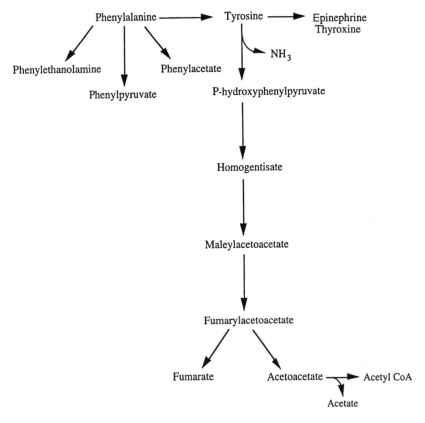

FIGURE 6   Phenylalanine and tyrosine catabolism. This pathway has a number of mutations resulting in a variety of genetic diseases.

ANDROGENS

Male sex hormones.

ANDROID OBESITY

A form of obesity where fat distribution is mainly in the shoulders and abdominal area.

ANEMIA

Below normal levels of red blood cells and/or hemoglobin due to one or more problems in hemoglobin synthesis and/or red blood cell maturation. The many forms are listed in Table 8 (pages 34 and 35) and the various features of anemia are listed in Table 9.

ANERGY

Decreased reaction to specific antigens.

ANEURINE

Thiamin.

ANEURYSM

A bulge in the vascular tree (usually arterial); if the vessel ruptures, hemorrhage or internal bleeding occurs, and unless treated promptly, death can result.

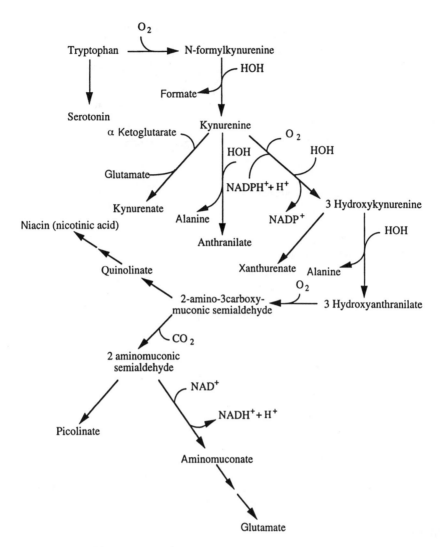

FIGURE 7 Catabolism of tryptophan showing conversion to the vitamin niacin. This conversion is not very efficient, taking approximately 60 molecules of tryptophan to produce 1 molecule of niacin. Tryptophan catabolism also results in picolinate which is believed by some to play a role in trace mineral conservation.

ANGINA PECTORIS

Sharp pain emanating from the breastbone to the left arm and fingers, due to inadequate oxygen supply to the heart muscle. If the vascular tree of the heart has lost its elasticity because of atherosclerosis the circulation of oxygenated blood will be impaired.

ANGIOTENSIN

A vasoconstrictor; precursor form is angiotensinogen which is synthesized in the liver.

ANGULAR STOMATITIS

Cracks in the corners of the mouth; sometimes regarded as a symptom of riboflavin deficiency. May occur for other reasons as well.

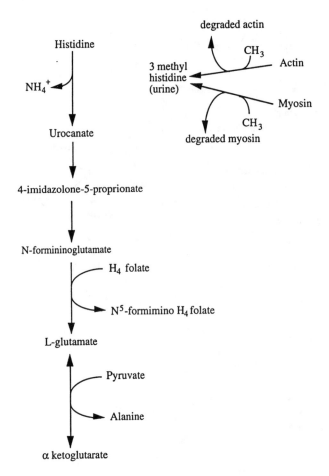

FIGURE 8   Catabolism of histidine. Note that 3 methyl histidine is not a part of the pathway. This metabolite is formed in the muscle when the contractile proteins actin and myosin are degraded.

ANIMAL FAT

Fat stored in animals; this fat contains cholesterol and its esters, and the triacylglycerides contain more saturated fatty acids of 16 and 18 carbons than unsaturated fatty acids.

ANIMAL MODELS FOR HUMAN DISEASE

Numerous small animals have some characteristics in common with diseased humans. These can be used to study the disease process. Some of the more common ones are listed in Table 10.

ANION

A negatively charged electrolyte or ion.

ANNATTO

An additive involved in idiosyncratic food intolerance reactions. It is a coloring agent of natural origin that is added to cheese, butter, dressings, syrups, and some types of oil. Some investigators have demonstrated that symptoms may worsen in patients with urticaria and/or angioedema after ingestion of annatto (see Table 4, Additives).

TABLE 6
Characteristic Chemical Reactions of Amino Acids

Reaction Name	Reagent	Use
Ninhydrin reaction	Ninhydrin	To estimate amino acids quantitatively in small amounts
Sanger reaction	1-fluoro.2,4-dinitrobenzene	To identify the amino terminal group of a peptide
Dansyl chloride reaction	1-deimethylamino-naphthalene (also called dansylchloride)	To measure very small amounts of amino acids quantitatively
Edmann degradation	Phenylisothiocyanate	To identify the terminal NH_2 group in a protein
Schiff base	Aldehydes	Labile intermediate in some enzymatic reactions involving α-amino acid substrates

From National Research Council, Food and Nutrition Board, 1989, 10th ed., National Academy Press, Washington, D.C.

TABLE 7
Recommended Daily Dietary Allowances (RDA) for Protein (United States, 1993)

Age Group		Recommended Protein Intake g/day
Infants to 6 months		kg × 2.2
Infants, 6 months to 1 year		kg × 2.0
Children,	1–3	23
	4–6	30
	7–10	34
Males	11–14	45
	15–18	56
	19–22	56
	23–50	56
	51+	56
Females	11–14	46
	15–18	46
	19–22	44
	23–50	44
	51+	44
Pregnant		add 30
Lactating		add 20

From National Research Council, Food and Nutrition Board, 1989, 10th ed., National Academy Press, Washington, D.C.

TABLE 8
Types of Anemias

Type	Description	Effects on the Body
A. Nutritional in Origin		
Hemolytic anemia resulting from Vitamin E deficiency	Red blood cells have an abnormal membrane which makes them extra sensitive to hemolysis. Most often found in premature infants given milk formulas containing polyunsaturated fats without adequate Vitamin E. Also found in adults with a deficiency of the vitamin.	An increased rate of destruction of red cells, resulting in anemia. Edema and some of its consequences (swollen legs, noisy breathing, and puffy eyelids). Severe deficiency of Vitamin E in infants may also be accompanied by encephalomalacia (softening of the brain).
Iron-deficiency anemia	The most common form of anemia. Red cells are reduced in size (microcytic) and contain a subnormal amount of hemoglobin (hypochromic). Also, the cell count is subnormal, due to a decreased production of hemoglobin. Most prevalent in infants, children, and pregnant women.	Deficiency of hemoglobin and its consequences (paleness of skin and mucous membranes, fatigue, dizziness, sensitivity to cold, shortness of breath, rapid heartbeat, and tingling in fingers and toes).
Megaloblastic anemia	Abnormal maturation of red cells resulting in enlarged cells (megaloblasts or macrocytes) with normal concentrations of hemoglobin (normochromic). Subnormal cell count. Caused by deficiency of folic acid and/or Vitamin B-12.	Blood cells fail to mature. Macrocytic anemia. Vitamin B-12 deficiency may lead to gastrointestinal and neural disorders. (Also see effects given below under pernicious anemia.)
Pernicious anemia	Same as above description of megaloblastic anemia. Additionally, there are gastrointestinal disorders (glossitis, achlorhydria, and lack of intrinsic factor for Vitamin B-12 absorption) and neurologic damage (shown by abnormal electroencephalogram).	Megaloblastic anemia. Abnormalities of cells lining the gastrointestinal tract. Atrophy of gastric parietal cells and achlorhydria. Synthesis of abnormal fatty acids and their deposition in nerve tissue. Mental dysfuncion.
Pica associated with iron-deficiency anemia	Abnormal craving for nonfood items leads to the eating of clay, dirt, plaster, paint chips, and ice. Iron deficiency often develops in this disorder.	Certain nonfood items (some types of clays) interfere with iron absorption.
Pregnancy anemia	The added requirements of a developing fetus produce in most cases an iron-deficiency anemia, although there may also be a folic acid deficiency.	Effects are the same as those of iron deficiency, except that the anemia may develop more rapidly in the pregnant woman.
Siderotic anemia due to deficiency of pyridoxine (Vitamin B-6)	Microcytic, hypochromic anemia similar to that caused by iron deficiency, except that serum iron is normal or at an elevated level. Vitamin B-6 deficiency impairs synthesis of hemoglobin.	(See effects given above for iron-deficiency anemia.)
B. Nonnutritional in Origin		
Aplastic anemia	Cessation of blood cell production in the bone marrow due to toxic agents, reaction to drugs, and unknown causes.	Great decrease in all blood cells produced in the bone marrow (red cells, white cells, and platelets). All the complications of anemia plus hemorrhages (due to lack of platelets needed for clotting).
Blood loss	Restoration of the full complement of red cells after blood loss is slower than repletion of other constituents of blood.	Effects are the same as those of iron deficiency but may be more severe, depending upon extent of blood loss.

TABLE 8 (CONTINUED)
Types of Anemias

Type	Description	Effects on the Body
Familial hemolytic jaundice (spherocytic anemia)	A hereditary disorder in which red cells are shaped like spheres instead of being toroidal (donutlike) shape. Jaundice results from the excessive destruction of the abnormal cells by the spleen.	Yellowish color of the skin and whites of the eyes (jaundice). Reduction in the number of circulating red cells.
Hemolytic anemia due to deficiency of G6PD enzyme	Increased hemolysis of red cells due to the effects of drugs, toxic agents, and compounds in foods such as fava beans. May also be the result of a mutation in the gene for G6PD.	Anemia and jaundice (due to excessive hemolysis). The trait is sex-linked.
Hemolytic anemia of the newborn due to Rh factor incompatibility	Rh-negative mothers who develop antibodies against Rh-positive blood toward the end of pregnancy with an Rh-positive fetus (due to some transfer of maternal blood to the fetus).	Destruction of red cells in the newborn infant. In severe cases, there may be almost complete destruction of the infant's red cells and damage to the brain by the accumulation of bilirubin (pigment resulting from the breakdown of hemoglobin).
Hookworm or tapeworm infestation	Infestation of the gastrointestinal tract by parasitic worms which feed on blood (hookworm) or nutrients (tapeworm). Anemia may be due to blood loss, deficiencies of folic acid, iron, and/or Vitamin B-12.	Anemia, fatigue, irritability, fever, abdominal discomfort, nausea, or vomiting.
Infection	The production of red cells by the marrow is sometimes inhibited by toxins from an infectious agent.	Anemia and weakness.
Leukemia	A form of cancer in which there is over-production by the body of white cells. Normal production of other blood cells (red cells, platelets, and normal white cells) is prevented by the overgrowth of abnormal leukocytes in the bone marrow and other blood-forming organs (liver, spleen, and lymphatic tissues).	Grayish-white color of blood with a large excess of leukocytes. Death often results from the acute form of the disease and from the chronic form when it is not treated.
Mediterranean anemia (also called thassalemia and Cooley's anemia)	A hereditary disease most prevalent in persons whose ancestors came from the Mediterranean basin (Italy, Sicily, Sardinia, Greece, Crete, Cyprus, Syria, and Turkey). Red cells are fragile and contain abnormal hemoglobin.	An increased rate of destruction of red cells. Bone abnormalities, enlargement of the spleen, leg ulcers, and jaundice.
Sickle cell anemia	A hereditary disease in which the red cells have a sickle shape due to the presence of an abnormal hemoglobin. Sickle cells cannot carry as much oxygen as normal red cells, and they have a shorter than normal lifetime.	Anemia. Pain in the joints and extremities. Limited ability to perform strenuous exercise. Death may occur if sickle cells clump together and clog blood flow in tissues, such as the brain.

Source: Adapted from Ensminger et al., *Foods and Nutrition Encyclopedia*, 2nd ed., CRC Press, Boca Raton, FL, 1994, 78–80.

TABLE 9
Normal Blood Values for Measurements Made to Assess the Presence of Anemia

Measurement	Normal Values	Iron Deficiency Anemia	Chronic Disease	B$_{12}$ or Folic Acid Deficiency
Red blood cells (million/cu mm)	Males: 4.6–6.2; females: 4.2–5.4	Low	Low	Low
Hemoglobin (g/dl)	Males: 14–18; females: 12–16	Low	Low	Low
Hematocrit (vol %)	Males: 40–54%; females: 37–47%	Low	Low	Low
Serum iron	60–280 ug/dl	Low	Low	Normal
TIBC[a]	250–425 ug/dl	High	Low	Normal
Ferritin	60	Less than 12	Normal	Normal
Percent saturation	90–100%	Low	Normal to high	Normal
Hypochromia	No	Yes	Slight	None
Microcytes	Few	Many	Slight	Few
Macrocytes	Few	Few	None	Many
RDW (RBC size)	High	High	Normal to low	Very high
Red cell folate	>360 nmol/l	Normal	315–358	<315
Serum folate	>13.5 mg/ml	Normal	Normal	Low (<6.7 mg/ml)
Serum B$_{12}$	200–900 pg/ml	Normal	Normal	Low
MCV[b]	82–92 cu μ	<80	Normal	>80–100

[a] Indirect measure of serum transferrin; iron binding capacity.

[b] Mean cell volume. When volume increases, the size of the red cell has increased (↑ % of megaloblasts).

ANOMERIC CARBON
A carbon atom to which four different groups are attached.

ANOREXIA
Loss of desire to eat.

ANOREXIA NERVOSA
Chronic condition of voluntary inadequate (or total abstinence of) food consumption. Frequently observed in adolescent females and is related to their inaccurate perception of their body fatness. They become obsessed with the desire to be thin and either refuse to eat and adequately nourish their bodies or they eat but after eating, force themselves to regurgitate food. Self-induced vomiting is called bulimia. Additional behavior related to an obsession with body image includes the regular use of laxatives and diuretics and the extensive participation in exercise designed to increase energy expenditure. Although the patients may be eating some food, these patients are not consuming enough food to meet their macro- and micronutrient requirements. Because of this, they are in negative energy and protein balance. These patients are characterized by little body fat. Because ovulation requires a minimal amount of fat in the body, ovulation ceases. Amenorrhea, hypothermia, and hypotension also develop and, if untreated, anorexics will starve to death. Their catabolic hormone levels are high, and their body energy stores are being raided as a result. Insulin resistance due to an excess of the catabolic hormones is observed. Liver and muscle glycogen levels are low. Fat

TABLE 10
Small Animal Analogs for Human Degenerative Diseases

Insulin-Dependent Diabetes Mellitus (IDDM)
Streptozotocin treated animals of most
  species
Alloxan can be substituted for streptozotocin.
Pancreatectomy will also produce IDDM.
BB rat (autoimmune disease)
db/db mouse
NOD mouse
FAT mouse
NZO mouse
TUBBY mouse
Adipose mouse
Chinese hampster (*cricetulus griseus*)
South African hampster (*mystromys alb*)
Tuco-Tuco (*clenomys tabarum*)

Noninsulin Dependent Diabetes Mellitus
ob/ob mouse
KK, yellow KK mouse
A^{vy}, A^y yellow mouse
P, PB13/Ld mouse
db PAS mouse
BHE/cdb rat
Zucker diabetic rat
SHR/N-cp rat
Spiny mouse
HUS rat
LA/N-cp rat
Wistar Kyoto rat

Obesity
Zucker rat
SHR/N-cp rat
LA/N-cp rat
ob/ob mouse
Ventral hypothalamus lesioned animals
Osborne-Mendel rats fed high fat diets

Hypertension
SHR rats
JCR:LA rats
WKY rats
Transgenic rats

Gallstones
The rat does not have a gall bladder nor does it
  have stones.
Gerbil fed a cholesterol rich, cholic acid rich diet
Hamster, prairie dog, squirrel monkey, or tree
  shrew fed a cholesterol rich diet

Lipemia
Zucker fatty rat
BHE/cdb rat
NZW mouse
Transgenic mice given gene for atherosclerosis

Atherosclerosis
Transgenic mice given gene for atherosclerosis
NZW mouse
JCR:LA cp/cp rat

stores are minimal. As the weight loss proceeds further, these individuals have a reduced bone mass, a decreased metabolic rate, decreased heart rate, hypoglycemia, hypothyroidism, electrolyte imbalance, elevated free fatty acid and cholesterol levels, peripheral edema, and lastly, cardiac and renal failure. When their body fat content falls below 2% of total body weight, they will die. This 2% represents the lipids essential to the structure and function of membranes as well as those complex lipids that comprise the central nervous system. Reversal is difficult in some patients. Mortality is estimated at 6% of cases. Included in the mortality figure of 6% are those who commit suicide. Aggressive treatment can achieve reversal in 50% of the cases. Approximately 44% are those who recover spontaneously without medical intervention. Treatment success also depends on the degree of self-prescribed food intake restriction. Total food abstinence is far more threatening than mild abstinence. Restoring the weight loss of the anorexic patient is difficult. The caloric requirements for weight regain in anorexic patients are highly variable and depend largely on the physiological status of the patient at the time of intervention and on the pre-anorexia body weight. Those patients who were obese prior to their self-induced anorexia regain their lost weight faster than patients who were of normal body weight.

ANOSMIA

Loss of the sense of smell.

ANOXIA

Lack of oxygen in blood or tissues; may be local due to inadequate oxygen delivery to a localized area or may be global (whole body).

ANTABUSE®

Drug used to help alcoholics resist alcohol consumption. When used, the patient will experience severe gastrointestinal distress if alcohol is consumed.

ANTACIDS

Nonabsorbable bases or buffers that combat excessive gastric acidity by neutralizing the acid. Among the more common are: aluminum hydroxide, aluminum oxide, calcium carbonate, calcium-magnesium carbonate, dihydroxy-aluminum amino acetate, glycine, magnesium carbonate, magnesium phosphate, magnesium trisillicate, sodium bicarbonate, sodium citrate, and urea (carbamide).

ANTECEDENTS

Events that precede or are causally linked to an event.

ANTHROPOMETRY

Measurement of body features, i.e., weight, height, etc.

ANTIBIOTICS

Chemical substances that inhibit growth or kill pathogenic micro-organisms.

ANTIBODY

A protein synthesized in response to a specific antigen that the immune system recognizes as "foreign."

ANTICOAGULANTS

Compounds which interfere with the normal blood clotting process. Heparin is one such substance.

ANTICODON

A sequence of three bases in the transfer RNA which is complimentary to that in the messenger RNA.

ANTIDIURETIC HORMONE (ADH)

Also known as vasopressin. A hormone that is released by the pituitary and promotes water conservation by the kidney. It also raises blood pressure.

ANTIGEN

A compound that elicits or stimulates the production and release of antibodies.

ANTIHEMORRHAGIC VITAMIN

Vitamin K.

ANTIHISTAMINES

Compounds that inhibit the release and/or synthesis of histamines.

ANTIHYPERTENSIVE AGENTS

Drugs that serve to maintain normal blood pressure. They can block the receptors for the vasoconstrictor hormones, promote water loss by decreasing the renal water reabsorption process, or interfere with the calcium ion second messenger systems.

ANTI-INFLAMMATORY DRUGS

Two types. Steroids and nonsteroids. The steroids, hydrocortisone, prednisone, and other similar compounds, are prescription drugs which act by inhibiting the enzyme phospholipase A_2. Phospholipase A_2 stimulates the release of arachidonic acid from the membrane phospholipids. Hence, inhibition of this reaction will result in a decreased supply of arachidonic acid for eicosanoid synthesis (see nonsteroidal anti-inflammatory drugs).

ANTIMETABOLITE

A compound similar to a naturally occurring metabolite but which interferes with metabolic processing because it is not identical in all respects to the metabolite.

ANTIMICROBIAL

See antibiotics. Antimicrobial also refers to any treatment that kills micro-organisms regardless of where these organisms reside. Cleaning solutions, for example, can be antimicrobial solutions.

ANTIMINERALS

See type B antinutritives. Minerals that interfere with the absorption or use of other required minerals or minerals that, in any amount, are toxic. Examples of the former are the zinc, copper, and iron interactions. If any one is in excess it serves as an antimineral for the others. Examples of the latter are lead, antimony, cadmium, and mercury.

ANTINEURITIC FACTORS

Factors needed for normal nerve development, usually included are the B vitamins; an antineuritic factor is one which prevents an inflammation of the neuron or axon.

ANTINUTRITIVES

Compounds which are capable of producing nutritional deficiency or interfering in the utilization and function of nutrients. They can interfere with food components before intake, during digestion in the gastrointestinal tract, and after absorption in the body. The conditions under which they may have important effects are malnutrition or a marginal nutritional state. Antinutritives can be characterized as type A, type B or type C antinutritives.

ANTIOXIDANTS

Agents that prevent or inhibit oxidation reactions; in particular they are agents that prevent the oxidation of unsaturated fatty acids. Vitamins A, E, and C act as antioxidants. Some food additives prolong product freshness by acting as antioxidants.

ANTIPROTEINS

See type A antinutritives.

ANTIPYRIDOXINE FACTORS

See type C antinutritives.

ANTIRACHITIC FACTORS

Nutrients which are required for normal bone growth and development. Includes Vitamins C and D and minerals (Ca, phosphorous, magnesium, manganese, potassium, etc.). These nutrients are called antirachitic because they prevent the development of rickets. Vitamin K is also required for normal bone development but is not usually included in this group of nutrients.

ANTITHIAMINE FACTORS

See type C antinutritives.

ANTIVITAMINS

Substances that interfere with normal vitamin action.

ANURIA

Lack of urine secretion.

AORTA

The vessel that carries blood from the left ventricle of the heart to the vessels that serve the rest of the body.

AORTIC ANEURYSM

Aneurysm affecting any part of the aorta.

AORTIC INSUFFICIENCY

Condition in which blood regurgitates into the ventricle through a compromised aortic valve resulting in left ventricle dilation and hypertrophy.

AORTIC STENOSIS

Condition in which the diameter of the aortic valve opening narrows causing left ventricular hypertrophy and leading to congestive heart failure.

ANUS

Opening at the posterior end of the digestive tract.

APATHY

Indifference.

APHRODISIACS

Substances thought to increase sexual desire as part of a cultural belief about sexual performance. There is little scientific evidence to support these beliefs.

APOENZYME

The inactive part or "backbone" of the enzyme protein.

APOPROTEINS

Blood proteins that can carry lipid (or some other compound). The lipid carrying proteins are listed in Table 11. The term apoprotein can also refer to other proteins that are components of other transport or enzyme systems.

APPESTAT THEORY

Also referred to as the set-point theory which hypothesizes that the body establishes a preferred weight and defends that weight under varying food intake conditions.

APPETITE

Desire for food.

TABLE 11
Proteins Involved in Lipid Transport

Protein	Function
apo A-II	Transport protein in HDL
apo B	Transport protein for chylomicrons
High density lipoprotein binding protein (HDLBP)	Binds HDL and functions in the removal of excess cellular cholesterol
apo D	Transport protein similar to retinol-binding protein
apo (a)	Abnormal transport protein for LDL
apo A-I	Transport protein for chylomicrons and HDL
apo C-III	Transport protein for VLDL
apo A-IV	Transport protein for chylomicrons
CETP	Participates in the transport of cholesterol from peripheral tissue to liver; reduces HDL size
LCAT	Participates in the reverse transport of cholesterol from peripheral tissues to the liver
apo E	Protein remnant transferred from HDL to chylomicron remnant. Required for clearance of chylomicron remnant
apo C-I	Transport protein for VLDL
apo C-II	Chylomicron transport protein required cofactor for LPL activity

Adapted from Berdanier, C.D., Ed., *Nutrients and Gene Expression. Clinical Aspects*, CRC Press, Boca Raton, FL, 1996, 104.

ARACHIDONIC ACID

Long chain fatty acid having four double bonds and 20 carbons.

ARACHIS OIL

Peanut oil.

ARCHIMEDES PRINCIPLE

An object's volume when submerged in water equals the volume of the water it displaces. If the mass and volume are known, the density can be calculated.

ARGINASE

An enzyme which catalyzes the cleavage of arginine to urea and ornithine.

ARGINEMIA

A genetic disease where a mutation in the gene for arginase has occurred, characterized by high blood levels of arginine.

ARGININE

An essential amino acid for growing animals (see Table 5). Precursor of nitric oxide, a vasoactive compound; precursor of urea in the urea cycle (see urea cycle).

ARM CIRCUMFERENCE

See midarm circumference.

AROMATIC AMINO ACIDS

Amino acids that have a ring structure. Included are phenylalanine, tyrosine, and tryptophan (see Table 5).

ARRHYTHMIA

Condition resulting from abnormal cardiac impulse initiation and/or conduction causing the heart to pump irregularly.

ARTERIAL BLOOD GAS (ABG) STUDIES

Group of laboratory tests used to reflect the acid/base balance of the body. Included in arterial blood gas analysis are tests that provide information on pH, partial pressure of carbon dioxide ($PaCO_2$), partial pressure of oxygen (PaO_2), oxygen saturation (SaO_2), bicarbonate (HCO_3), and base excess.

ARTERIOGRAPHY

A method of examining the arteries using x-rays and an infusion of a radio-opaque dye solution.

ARTERIOSCLEROSIS

General term for degeneration of the arteries resulting in thickening and hardening of the arterial wall; referred to as "hardening of the arteries."

ARTERIOSCLEROSIS OBLITERANS
Proliferation of the intima of an artery resulting in complete blockage of that artery.

ARTIFICIAL SWEETENERS
Substances that elicit a sweet taste but which have little or no energy value.

ASCITES
Characterized by accumulation of fluid in the abdomen.

ASCORBIC ACID
Vitamin C; a simple compound needed to prevent scurvy; important for connective tissue synthesis, serves as an antioxidant (see vitamins, Table 49).

ASCORBIC ACID OXIDASE
See type C antinutritives.

ASEPTIC
Sterile; absence of pathogens.

ASPARAGINE
A nonessential amino acid containing two amino groups, four carbons, and two carboxy groups (see Table 5, Amino Acids).

ASPARTAME
A non-nutritive sweetener composed of two amino acids, aspartate, and phenylalanine (see also non-nutritive sweeteners).

ASPARTATE (ASPARTIC ACID)
A nonessential amino acid containing two carboxyl groups (see Table 5, Amino Acids).

ASPIRATION
The process of withdrawing fluids by suction. Can also refer to the inspiration of food or food particles into the trachea.

ASSIMILATION
See absorption.

ASTHENIA
Loss of strength.

ATAXIA
Lack of coordination of muscle movement.

ATHEROGENIC
Atherosclerosis producing.

ATHEROSCLEROSIS

A progressive degenerative condition occurring within the vascular tree and resulting in occlusions and loss of elasticity.

ATP

The energy rich compound that serves as the energy coinage in the cell.

ATPASE

A group of enzymes which catalyze the removal or addition of a single phosphate group to the high energy compound containing adenine. In the direction of cleavage $ATP \rightarrow ADP + Pi$; in the reverse $ADP + Pi \rightarrow ATP$.

ATRIAL FIBRILLATION

An arrhythmia characterized by a rapid atrial rate of 350–600 beats/minute, with a ventricular rate of 160–200 beats/minute.

ATROPHY

Reduced size of an organ or tissue.

ATTENTION DEFICIT HYPERACTIVITY DISORDER

Term used to describe previously accepted terminology such as minimal brain dysfunction, hyperkinetic behavior syndrome, or learning disabled. Characterized by age inappropriate behaviors involving attention, impulsiveness, hyperactivity, or restlessness.

ATTENUATED

Weakened; lessened.

ATTRIBUTABLE PROPORTION (AP)

An effect parameter, indicating the proportion of diseased persons (cases) which can be attributed to exposure. This proportion (AP_e) is obtained by dividing the rate difference by the rate among the exposed: $AP_e = (I_1 - I_0)/I_1$. This is also a parameter for the proportion of cases in the total population which can be attributed to exposure. The total population can be divided in a proportion unexposed individuals (P_0) and a proportion exposed individuals (P_1). The incidence rate in the total population (I_t) can be calculated from $I_t = P_0I_0 + P_1I_1$. The attributable proportion among the total population (AP_t) is defined as: $AP_t = (I_t - I_0)/I_t$.

ATTRIBUTABLE RATE

See rate difference.

AUTOIMMUNITY

The destruction of self through the development of antibodies to the body's own components. It is a disorder of immunologic recognition resulting in excessive B-cell reactivity with autoantibodies produced in combination with autoreactive T cells. The T cells are the ultimate effectors of the target cell destruction. A number of diseases are thought to be autoimmune diseases. Among these are insulin-dependent diabetes, rheumatoid arthritis, and lupus. Autoimmunity is genetically controlled. In insulin-dependent diabetes mellitus, three groups of genes found in the MHC region of the DNA in chromosome 6 have been implicated as being sites for mutation. The first group, called class 1 genes include the HLA-A, HLA-B, and HLA-C genes. These genes code for single chain glycoproteins which are recognized by the cytotoxic T cells. T-cell activation is initiated by the T-cell receptor which recognizes an antigen as part of a cell (whether a foreign cell or not). Autoimmunity involves macrophages as well as the B cells and T cells. The role of the macrophage is to process the antigen so that the T cells and B cells can react to it. Autoimmune disease is a disease of mistaken identity where the antibodies lack specificity and react with self antigens.

AUTOSOMAL RECESSIVE TRAIT

A genetic trait which will express itself only if the individual inherits two identical copies of the same gene (one from each parent).

AUTOSOMAL TRAIT

A genetic characteristic carried on any pair of chromosomes except the xx or xy chromosome pair which determines the sex of the individual.

AUTOXIDATION

Reaction of an organic compound with elemental oxygen under mild conditions. Compounds of many types, including hydrocarbons, such as (poly)unsaturated fatty acids, alcohols, phenols, and amines, may undergo autoxidation. Free fatty acids are more susceptible to oxidation than the fatty acid moieties in glycerides.

AVIDIN

A glycoprotein found in egg white that binds biotin rendering this vitamin unavailable to the consumer. If the egg is cooked, the avidin is denatured and no longer binds biotin. Avidin is an antinutrient.

AVITAMINOSIS

Condition resulting from a vitamin deficiency.

AZO DYES

Additives involved in idiosyncratic food intolerance reactions. Tartrazine is a yellow dye which is, of all azo dyes, most frequently associated with certain symptoms. In Europe, it is used in lemonades, puddings, ice cream, mayonnaise, sweets, and preservatives. Some authors claim that it can cause hyper-reactivity in children. However, this remains controversial. Asthma has also been related to tartrazine intake, although recent studies have failed to identify sensitive patients in double-blind challenges. Other symptoms which are attributed to tartrazine are urticaria and angioedema, but these are extremely rare.

AZOTEMIA

Elevation of urea and other nitrogenous waste compounds in blood due to renal failure.

B

B CELLS

Lymphocytic cells produced in the bone marrow that are not further processed by the thymus gland.

B VITAMINS

A group of vitamins that are water soluble. These include thiamin (B_1), riboflavin (B_2), niacin (B_3, nicotinic acid, nicotinamide), pyridoxine (B_6, pryridoxal, pyridoxamine), folacin (folate, folic acid), vitamin B_{12} (cobalamin), pantothenic acid (pantothenate), and biotin (see vitamins, Table 49).

BABY BOTTLE SYNDROME

Extensive dental caries that form in children allowed to nurse on bottles of fluid that contain carbohydrate. Usually the syndrome is noted in children less than two years of age that have been habitually put to bed with a bottle of milk or juice.

BACTERIAL TOXINS

Toxins produced by bacteria. According to the mechanisms underlying the effects of bacterial toxins, they can be classified as follows:

1. subunit bacterial toxins;
2. membrane-affecting bacterial toxins;
3. lesion-causing bacterial toxins;
4. immuno-active bacterial toxins.

BACTERIOPHAGE

Bacteria eater.

BAKING SODA

Leavening agent that releases CO_2 when wet. The gas then is trapped in the dough mix, giving volume and fragility or tenderness to the mix when baked.

BALANCE METHOD

Intake, use, and excretion of a given nutrient is quantitated. When balance is positive, intake exceeds excretion; when negative, excretion exceeds intake.

BARBITURATES

Sedatives that can be habit forming if misused.

BARIATRICS

A medical term referring to the management of people who are overfat or obese.

BARIUM

A radio opaque mineral used in the x-ray examination of the gastrointestinal tract.

BAROCEPTORS

Sensory nerve endings in the walls of the auricles of the heart, carotid artery sinus, vena cava, and aortic arch that respond to changes in pressure.

BASAL ENERGY EXPENDITURE (BEE)

Estimated energy used by the body at rest in a fasting state to maintain essential body functions. The BEE is then adjusted for activity, injury or disease, and thermic effect of food to predict the total daily energy expenditure. This is then used to estimate the energy intake requirement (see Table 12).

BASAL METABOLISM

The minimum activity of metabolic processes occurring in the body. With reference to energy, it is the least amount of energy used by the body to sustain itself. When measured, the individual is at rest (not asleep), in a comfortable environment (neither shivering nor sweating), free of emotional, mental, and physical stress, and at sexual repose. The basal metabolic rate can be measured as the heat produced by the body under these conditions or as the oxygen consumed. Oxygen consumption is considered the indirect measure of basal metabolism under the assumption that energy consuming reactions which produce heat also use oxygen. Other indirect measures have been devised that relate to either heat production or oxygen use. Table 12 lists some of these methods.

BASEDOW'S DISEASE

Excess thyroid hormone production. Also called Grave's Disease or hyperthyroidism.

BASIC AMINO ACIDS

Amino acids whose side chains have positively charged amino groups. These are histidine, lysine, and arginine.

BASIC LIFE SUPPORT (BLS)

Resuscitation techniques involving evaluation and intervention with regard to breathing status, airway obstruction, heart action, and circulation.

BAT THERMOGENESIS

Heat produced by special fat pads called brown adipose tissue (BAT) located at the base of the neck, beneath the sternum, and under the shoulder blades. Brown adipose tissue is brown because its cells contain many more mitochondria than white fat cells. This tissue is more highly vascularized than white fat tissue. BAT mitochondria when stimulated by catecholamines become uncoupled and produce heat when fatty acids are oxidized. This uncoupling is due to the presence of uncoupling protein. There are several of these proteins found in different tissue types.

BCAA

Branched chain amino acids (See Table 5, Amino Acids). These are valine, leucine, and isoleucine.

BEEF TEA

Beef broth.

TABLE 12
Methods and Equations Used for Calculating Basal Energy Need

Method	
1. Heat production, direct calorimetry	kcal (kJ)/m² (surface area)
2. Oxygen consumption; indirect	O_2 cons/$w^{0.75}$
3. Heat production; indirect	Insensible Water Loss (IW) = Insensible weight loss (IWL) + (CO_2 exhaled – O_2 inhaled) Heat production = IW × 0.58 × $\dfrac{100}{25}$ (0.58 = kcal to evaporate 1 g water)
4. Energy used; indirect	Basal energy = $\dfrac{\text{Creatinine N (mg/day)}}{0.00482 \, (W)}$
5. Estimate (energy need not measured)	BMR = 66.4730 + 13.751W + 5.0033L. 6.550A (men) BMR = 655.0955 + 9.463W + 1.8496 L. 4.6756A (women)
6. Estimate (energy need not measured)	BMR = $71.2W^{0.75}$ $\left(1 + 0.004\,[30 - A] + 0.010\left[\dfrac{L}{w^{0.33}} - 43.4\right]\right)$(men) BMR = $65.8W^{0.75}$ $\left(1 + 0.004\,[30 - A] + 0.018\left[\dfrac{L}{w^{0.33}} - 42.1\right]\right)$(women)

Note: Abbreviations are as follows: W = weight in kg; L = height in cm; A = age in years.

From Berdanier, C.D., *Advanced Nutrition: Macronutrients*, CRC Press, Boca Raton, FL, 1994, 46.

BEHAVIOR MODIFICATION
Self-monitoring techniques useful in weight control that provide individuals with new methods to apply to current overeating situations.

BENZEDRINE
A member of the amphetamine family of drugs which are stimulants and appetite suppressants.

BERIBERI
Thiamin deficiency disease characterized by neural disorders, accumulation of fluid in the heart sac, impaired heart action, anorexia, and muscle pain.

β ADRENERGIC BLOCKERS
Drugs used to control blood pressure.

β ALANINE
A naturally occuring form of alanine which is not incorporated into protein but which is an essential component of coenzyme A, pantothenic acid, and carnosine.

β-CAROTENE

Precursor of active vitamin A. β carotene provides some of the rich yellow and orange color of vegetables rich in this substance. Carrots are an example.

β CELLS

Cells in the Islets of Langerhans of the pancreas which produce and release insulin. When these cells are destroyed either through autoimmune destruction, viral-mediated destruction, or through chemicals such as alloxan or streptozotocin, insulin-dependent diabetes mellitus results.

β HYDROXYBUTYRATE, β HYDROXYBUTYRIC ACID

One of the ketone bodies. The result of the reduction of acetoacetate via β hydroxybutyrate dehydrogenase with NAD^+ as hydrogen acceptor.

β OXIDATION

Process in the mitochondria for the oxidation of fatty acids (see fatty acid oxidation).

BETAINE

Precursor of choline.

BETEL NUTS

Nuts from the areta palm; when chewed, these nuts have a stimulant effect.

BIAS

A measure of inaccuracy or departure from accuracy.

BICARBONATE

Any salt containing HCO_3; bicarbonate in the blood is indicative of the alkali reserve.

BIFIDUS FACTOR

Compound in human milk that inhibits growth of particular bacteria in the digestive tract.

BILE

Fluid produced by the liver and stored in the gall bladder which releases this fluid in response to a variety of gut hormonal signals (primarily cholecystokinen). Bile contains bile salts.

BILE ACID SEQUESTRANTS

Group of medications used to treat hypercholesterolemia.

BILE ACIDS

Cholic and chenodeoxycholic acid synthesized by the liver from cholesterol. These acids are present as anions and are referred to as bile salts. At pH values above 7.4, bile salts form aggregates with fats at concentrations above 2–5 mM. These aggregates are called micelles. The primary bile acids are secreted into the intestine, and the intestinal flora convert these acids to their conjugated forms by dehydroxylating carbon 7. Further metabolism occurs at the far end of the intestinal tract where lithocholate is sulfated. While the dehydroxylated acids can be reabsorbed and sent back to the liver via the portal blood, the sulfated lithocholate is not. It appears in the feces. All four of the bile acids, the primary and dehydroxylated forms, are recirculated via the entero-hepatic system such that very little of the bile acids is lost. It has been estimated that the bile acid lost in the feces (~0.8 g/day) equals that newly synthesized by the liver such that the total pool remains between 3–5 g. The amount secreted per day is on the order of 16–70 g. Since the pool size is only 3–5 g, this means that these acids are recirculated as much as 14 times a day. The function of the bile acids is thus quite similar to that of enzymes. Neither are "used up" by the processes they participate in and facilitate. In the instance of fat absorption, the bile acids facilitate the formation of micelles which in turn facilitate the uptake of the dietary fatty acids, monoglycerides, sterols, phospholipids, and other fat-soluble nutrients by the enterocyte of the small intestine.

BILE PIGMENTS

Breakdown product of the heme portion of hemoglobin, myoglobin, and the cytochromes (see also bilirubin, biliverdin, and heme).

BILE SALTS

Anionic forms of bile acids. Glycocholate is a combination of cholyl CoA with glycine; taurocholate is a combination of cholyl CoA with taurine.

BILIARY CALCULI

Stones in the biliary tree. If vessels are blocked by these stones biliary cirrhosis results.

BILIRUBIN

A bile pigment resulting from the breakdown of heme, the nonprotein, iron-containing portion of hemoglobin. In excessive hemoglobin breakdown, bilirubin may spill into the blood and produces a deep yellow color in the skin. This is called jaundice. Excess billirubin in the blood is called bilirubinemia.

BILIVERDIN

The product of the first step in heme catabolism.

BIOAVAILABILITY

Quantity of nutrient available to the body after absorption. Bioavailability is a particular concern in the absorption of essential minerals. In this setting, bioavailability is defined as the percent of the consumed mineral that enters via the intestine and is used for its intended purpose.

BIOELECTRICAL IMPEDANCE

The measure of resistance to an alternating current in a body. Used to estimate percent body fat and body water.

BIOFLAVONOIDS

A group of yellow pigments in plants that have biological activity but are not considered essential nutrients. At one time they were called vitamin P.

BIOGENIC AMINES

Formed in the body by decarboxylation of amino acids. Can be found in food plants. Biogenic amines of plant origin include dopamine (occurrence [in mg per 100 g fresh weight]: avocado

[0.4–0.5], banana pulp [66–70], orange [0.1], date [<0.08], fig [<0.02], pawpaw [0.1–0.2]); epinephrine (occurrence: banana pulp [<0.25], date [<0.08], fig [<0.02]); norepinephrine (occurrence: banana pulp [10.8], potato [0.01–0.02], date [<0.08], fig [<0.02], plantain [green: 0.2, ripe: 0.25]); serotonin (occurrence: avocado [1.0], banana pulp [2.5–8.0], eggplant [0.2], red plum [1.0], ripe tomato [1.2], date [0.9], fig [1.3], pawpaw [0.1–0.2], pineapple [green: 5.0–6.0, ripe: 2.0, juice: 2.5–3.5], plantain [green: 2.0–6.0, ripe: 4.0–10.0, cooked: 4.7]); and tyramine (occurrence: avocado [2.3], banana pulp [6.5–9.4], eggplant [0.3], orange [1.0], red plum [0.6], ripe tomato [0.4], potato [0.1]). Large dietary intakes of foods containing these amines can pose some risk of harm. An example is the consumption of food combinations containing dopamine, norepinephrine, and tyramine. When combined with ingestion of monoamine oxidase inhibitors, mediating the oxidative deamination of these phenethyl-amines, hypertension can result.

Biogenic amines in food can also originate from fermentation or bacterial contamination. The main producers of biogenic amines in foods are Enterobacteriaceae and Enterococci. Examples of biogenic amines include ethylamine (precursor: alanine), putrescine (precursor: ornithine), histamine (precursor: histidine), cadaverine (precursor: lysine), tyramine (precursor: tyrosine), phenylethylamine (precursor: phenylalanine), and tryptamine (precursor: tryptophan). Symptoms of biogenic amine intoxication, persisting for several hours, include burning throat, flushing, headache, nausea, hypertension, numbness and tingling of the lips, rapid pulse, and vomiting. Especially histamine has been indicated as the causative agent in several outbreaks of food intoxication. The toxicity of histamine seems to be enhanced by the presence of other biogenic amines found in foods that can inhibit histamine-metabolizing enzymes in the small intestine. Factors stimulating the formation of biogenic amines include: (1) presence of free amino acids, acting as precursors; (2) low pH of the product; (3) high NaCl concentration; and (4) microbial decarboxylase activity. Occurrence of biogenic amines has been reported in lactic fermented products, in particular wine, cheese, fish, and meat, and at low levels in fermented vegetables. Natural occurrence of biogenic amines (produced by microbial decarboxylase activity) has been reported in fruits, vegetables, and fish. Pasteurization of cheese and milk, good hygienic practice, and selection of starters with low decarboxylase activity are measures to prevent the accumulation of biogenic amines.

BIOLOGICAL VALUE OF PROTEINS

A measure of the quality of a dietary protein with respect to its availability and its amino acid composition which meet the amino acid needs of the consumer. Foods containing high quality proteins are usually from animal sources (milk, eggs, meat, cheese, etc.) while poor quality proteins are usually (but not always) from plants.

BIOMARKER

A measurement of a particular enzyme or substrate or specific characteristic of cells, tissues, or whole animals that characterizes and identifies that particular biological system.

BIOPSY

The removal of a very small amount of tissue from a selected site.

BIOTIN

A vitamin of the B family. An important coenzyme in fatty acid synthesis and in pyruvate metabolism. Carboxylases require biotin attached to a lysine residue for activity. The oxidation of odd chain fatty acids also requires biotin, as does gluconeogenesis (see vitamins, Table 49).

BITOT'S SPOTS

Shiny foam-like spots on the white of the eye; often observed in malnutrition.

BLACK TONGUE

A disease seen in dogs due to niacin deficiency; the canine equivalent of pellegra.

BLANCHING

A processing technique involving brief exposure to boiling water. Blanching wilts the leaf structure of plants, may inhibit peroxidation of fats and oils, and results in inactivation of a variety of enzymes that contribute to food spoilage.

BLAND DIET

Diet designed to potentially avoid irritation of the gastrointestinal tract and to decrease peristalsis. Considerable variability exists among diet manuals for foods allowed on a bland diet; many health care facilities do not use a bland diet, for the diet does not decrease gastric acid secretion or increase healing rate of peptic ulcers.

BLEPHARITIS

Inflammation of the eyelids.

BLIND LOOP SYNDROME

Condition resulting from an undesirable change in the anatomy of the small intestine where a loop is formed in which intestinal contents enter but cannot leave.

BLOOD CLOTTING

See Vitamin K.

BLOOD GLUCOSE LEVEL

Normally ranges between 80–120 mg/dl or 4–6 mmol/l.

BLOOD PRESSURE

The pressure exerted on the vascular tree by the pumping action of the heart. Normal blood pressure is 120 (systolic) over 80 (diastolic) mm mercury. Pressure is measured by a syphignomanometer.

Hypotension — low blood pressure.
Hypertension — high blood pressure.

BLOOD UREA NITROGEN (BUN)

Biochemical test used to evaluate renal excretory capacity and to diagnose renal disease. The level of urea in the blood is 8–20 mg/dl or 2.86–7.14 mmol/l.

BMI

Body mass index = body weight (kg)/height (cm)^2.

BMR

Basal metabolic rate. The minimal amount of energy needed to sustain the body's metabolism. Frequently expressed in terms of the amount of oxygen used to sustain this metabolism because of the constancy between energy flux and oxygen use.

BODY CELL MASS

The metabolically active, energy requiring mass of the body.

BODY DENSITY

Weight (mass) per unit volume.

BODY FRAME SIZE

Determined by measuring wrist circumference at the smallest circumference distal to the styloid process of the radius and ulna and comparing to established classifications as small, medium, or large body frame.

BODY-ORIENTED FOOD CHEMICALS

Food chemicals in the form of nutrients, which are necessary for growth, maintenance, and reproduction of living organisms. They are divided into two groups: (1) macronutrients (fats, carbohydrates, and proteins) and (2) micronutrients (vitamins and minerals, including trace elements). For the intake of nutrients recommended dietary allowances (RDAs) are set by official committees. These allowances are set in broad terms to allow for individual variation.

BOLUS

Single large dose of a substance sometimes administered as a pill, sometimes as a solution.

BOMBESIN

A 14 amino acid peptide hormone found in the central nervous system, the thyroid gland, lung, adrenal, and skin and which has a broad spectrum of action. It raises blood glucose level, lowers body temperature, increases locomotor activity, and raises the pain threshold. It also induces satiety and thus plays a role in food intake regulation. As a neuropeptide, bombesin is found in all neurons of the CNS. It is found in large quantities in the hypothalamus where it functions as a modulary agent altering dopamine metabolism in this tissue as well as in other brain regions. Bombesin is also known as gastrin-releasing peptide. In the intestinal tract, the action of bombesin opposes that of somatostatin. It directly stimulates pancreatic enzyme release and gastric acid secretion.

BORON

A mineral needed in very small amounts. Found in the bone mineral.

BOTULISM

One of the diseases caused by "food poisoning" (see food borne disease). A bacterial intoxication caused by ingestion of food contaminated by toxins of *Clostridium botulinum* or *Clostridium parabotulinum*. Because of its lethality and severity of symptoms, botulism is a dreaded disease. Outbreaks of the disease have been reported from various countries since the early part of the nineteenth century. Recent outbreaks have been reported after consumption of yoghurt with hazelnut (1989: 27 cases, 1 death), fermented seal oil (1989: 4 cases, 2 deaths), white fish (1989: 8 cases, 1 death), traditional Eskimo fish product (1984, 1989), and infant botulism (1987–1989: 68 cases).

BOWEL

Synonym for large intestine; sometimes includes the small intestine as well.

BRADYCARDIA

A slow heart rate characterized by a pulse less than 60 beats per minute.

BRANCHED CHAIN AMINO ACIDS

A group of amino acids (leucine, isoleucine, valine) metabolized by muscle tissue rather than the liver.

BRIGHT'S DISEASE

Kidney disease.

BROWN ADIPOSE TISSUE (BAT)

Highly vascularized adipose tissue with mitochondria-rich adipocytes (see BAT thermogenesis).

BTU

British thermal unit. Amount of energy needed to raise the temperature of one pound of water one degree Farenheit.

BUFFER

A compound that resists a change in hydrogen ion concentration in solution.

BULIMIA

Habitual self-induced vomiting. Frequently accompanies anorexia nervosa.

BUTYLATED HYDROXYANISOL (BHA)

A food additive similar in function to BHT.

BUTYLATED HYDROXYTOLUENE (BHT)

A food additive that serves as an antioxidant, particularly useful in preventing the auto-oxidation of unsaturated fatty acids.

C

CACHEXIA

Tissue wasting as in disease or overwhelming trauma or starvation.

CACOGEUSIA

The presence of a bad taste in the mouth.

CADMIUM

A mineral that is toxic.

CAFFEIC ACID

See type C antinutritives.

CAFFEINE

An alkaloid present in coffee. Has diuretic properties as well as stimulatory effects on circulation and respiration.

CALCIDIOL

A metabolite of vitamin D; 25-hydroxyvitamin D used to make the active form, 1,25 dihydroxy vitamin D (see vitamins, Table 49).

CALCIFEROL

Synonym for vitamin D.

CALCIFICATION

Deposition of calcium as a salt of phosphate in the ground substance of bone.

CALCITONIN

Hormone secreted by the thyroid gland; functions in the maintenance of calcium homeostasis by opposing the calcium mobilizing action of parathormone.

CALCITRIOL

Synonym for the active form of vitamin D; 1,25 dihydroxy vitamin D; 1,25 dihydroxy cholecalciferol (see vitamins, Table 49).

CALCIUM

An essential mineral; important as a second messenger for a variety of hormones; essential in the regulation of oxidative phosphorylation and for bone mineralization (see minerals, Table 29).

CALCIUM CHANNEL BLOCKERS

Drugs used to increase the pumping action of the heart.

CALCIUM GLUCONATE

Water-soluble salt of calcium.

CALCIUM TETANY

Muscle spasms which occur when calcium is absent or deficient in the tissue.

CALCULUS

Synonym for gallstones or kidney stones; complex mineral precipitants.

CALMODULIN

Calcium-dependent regulatory protein. It has four calcium binding sites and full occupancy of these leads to a marked conformational change which in turn is related to its ability to activate or inactivate enzymes. Calmodulin is an intracellular calcium transport protein which carries calcium from the endoplasmic reticulum (where calcium is stored) to sites for its use.

CALORIE (KILOCALORIE)

Classical nutritionists use the term Calorie or kilocalorie (kcal) to represent the amount of heat required to raise the temperature of 1 kilogram of water 1°C. The international unit of energy is the joule. One Calorie or kcal is equal to 4.184 kilojoules or 4.2 kJ. The joule is 10^7 ergs where 1 erg is the amount of energy expended in accelerating a mass of 1 g by 1 cm/s. The international joule is defined as the energy liberated by one international ampere flowing through a resistance of one international ohm per second.

CALORIMETRY

The measurement of heat produced by the body or by food.

cAMP

Cyclic 3′5′ adenosine monophosphate. An activator of protein kinase; serves as a second messenger for certain hormones.

CANCER

A group of diseases characterized by abnormal growth of cells which, because it is uncontrolled, subsume the normal functions of vital organs and tissues.

CANOLA OIL

An oil extracted from a variety of the rapeseed plant renamed canola; contains unsaturated fatty acids of the omega 3 family and no erucic acid.

CARBOHYDRATE

Polyhydroxy aldehydes or ketones and their derivatives. The carbohydrates are divided into three major classes: monosaccharides, oligosaccharides, and polysaccharides. A monosaccharide consists of a single polyhydroxy aldehyde or ketone unit. An oligosaccharide contains two to ten monosaccharide units (the upper limit on the number of monosaccharides in an oligosaccharide is not rigorously defined). Disaccharides, composed of two monosaccharides, are the most prevalent oligosaccharides. A polysaccharide is composed of very long chains of monosaccharides.

Structure and Nomenclature

Monosaccharides

Monosaccharides, called simple sugars, have the empirical formula $(CH_2O)_n$, where $\underline{n}$ is 3 or more. Although monosaccharides may have as few as three or as many as nine carbon atoms, the ones of interest to the nutritionist have five or six. The carbon skeleton is unbranched, and each carbon atom, except one, has a hydroxyl group and a hydrogen atom. At the remaining carbon atom, there is a carbonyl group. If the carbonyl function is on the last carbon atom, the compound is an aldehyde and is called an <u>aldose</u>; if it occurs at any other carbon, the compound is a ketone and is called a <u>ketose</u>. These structures are illustrated in Figure 9.

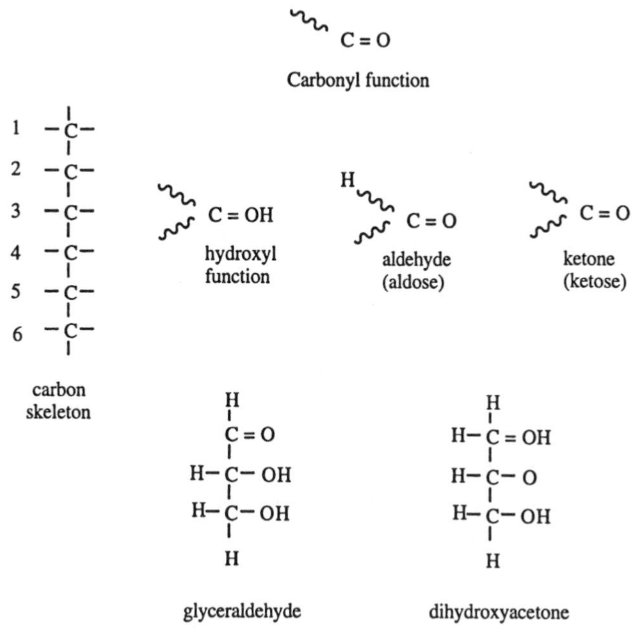

FIGURE 9   Structures of monosaccharides.

The simplest monosaccharide is the three-carbon aldehyde or ketone, <u>triose</u>. Glyceraldehyde is an aldotriose; dihydroxyacetone is a ketotriose. Successive chain elongation of trioses yields <u>tetroses</u>, <u>pentoses</u>, <u>hexoses</u>, <u>heptoses</u>, and <u>octoses</u>. In the aldo-series these are called: aldotriose, aldotetrose, aldopentose, aldohexose, etc.; in the keto-series; ketotriose, ketotetrose, ketopentose, ketohexose, etc.

Hexoses are white crystalline compounds, freely soluble in water but insoluble in such nonpolar solvents as benzene and hexane. Most of them have a sweet taste and are by far the most abundant of the monosaccharides. Of these, glucose, fructose, and galactose are most often found in foods, frequently as components of disaccharides or polysaccharides. Mannose is occasionally found but only in complexes that are poorly digested. Aldopentoses are important components of nucleic acid; derivatives of triose and heptose are intermediates in carbohydrate metabolism.

The monosaccharides in the body undergo a number of reactions which will be detailed in the section on metabolism. These reactions produce five general groups of products as shown in Table 13.

Oligosaccharides
Oligosaccharides consist of two to ten monosaccharides joined with a glycosidic bond.

The bond is formed between the anomeric carbon of one sugar and any hydroxyl function of another sugar. If two monosaccharides are bonded in this manner, the resulting molecule is a disaccharide; if three, a trisaccharide; if four, a tetrasaccharide, etc.

TABLE 13
Characteristic Reaction Products of
Carbohydrates in the Body

Product	Example
Phosphoric acid esters	Glucose 6 phosphate
Polyhydroxy alcohols	Sorbitol
Deoxy sugars	Deoxyribose
Sugar acids	Gluconic acid
Amino sugars	Glucosamine

Disaccharides

Of the oligosaccharides, by far the most prevalent in nature are the disaccharides. Of dietary significance are the disaccharides, lactose, maltose, and sucrose.

Lactose, the sugar found in the milk of most mammals (it is lacking in the milk of the whale and the hippopotamus), consists of a D-galactose and D-glucose joined with a glycosidic linkage at carbon one of galactose and carbon four of glucose. The glucose residue of lactose possesses a free anomeric carbon; the α form is the most predominant. Lactose is a reducing sugar. The glycosidic linkage between galactose and glucose is symbolized by α (1 → 4).

An important characteristic of lactose is its ability to promote, in the intestinal tract, the growth of certain beneficial lactic acid-producing bacteria. These bacteria have a possible role in the displacement of undesirable putrefactive forms of bacteria. Lactose also appears to enhance the absorption of calcium.

Maltose, also known as malt sugar, contains two glucose residues. The glycosidic linkage is α (1 → 4).

Cellobiose, the repeating disaccharide unit of cellulose, and gentiobiose are two other disaccharides that have as their repeating units D-glucose. In cellobiose the glycosidic linkage is β (1 → 4); in gentiobiose it is β (1 → 6). Since all have free anomeric carbons, they are reducing sugars.

Sucrose, also known as table sugar, cane sugar, beet sugar, and grape sugar, is a disaccharide of glucose and fructose linked through the anomeric carbon of each monosaccharide. Because neither anomeric carbon is free, sucrose is a nonreducing sugar. When sucrose is used in the preparation of acidic foods, some inversion (hydrolysis of sucrose to glucose and fructose) invariably takes place. For instance, if it is used to sweeten fruit drinks, it is completely inverted within a few hours. In soft drinks there is also a considerable amount of inversion. Invert sugar is sweeter than sucrose. Honey is, in large part, invert sugar. The bees collect sucrose from flowers and the bee's enzymes invert the sucrose. Honey, however, is not pure glucose and fructose; its other major constituents are sucrose, water, and small quantities of flavor extract peculiar to the flower from which it is obtained. The development of an enzyme which will isomerize D-glucose to D-fructose has proved to be commercially valuable. It provides a method of obtaining a product known as high-fructose corn syrup, which is sweeter than an equimolar sucrose solution.

In general, the disaccharides, while of importance as dietary sources of carbohydrates, have few metabolic functions. They are hydrolyzed into their component monosaccharides in the enterocyte and converted to glucose which is the body's primary metabolic fuel.

A few oligosaccharides with more than two monosaccharide moieties are of nutritional significance. Stachyose, a tetrasaccharide composed of two molecules of D-galactose, one of D-glucose, and one of D-fructose, is found in certain foods, particularly those of legume origin. It is usually found with raffinose (fructose, glucose, and galactose) and sucrose. The human digestive tract does not possess an enzyme which can hydrolyze stachyose or raffinose. Evidently, however, these sugars are fermented in the lower intestinal tract by the intestinal flora. This further metabolism is thought to be at least primarily responsible for the unwanted flatus (gas produced and released by the intestinal tract) that frequently follows the ingestion of many legumes.

Polysaccharides

Polysaccharides (also known as glycans) are compounds consisting of large numbers of monosaccharides linked by glycosidic bonds; they are analogous in structure to oligosaccharides. Some possess low molecular weights, corresponding to 30–90 monosaccharides. However, most of the carbohydrates found in nature exist as polysaccharides with a high molecular weight; they may contain several hundred or even thousands of monosaccharide units. Polysaccharides differ from one another in the nature of their repeating monosaccharide units, in the number of such units in their chain, and in the degree of branching.

The polysaccharides which contain only a single kind of monosaccharide or monosaccharide derivative are called **homopolysaccharides**; those which have two or more different monomeric units are called **heteropolysaccharides**. Often homopolysaccharides are given names which indicate the nature of the building blocks: for example, those which contain mannose units are mannans; those which contain fructose units are called fructans. The important biological polysaccharides are the **storage polysaccharides**, the **structural polysaccharides**, and the **mucopolysaccharides**.

Storage polysaccharides

Among plants the most abundant storage polysaccharide is starch. It is deposited abundantly in grains, fruits, and tubers in the form of large granules in the cytoplasm of cells; each plant deposits a starch characteristic of its species. Starch exists in two forms: α-amylose and amylopectin. α-Amylose makes up 20–30% of most starches and consists of 250–300 unbranched glucose residues bonded by α (1 → 4) linkages. The chains vary in molecular weight from a few thousand to 500,000. The molecule is twisted into a helical coil. Amylopectin, which comprises the remainder of the starch in a plant, is highly branched. Its backbone consists of glucose residues with α (1 → 4) glycosidic linkages; its branch points are α (1 → 6) glycosidic bonds. Although the structure of amylopectin is shown in Figure 13 as being linear, it too exists as a helical coil.

When amylose is broken down in successive stages by either the enzyme amylase or by the action of dry heat, as in toasting, the resulting polysaccharides of intermediate chain length are called **dextrin**. Amylopectin, when broken down by the same methods, does not cleave at its branch points. This end product is a large, highly branched product called **limit dextrin**.

Other homopolysaccharides are found in plants, bacteria, yeast, and mold as storage polysaccharides. Dextrans, found in yeast and bacteria, are branched polysaccharides of D-glucose with their major backbone linkage α (1 → 6). Inulin, found in artichokes, consists of D-fructose monomers with β (2 → 1) glycosidic linkages. Mannans are composed of mannose residues and are found in bacteria, yeasts, mold, and higher plants.

Among animals, the storage polysaccharide is glycogen. Glycogen is stored primarily in the liver and muscles. Like amylopectin, glycogen is a branched polysaccharide of D-glucose with a backbone glycosidic linkage of α (1 → 4) and branch points of α (1 → 6). However, its branches occur every 8 to 10 residues, as compared to every 12 for amylopectin. For muscle glycogen, the molecular weight has been estimated to be about 10^6; for liver, 5×10^6 (corresponding to about 30,000 glucose residues). Glycogen is of no importance as a dietary source of carbohydrate. The small amount of glycogen in an animal's body when it is slaughtered is quickly degraded during the postmortum period.

Structural polysaccharides

Cellulose is the most abundant structural polysaccharide in the plant world. Of the carbon in vegetables, 50% is cellulose; wood is about one-half cellulose, and cotton is nearly pure cellulose. It is a straight chain polymer of D-glucose with β (1 → 4) glycosidic linkages between the monosaccharides. Cellobiose, a disaccharide, is obtained on partial hydrolysis of cellulose. The molecular weight of cellulose has been estimated to range from 50,000 to 500,000 (equivalent to 300 to 3000 glucose residues). Cellulose molecules are organized in bundles of parallel chains, called fibrils, which are cross-linked by hydrogen bonding; these chains of glucose units are relatively rigid and are cemented together with hemicelluloses, pectin, and lignin.

Hemicellulose bears no relation structurally to cellulose. It is composed of polymers of D-xylose with β (1 → 4) glycosidic linkages and side chains of arabinose and other sugars. Pectin is a polymer of methyl D-galacturonate. Pectin is found in fruit and is the substance needed to make jelly out of cooked fruit. The juice plus sucrose plus the pectin form a gel that is stable for many months at room temperature. Pectin is a nonabsorbable carbohydrate that has pharmacological use as well. It is a key component together with kaolin of an antidiarrheal remedy.

There are other structural polysaccharides found in nature. Chitin is a polysaccharide which forms the hard skeleton of insects and crustaceans and is a homopolymer of N-acetyl-D-Glucosamine. Agar, derived from sea algae, contains D- and L-galactose residues, some esterified with sulfuric acid, primarily with 1 → 3 bonds; alginic acid, derived from algae and kelp, contains monomers of D-mannuronic acid; and vegetable gum (gum arabic) contains D-galactose, D-glucuronic acid, rhamnose, and arabinose. These are used as food stabilizers by the food processing industry. Algin derivatives, for example, are used to stabilize the emulsions made in salad dressings; gum arabic is frequently used to stabilize processed cheese products, where it acts to retard the separation of the solids from the fluid component in such products.

Mucopolysaccharides

The mucopolysaccharides are heteropolysaccharides which are components of the structural polysaccharides found at various places in the body. Mucopolysaccharides consist of disaccharide units in which glucuroic acid is bound to acetylated or sulfurated amino sugars with glycosidic β (1 → 3) linkages. Each disaccharide unit is bound to the next by a β (1 → 4) glycosidic linkage. Thus they are linear polymers with alternating β (1 → 3) and β (1 → 4) linkages.

Hyaluronic acid is the most abundant mucopolysaccharide. It is the principal component of the ground substance of connective tissue and is also abundant in the synovial fluid in joints and the vitreous humor of the eye. The repeating unit of hyaluronic acid is a disaccharide composed of D-glucuronic acid and N-acetyl-D-glucosamine; it has alternating β (1 → 3) and β (1 → 4) glycosidic linkages. The molecular weight is several million.

Another mucopolysaccharide which forms part of the structure of connective tissue is chondroitin. It differs from hyaluronic acid only in that it contains N-acetyl-D-galactosamine residues rather than N-acetyl-D-glucosamine ones. The sulfate ester derivatives of chondroitin, chondroitin sulfate A and chondroitin sulfate C, are major structural components of cartilage, bone, cornea, and other connective tissue. Types A and C have the same structure as chondroitin except for a sulfate ester at carbon atom 4 of the N-acetyl-D-galactosamine residue on type A and one at carbon atom 6 of type C. Heparin (β-heparin), an anticoagulant, is a mucopolysaccharide which is similar in structure to hyaluronic acid because it contains residues of D-glucuronic acid, sulfate, and acetyl groups. Its structure is not entirely known.

CARBOHYDRATE DIGESTION

Once a carbohydrate-rich food is consumed, digestion begins. As the food is chewed it is mixed with saliva which contains α amylase. This amylase begins the digestion of starch by attacking the internal α 1,4-glucosidic bonds. It will not attack the branch points having α 1,4 or α 1,6-glucosidic bonds, hence the salivary α amylase will produce molecules of glucose, maltose, α-limit dextrin, and maltotriose. The α amylase in saliva is an isozyme with the same function as that in the pancreatic juice. The salivary α amylase is denatured in the stomach as the food is mixed and acidified with the gastric hydrochloric acid. As the stomach contents move into the duodenum, it is called chyme. The movement of chyme into the duodenum stimulates cholesystokinin release. This gut hormone acts on the exocrine pancreas stimulating it to release pancreatic juice into the duodenum and on the gall bladder to release bile. Cholesystokinin is secreted by the epithelial endocrine cells of the small intestine, particularly the duodenum. Its release is stimulated by amino acids in the lumen and by the acid pH of the stomach contents as it passes into the duodenum. The low pH of the chyme also stimulates the release of secretin which, in turn, stimulates the exocrine pancreas to release bicarbonate and water so as to raise the pH of the chyme. This is necessary to maximize the activity of the digestive enzymes located on the surface of the luminal cell. Starch digestion begins in the mouth with salivary amylase. It pauses in the stomach as the stomach contents are acidified but resumes when the chyme enters the duodenum and the pH is raised. The amylase of the pancreatic juice is the same as that of the saliva. It attacks the same bonds in the same locations and produces the same products, maltose, maltotriose, and the small polysaccharides (average of 8 glucose molecules) called α-limit dextrins. The limit dextrins are further hydrolyzed by α glucosidases on the surface of the luminal cells. The hydrolysis of the bonds not attacked by α amylase, α glucosidase, or the disaccharidases, maltase, lactase, or sucrase, are passed to the lower part of the intestine where they are attacked by the enzymes of the intestinal flora. Most of the products of this digestion are used by the flora themselves; however, the microbial metabolic products may be of use. The flora can produce useful amounts of short-chain fatty acids and lactate as well as methane gas, carbon dioxide, water, and hydrogen gas. The carbohydrates of legumes typify the substrates these flora use. Raffinose, which is an α galactose 1 → 6 glucose 1 → 2 β fructose, and trehalose, an α glucose 1 → 1 α glucose, are the typical substrates from legumes for these flora. The flora will also attack portions of the fibers and celluloses that are the structural elements in fruits and vegetables. Again, some useful products may be produced, but the bulk of these complex polysaccharides having β linkages and perhaps other substituent groups as part of their structure are largely untouched by both intestinal and bacterial enzymes. These undigested unavailable carbohydrates serve very useful functions:

1. They provide bulk to the diet which in turn helps to regulate the rate of food passage from mouth to anus.
2. They act as adsorbants of noxious or potentially noxious materials in the food.
3. They assist in the excretion of cholesterol and several minerals, thereby protecting the body from overload.

Populations consuming high fiber diets have a lower incidence of colon cancer, fewer problems with constipation, and lower serum cholesterol levels.

The disaccharides in the diet are hydrolyzed to their component monosaccharides by enzymes also located on the surface of the luminal cell. Lactose is hydrolyzed to glucose and galactose by lactase; sucrose is hydrolyzed to fructose, and glucose and maltose is hydrolyzed to two molecules of glucose. Table 14 lists these enzymes together with their substrates and products.

TABLE 14
Enzymes of Importance to Carbohydrate Digestion

Enzyme	Substrate	Products
α Amylase	Starch, amylopectin, glycogen	Glucose, maltose, maltotriose, α-limit dextrin
α Glucosidase	α limit dextrin	Glucose
Lactase	Lactose	Galactose, glucose
Maltase	Maltose	Glucose
Sucrase/isomaltase	Sucrose/α-limit dextrin	Glucose, fructose

From Berdanier, C.D., *Advanced Nutrition: Macronutrients*, CRC Press, Boca Raton, FL, 1994, 174.

CARBOHYDRATE LOADING (GLYCOGEN LOADING)

A technique used by endurance athletes to increase their muscle glycogen content. This technique dictates the exhaustion of the muscle glycogen store followed by rest and glycogen repletion just prior to the competitive event. The rest/repletion routine results in an increased store of glucose from glycogen within the muscle. Since the first phase of glycolysis is anaerobic, an enlarged supply of glucose from glycogen which can be oxidized in the absence of oxygen thus delays exhaustion.

CARBONYL GROUP

An aldehyde group or ketone group

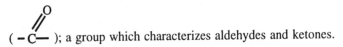 ($-C-$); a group which characterizes aldehydes and ketones.

CARBOXYLASE

An enzyme which catalyzes the addition of a carboxyl group to a carbon chain. This enzyme class usually requires thiamin as thiamin pyrophosphate (TPP) as a coenzyme.

CARBOXYLATION

The addition of a carboxyl group

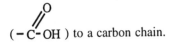 ($-C-OH$) to a carbon chain.

CARCINOGENESIS

The process of developing cancer.

CARDIAC CATHETERIZATION

Procedure used to identify coronary artery blockage in which a catheter or probe is introduced into the vascular system and heart.

CARDIAC FAILURE

Heart ceases to pump or pumps inadequately.

CARDIAC HYPERTROPHY

Enlarged heart.

CARDIAC OUTPUT

The quantity of blood discharged from the left ventricle per minute. Normal cardiac output at rest is 3.0 liter per square meter of body surface per minute.

CARDIOMYOPATHY

Structural or functional disease of the heart muscle (the myocardium).

CARDIOPULMONARY ARREST

Sudden cessation of ventilation and circulation.

CARDIOPULMONARY BYPASS

A procedure used to divert blood from the heart and lungs while maintaining perfusion and oxygenation to the rest of the body through the use of a heart-lung machine.

CARDIOVASCULAR DISEASE

A group of diseases characterized by a diminution of heart action. The oxygen and nutrient supply to the heart may be impeded and/or the heart muscle degenerated or the vascular tree which supplies the heart degenerated or occluded.

CARDIOVASCULAR TESTS AND THERAPIES

Cardiac catheterization
See above.

Electrophysiological studies
Various techniques that record electrical activity from the body surface and the endocardial surface of the heart.

Intravascular stents
Procedure in which a stainless steel stent, attached to a balloon-tipped catheter, is placed in a blocked area of a coronary artery to open it.

Laser angioplasty
Procedure in which a laser is used to open a partially occluded coronary artery. Laser angioplasty is often followed by balloon angioplasty to further open the artery.

Mechanical atherectomy
The process of mechanically removing a coronary artery blockage, usually with the aid of a drill-type catheter.

Percutaneous transluminal coronary angioplasty (PTCA)
A procedure in which an inflated balloon-tipped catheter is used to dilate a blocked coronary artery.

CARIOGENESIS

The process of tooth decay.

CARNITINE

An essential component of fatty acid oxidation; participates in the transport of fatty acids into the mitochondrion prior to oxidation as shown in Figure 10. Carnitine is synthesized from lysine and methionine as shown in Figure 11.

CARNOSINE

A dipeptide synthesized from β alanine and histidine. Found in muscle where it activates myosin ATPase. Carnosine also serves to buffer the acidic state that develops in working muscle.

CAROTENOIDS

A group of yellow-orange pigments some of which can be hydrolyzed to active vitamin A (see vitamins, Table 49). α, β, and γ carotene are considered provitamins because they can be converted to active vitamin A. The carotenes also have an antioxidant function.

CARRIER

A substance, usually a protein, which binds to a substrate and transports it from its point of origin to its point of use.

CASE-CONTROL STUDIES

Nonexperimental studies in which cases of a particular disease are selected and the patient's exposure in the past is compared with that of controls. This type of study is suitable for studying rare diseases. The numbers of subjects needed are small compared to those needed

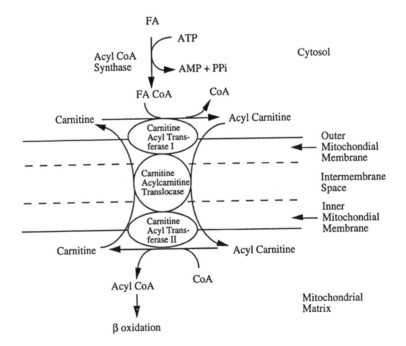

FIGURE 10   Mechanism for the entry of fatty acids into the mitochondrial β oxidation pathway.

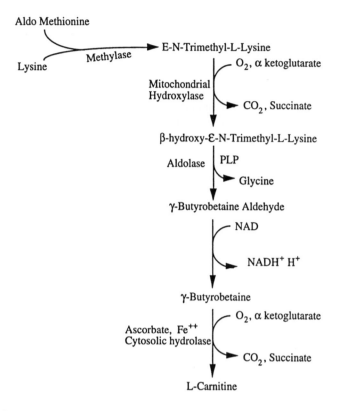

FIGURE 11 Synthesis of carnitine from lysine and methionine.

in cohort studies. Since the cases are selected without knowing the size of the source population at risk from which they arose, no information on the incidence rate of the disease in the population is obtained in these studies. Consequently, the relative risk cannot be calculated but is approximated by the odds ratio. The advantage of this study design is that exposure and disease are both measured at the same time, and therefore one does not have to wait as long as in the cohort design. In this type of study, however, valid assessment of exposure may be a problem, since exposure in the past is measured after the disease has occurred. The disease may have affected recollection of the exposure by the subject. For instance, the occurrence of the disease may be a stimulus to search for an explanation, leading to a more accurate recollection of exposure. Also, the disease may lead to denial of the exposure. For diseases with a long latency period and which influence the factor under investigation, information on exposure in the distant past is needed. This may be impossible.

CASSAVA

A starchy root that is a primary food source in tropical countries.

CATABOLISM

The totality of those reactions that reduce macromolecules to usable metabolites, carbon dioxide, and water.

CATALASE

An enzyme which catalyzes the conversion of peroxide to water and oxygen; this is a key enzyme in the cytoplasmic free radical suppression system.

CATALYST

A substance, usually a protein, in living (or nonliving) systems that enhances or promotes a chemical reaction without being a reactant. Enzymes are catalysts.

CATECHOLAMINES

Neurotransmitters (epinephrine, dopamine, and norepinephrine) which are produced in the adrenal medulla from tyrosine. These hormones are instrumental in orchestrating the "fight or flight" response to stress conditions. Synthesis is shown in Figure 12.

CATION

A positively charged ion.

CDP

Cytidine diphosphate. A nucleotide consisting of cytosine (a pyrimidine), ribose, and two high energy phosphate groups

CECUM

A blind appendage of the intestinal tract located at the juncture of the small and large intestine. Also called the appendix.

CELIAC DISEASE

A group of disorders characterized by diarrhea and malabsorption. Included is the disorder gluten-induced enteropathy.

CELL ANATOMY

The location of the various organelles of a eucaryotic cell is shown in Figure 13. The function of each component is listed in Table 15.

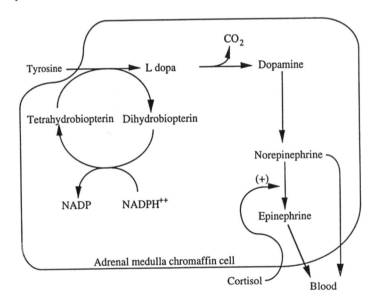

FIGURE 12   Biosynthesis of epinephrine and norepinephrine.

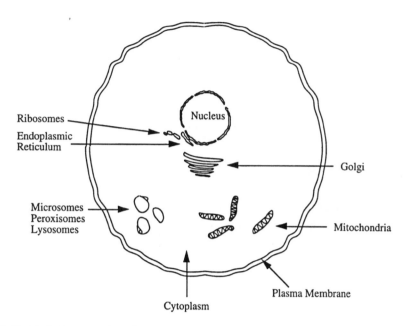

FIGURE 13 Typical eucaryotic cell showing representative intracellular structures. (From Berdanier, C.D., *Advanced Nutrition: Macronutrients*, CRC Press, Boca Raton, FL, 1994, 25.)

TABLE 15
Functions of the Organelles/Cell Fractions that Comprise the Typical Eucaryotic Cell

Organelle/Cell Fraction	Role in Cell	Processes Found
Plasma membrane	Cell boundary holds various receptors for a variety of hormones, substrates, and ions	Processes, exports, and imports substrates, ions, etc.; binds hormones to their respective receptors
Cytoplasm	Medium for a variety of enzymes, substrates, products, ions	Glycolysis, glycogenesis, glycogenolysis, lipogenesis, pentose shunt, urea synthesis (part) protein synthesis (part)
Nucleus	Contains DNA, RNA	Protein synthesis starts here with DNA transcription
Endoplasmic reticulum	Ca^{2+} stored here for use in signal transduction	Has role in many synthetic processes
Golgi apparatus	Sequesters and releases proteins	Export mechanism for release of macromolecules
Mitochondria	Powerhouse of cell	Krebs cycle, respiratory chain, ATP synthesis, fatty acid oxidation; first step of urea synthesis
Ribosomes	Site for completion of protein synthesis	Protein synthesis
Lysosomes	Intracellular digestion	Protein and macromolecule degradation
Peroxisomes	Suppression of oxygen free radicals	Antioxidant enzymes
Microsomes	Drug detoxification	Detoxification

From Berdanier, C.D., *Advanced Nutrition: Macronutrients*, CRC Press, Boca Raton, FL, 1994, 25.

CELL CULTURE

A technique for studying cells from specific tissues. After isolation, the cells are grown in media containing all the known ingredients essential for their support. Different cell types may have different requirements.

CELLULOSE

A structural polysaccharide found primarily in plants and composed of glucose units linked together with β 1,4 bonds (see carbohydrates).

CENTRAL STIMULANTS

Substances increasing the state of activity of the nervous system. A particular class of stimulants are the methylxanthines, which have effects on the peripheral and central nervous system. Examples of methylxanthines are caffeine (occurrence: coffee beans, tea leaves, cocoa beans, cocoanuts), theophylline (occurrence: tea), and theobromine (occurrence: cocoa beans, tea leaves, cola nuts).

CEPHALIN

A phospholipid, similar to lecithin, present in the brain.

CEREBROSIDE

A complex lipid in nerve and other tissues. A cerebroside is a sphingolipid.

CEREBROVASCULAR ACCIDENT

Also referred to as a stroke; sudden circulatory impairment in one or more blood vessels that supply the brain.

CEREBROVASCULAR DISEASE

Similar to cardiovascular disease in that the vascular tree of the brain has developed athero-sclerotic lesions which restrict or occlude the blood supply to this organ.

CERULOPLASMIN

A copper-containing globulin in blood plasma with a molecular weight of 150,000 and 8 copper atoms. It catalyzes the oxidation of amines, phenols, and ascorbic acid. It is reduced in amount in Wilson's disease (hepatolenticular disease).

CETOLEIC ACID ($CH_3(CH_2)_9CH = CH(CH_2)_9COOH$)

A toxic monounsaturated fatty acid, which occurs in herring oil. Its toxic effects are similar to those of erucic acid.

CHEILOSIS

Cracks at the corners of the mouth. Associated with inadequate riboflavin intake; however, it can also occur in the presence of adequate vitamin intake (see vitamins, Table 49).

CHELATE, CHELATION

A combination of metal ions chemically held within a ring of heterocyclic structures by bonds from each of these structures to the metal. Iron is held by heme in this fashion as part of the hemoglobin structure.

CHEMOTHERAPY

Treatment of illness using medication.

CHINESE RESTAURANT SYNDROME

See monosodium glutamate.

CHLORIDE

A major anion in the extracellular fluid. The major dietary source is table salt (NaCl). The normal concentration of chloride ions in serum is about 100 meq/l.

CHLORIDE SHIFT

Part of the system which maintains the blood acid-base balance. Chloride and bicarbonate ions exchange across the erythrocyte plasma membrane, "the shift."

CHLOROPHYLL

A heterocyclic iron/copper-containing green pigment in plants.

CHOLECALCIFEROL

A metabolite of cholesterol formed in the pathway for Vitamin D activation. Cholecalciferol is hydroxylated to 1,25 dihydroxy-cholecalciferol, the active Vitamin D. Also called Calcitrol.

CHOLECYSTITIS

Inflammation of the gallbladder.

CHOLECYSTOKININ (CCK)

A hormone released from duodenal cells and which stimulates the gall bladder to contract and release bile into the duodenum.

CHOLEDOCHOLITHIASIS

Obstruction of the common bile duct; presence of a stone in the duct.

CHOLELITHIASIS

Presence or formation of gallstones.

CHOLESTASIS

Arrest of bile excretion.

CHOLESTATIC JAUNDICE

Jaundice resulting from an abnormality (obstruction) in the flow of bile from the liver to the gall bladder to the intestine.

CHOLESTEROL

A four-ringed structure in the nonsaponifiable lipid class that is an important substrate for steroid hormone synthesis. Its synthesis is shown in Figure 14 and its metabolism in Figure 15.

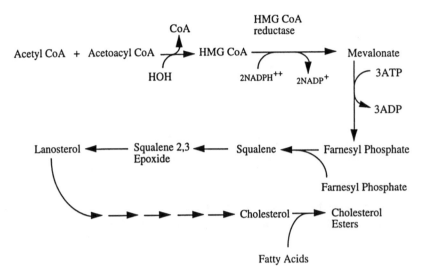

FIGURE 14　　Cholesterol biosynthesis

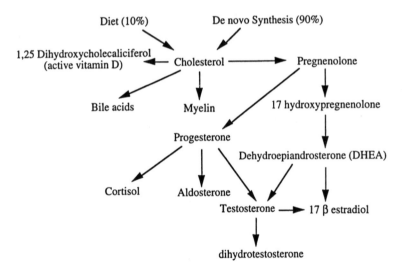

FIGURE 15　　Cholesterol metabolism

CHOLESYSTECTOMY

Surgical removal of gall bladder; the bile duct from the liver is connected directly to the small intestine.

CHOLINE

An amine. An essential nutrient when inadequate synthesis from the carboxylation of serine occurs; part of phospholipid lecithin; also an important component of the neurotransmitter, acetylcholine.

CHROMIUM

A trace mineral; may or may not be essential to the optimal use of glucose (see minerals, Table 29).

CHROMOSOMES

When DNA is extracted from the cell nucleus, it is not one continuous strand. Rather, it breaks up into fairly predictable arrangements called chromosomes. The chromosomes exist in pairs and have been numbered. Those determining the sex of the individual are labeled as X or Y. If the individual has one x and one y, he is a male. If the individual has two x chromosomes, she is a female. Many characteristics have been localized to particular chromosomes. There are species differences in the number of chromosomes. There are 23 sets of chromosomes (46 total) in the human.

CHRONIC DISEASE

A disease which takes years to develop.

CHRONIC LEAD INTOXICATION

Accumulation of lead in soft tissue and bone as a result of continuous exposure to this metal either in the air or in food or beverages.

CHRONIC OBSTRUCTIVE PULMONARY DISEASE (COPD)

Descriptive term characterized by chronic or recurring obstruction of air flow in the lungs resulting from chronic bronchitis, bronchial asthma, emphysema, or bronchiectasis.

CHRONIC RENAL FAILURE (CRF)

The irreversible loss of kidney function that develops over four progressive stages. The first stage is characterized by diminishing renal reserve as indicated by a 50% decrease in glomerular filtration rate. Progression to the second stage occurs when the glomerular filtration rate decreases further to between 20% and 50% of normal and azotemia, polyuria, and nocturia develop. The third stage, described as renal failure, occurs when the glomerular filtration rate drops below 20% of normal and uremia is present. In the final stage, referred to as end-stage renal disease, the glomerular filtration rate has decreased to less than 5% of the normal value and the individual is terminally uremic.

CHYLE

A turbid white or yellow fluid, taken up by the lacteals in the process of lipid digestion and absorption.

CHYLOMICRON

Fat-protein complex formed to carry absorbed dietary fats from the intestine to other tissues. Not normally found in the blood of a fasting individual.

CHYME

The semifluid mass of partly digested food extruded from the stomach into the duodenum of the small intestine.

CIGUATERA POISONING

A disease resulting from the consumption of contaminated fish, in which the toxin has accumulated via a food chain. The alga involved (the photosynthetic dinoflagellate *Gambierdiscus toxicus*) is consumed by a small herbivorous fish. Larger fish feeding on the smaller fish concentrate the toxin further in the chain. This kind of intoxication is found in the South Pacific and the Caribbean. The various ciguatera toxins do not all contribute to the poisoning to the same extent. The main cause is ciguatoxin. Symptoms of ciguatera poisoning are paresthesia in lips, fingers, and toes, vomiting, nausea, abdominal pain, diarrhea, bradycardia, muscular weakness, and joint pain. The mechanism underlying these symptoms may be based on the neuroactivity of ciguatoxin. It increases sodium permeability, leading to depolarization of nerves.

CILIA, CILIUM

Hair-like processes extending out from the surface of epithelial cells.

CIRRHOSIS

Chronic liver disease in which fatty deposits and fibrous connective tissue have replaced functioning liver cells. Cirrhosis may lead to loss of hepatic function and death.

CITRATE

An intermediate in the citric acid cycle; the essential starting metabolite for fatty acid synthesis in the cytosol.

CITRIC ACID CYCLE (KREBS CYCLE)

A cycle found in mitochondria which produces reducing equivalents for use by the respiratory chain and which also produces carbon dioxide. The cycle is shown in Figure 16.

CITRULLINEMIA

Excessive, high levels of citrulline in the blood. Citrulline is a metabolite formed from ornithine and carbamyl phosphate. Citrulline accumulates in a genetic disease caused by the mutation in the gene for arginosuccinate synthetase.

CLEAR LIQUID DIET

Therapeutic diet providing foods and beverages that are transparent and liquid at room temperature.

CLINICAL NUTRIENT DEFICIENCY SIGNS

Poor growth, skin lesions, lethargy, tissue wasting and/or malfunction.

CLINICAL TRIAL

An experiment using human subjects.

CMP

Cytidine monophosphate. A nucleotide consisting of cytosine (a pyrimidine), ribose, and one high energy phosphate group.

CoA

See coenzyme A.

CoQ

See coenzyme Q.

COALESCENCE

Irreversible destabilization of an emulsion.

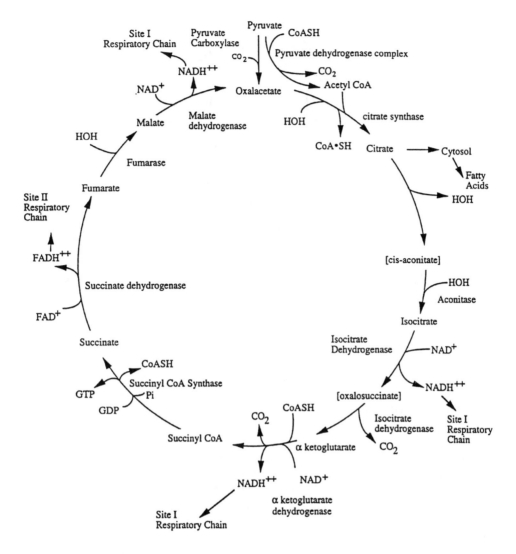

FIGURE 16 Krebs citric acid cycle in the mitochondria. This cycle is also called the tricarboxylate cycle.

COBALAMIN

Vitamin B_{12}. Essential to the metabolism of odd numbered fatty acids and to the synthesis of hemoglobin. B_{12} is a cobalt-containing coenzyme for two types of reactions. In the first, it participates in methyl group transfer as in the methylation of homocysteine to reform methionine. This reaction also requires folacin as N^5 methyltetrahydrofolate. Not only is methionine regenerated in this reaction but so too is tetrahydrofolate. This reaction is essential to hemoglobin synthesis. In the second reaction, 5' adenosylcobalamin is required for the action of methylmalonyl mutase which converts methylmalonyl-CoA to succinyl CoA. This is the final step in the oxidation of odd numbered fatty acids. The structure is shown in Figure 17 (see vitamins, Table 49).

COBALT

An essential mineral needed as a component of vitamin B_{12}.

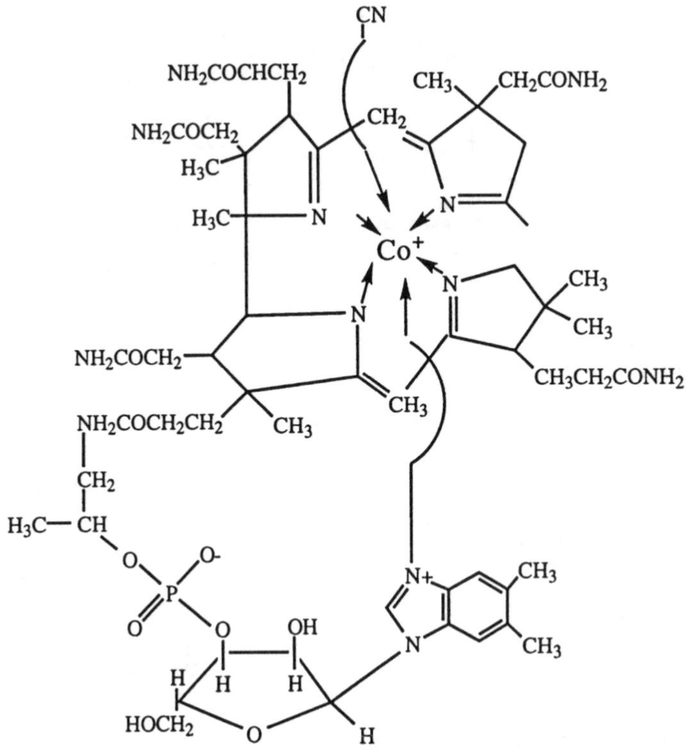

FIGURE 17 Structure of vitamin B_{12}.

CODON

A sequence of three bases (triplet) which specifies a particular amino acid in the sequence of reactions which comprise protein synthesis. The codons of the messenger RNA are matched by the anticodon of the transfer RNA which is bringing the amino acids to the ribosome for incorporation into the protein being synthesized.

COEFFICIENT OF DIGESTIBILITY

The percentage of a consumed food that is digested and absorbed and which does not appear in the feces.

COENZYME A

A coenzyme containing pantothenic acid. CoA forms a thio ester bond with acetyl and acyl groups and with amino acids and facilitates their metabolism. The structure is shown in Figure 18.

COFACTOR

An essential ingredient for an enzyme catalyzed reaction. Cofactors are usually minerals.

COHORT STUDIES

See follow-up studies.

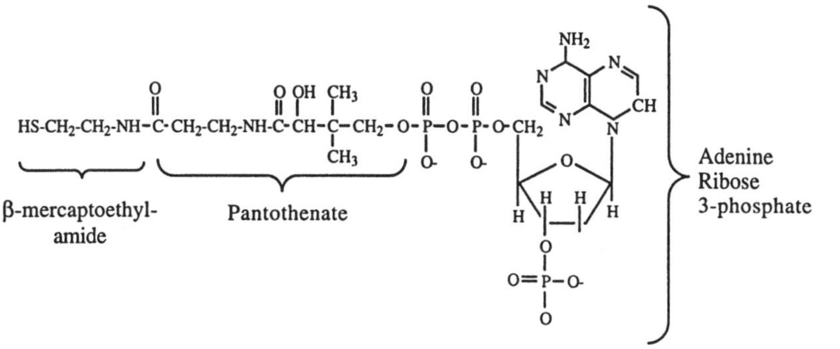

FIGURE 18 Structure of coenzyme A.

COLIC

Condition characterized by excessive flatus and belly pain.

COLITIS

Inflammation of the colon (see Crohn's disease).

COLLAGEN

The principle structural protein of bones, teeth, skin, cartilage, tendons, cornea, and blood vessels. Rich in proline and hydroxyproline. The synthesis of collagen *in vivo* is dependent on adequate intakes of Vitamin C. Collagen, when boiled, becomes partly soluble. The soluble portion can be separated from the insoluble portion and when separated is known as gelatin. Gelatin is deficient in tryptophan and thus is a poor quality dietary protein.

COLORINGS

See additives (Tables 3 and 4).

COLOSTOMY

Procedure in which a part of the colon is brought through the abdominal wall. The feces are then collected in an artificial collection container instead of being eliminated through the anus.

COLOSTRUM

The first milk of the lactating mother; rich in antibodies. This milk provides passive immunity to the newborn child.

COMPETITIVE INHIBITION

Inhibition of an enzymatic reaction which occurs when a substance, closely related to the substrate, binds to the active site of the enzyme yet is not catalyzed by it.

COMPLEMENTARY BASE PAIRS

The pairing of purine and pyrimidine bases of the DNA. Adenine is paired with thymine and cytosine with guanine. These pairs are linked together via hydrogen bonds which form the cross links between the two strands of DNA for the double helix typical of the nuclear genetic material. In RNA, adenine pairs with uracil. Figure 19 illustrates this pairing.

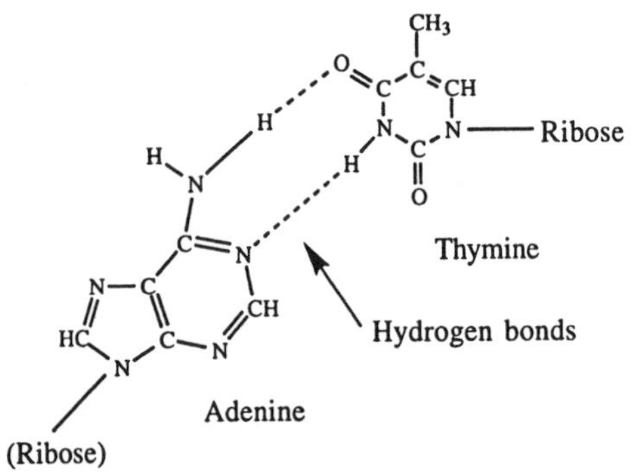

FIGURE 19 Hydrogen bonds form between complementary bases — adenine complements thymine; guanine complements cytosine.

COMPLETE PROTEIN

A dietary protein which contains all of the essential amino acids in amounts needed by the consumer.

COMPLEX CARBOHYDRATES

Polymers of simple sugars (monosaccharides) that are branched and which may contain lipid or protein or other substituents (SH groups, etc.) (see carbohydrates).

COMPLEX SIMILAR ACTION

Combination of substances with common sites of main action and interaction between the components. An example is the protection against goitrogens of the thiocarbamate type (e.g., goitrin) by iodine treatment through the diet. These goitrogens prevent the incorporation of iodine into tyrosine, the first step in thyroid hormone biosynthesis.

COMPONENT PUREEING

Meal preparation technique in which each menu item is individually pureed and then presented either separately or in a casserole.

CONCORDANCE

The chance that an identical mutation will occur in related family members.

CONFOUNDING

The combined effect of the factor under investigation and other factors. A factor can only be a confounder, if the occurrence of the disease as well as the exposure under investigation is associated with it. There is an essential difference between confounding and information or selection bias. If information on the confounder is collected during the study, it can be adjusted for in the statistical analyses. Sometimes, however, an unknown or not measured confounder is present. Such a confounder cannot be adjusted for in the statistical analyses and gives rise to bias in the study results.

CONGENITAL HEART DISEASE

Heart disease present at birth.

CONGESTIVE HEART FAILURE

Heart failure accompanied by venous congestion, or edema, noted in the lungs and peripheral venous system.

CONSTIPATION

Condition resulting in difficulty with defecation of feces, typically from prolonged retention of feces in the colon.

CONTAMINANT

A chemical contaminant in a food is a substance which is not normally present in that food in its natural form or which is present in concentrations not normally found or which is not permitted under the food regulations to be present, or, being an additive as defined under the regulations, exceeds the concentration permitted.

CONTAMINATION OF FOOD WITH METALS

Contamination of food with inorganic contaminants, including the corresponding organome-tallic complexes.

The most important contaminants are mercury, cadmium, and lead. The widespread use of mercury and its derivatives in industry and agriculture has resulted in an increased level of this contaminant in foodstuffs. The major types of food involved are cereal grains (bread, flour), meats (beef, pork, beef liver, canned meats, sausages), fish (canned salmon, shellfish, whitefish), dairy products (milk, cheese, butter), fruits, vegetables (fresh and canned), eggs (white and yolk), and beer. Fish and other seafoods are particularly affected, as the mercury in fish occurs in its most toxic form, the methyl form. Mercury can be observed in various forms: the elemental form (Hg^0), the inorganic or ionic form (Hg^{2+}), or the organic complex form ($R - Hg^+$). Elemental mercury can be oxidized to the inorganic form in the blood and other animal tissues, a process which is mediated by the enzyme catalase. Outside the body, such as in sediments, the oxidation can take place nonenzymatically in the presence of oxygen and organic matter. The formation of organic mercury (by methylation) can occur under a variety of conditions, both in environmental systems and in the animal body. Exposure to organic complexes of mercury, especially methylmercury, is more toxic than exposure to elemental or inorganic mercury. The clinical signs of methylmercury poisoning in humans include numbness and tingling of the extremities, mouth, and lips; loss of hearing and coordination; gross narrowing of the visual fields; reflex changes; progressive psychologic and mental deterioration; sweating and salivation; and muscle fasciculation and atrophy. The total daily intake of mercury per individual in the United States and in Western Europe is estimated at 1–20 µg. The tolerable weekly intake is 300 µg, of which not more than 200 µg should be in the form of methylmercury.

The extensive technological uses of cadmium have resulted in a widespread contamination of the soil, air, water, vegetation, and food supply. Sewage sludge, which is used as fertilizer and soil conditioner, is an important source of soil pollution with cadmium. The major types of food involved are dairy products; meat, fish, and poultry; grains and cereals; potatoes; vegetables (leafy vegetables, legumes, root vegetables); garden and other fruits; oils and fats; sugars and adjuncts; and beverages. In foodstuffs, only inorganic salts of cadmium are present. Factors affecting the absorption and retention of cadmium include:

1. calcium deficiency (increases absorption and retention);
2. pyridoxine deficiency (decreases absorption);
3. iron deficiency (increases absorption);

4. milk (increases absorption);
5. age (infants absorb and accumulate more cadmium than adults, whereas retention of cadmium in the kidneys increases with age).

Cadmium has a remarkably low turnover rate in human tissues. The principle organs involved in cadmium accumulation are the kidneys and the liver, although it has also been found in the pancreas and the lungs. Two forms of cadmium poisoning can be observed: (1) acute poisoning (symptoms: nausea, vomiting) and (2) chronic poisoning (symptoms: hypertension, lumbar pains and myalgia in the legs, skeletal deformation, reduced body height, multiple fractures, proteinuria, glaucoma). The intake of cadmium is estimated at 0.14–0.21 mg per week, of which 90% is attributed to the diet. The tolerable weekly intake of cadmium is 0.4–0.5 mg.

The principal source of the total body burden of lead is considered to be the diet, including drinking water. The major types of food involved in lead contamination include cereal grains, seafood (raw and canned), meats, whole eggs, vegetables (leafy vegetables; raw, dried, frozen, or canned legumes), and milk. In foodstuffs, lead exists exclusively as salts, oxides, or sulfhydryl complexes. Most lead salts and oxides are quite insoluble; this property has a significant relationship to the oral toxicity of lead. Since most lead compounds have a very low water solubility, only 10% of the ingested lead is absorbed. Absorbed lead can be distributed into three compartments: (1) the freely diffusible lead, which probably includes blood lead and freely exchangeable lead of soft tissues; (2) the more firmly bound but exchangeable soft tissue lead; and (3) the hard tissue lead, such as in bones, teeth, hair and nails. Blood and soft tissue lead are most likely to be responsible for the symptoms of poisoning. However, hard tissue lead may be an important source of blood and soft tissue lead. Lead poisoning in humans is associated with deficits in the central and peripheral nervous system function, anemia, hemolysis of red blood cells, acute abdominal colic, constipation, vomiting, and progressive renal failure. The average lead intake in the United States varies from 0.7–3.5 mg per week. The tolerable weekly intake through food is 3 mg for adults and 25 μg per kg body weight for children.

CONTAMINATION OF MILK WITH PLANT TOXINS

Milk is readily contaminated when lactating animals or women ingest toxins. Contamination of milk with plant toxins (white snakeroot or rayless goldenrod, for example) has been observed in the United States in rural areas, where the inhabitants depend on the local milk supply. Especially during periods of drought, when grazing plants are scarce and the weeds are in flower, the milk may contain sufficient toxin (tremetone) to give rise to outbreaks of "milk sickness." Symptoms include weakness, followed by anorexia, abdominal pain, vomiting, muscle tremor, delirium, coma, and eventually death. A characteristic accompanying phenomenon is the presence of acetone in the expired air.

CONTAMINATION WITH ORGANIC CHEMICALS

Major types of organic substances occurring as food contaminants are pesticides, industrial chemicals like halogenated aromatic hydrocarbons, and antibiotics.

Pesticides are biocidal substances or mixtures of such substances together with so-called "inert ingredients," which are used to control or eliminate unwanted species of insects, ascarids, rodents, fungi, higher plants (weeds), unwanted birds, and other pests. Any substance remaining on foodstuffs together with their degradation products, other derivatives or metabolites, and other types of contaminants of toxicological significance arising from the use of a pesticide is called a pesticide residue. Common classes of pesticides include: (1) organochlorines (e.g., aldrin/dieldrin; captafol; captan; 4,4-dichlorodiphenyltrichloroethane

[DDT]; 2,3,7,8-tetrachlorodibenzo-p-dioxin [TCDD]); (2) organophosphorus compounds (e.g. malathion; [methyl]parathion); and (3) carbamates (e.g., carbaryl; thiram). Among the types of food involved in contamination with pesticide residues are dairy products, fruits, vegetables, cereals, grains and grain products, fish, meat and meat products, poultry, wines, and honey. The major health hazards of pesticide residues in foodstuffs include: carcinogenicity (pesticides which are carcinogenic after conversion to proximate carcinogenic metabolites; or pesticides which become carcinogenic by transformation into nitrosocompounds outside the body or in the alimentary tract in the presence of nitrites), mutagenicity, and teratogenicity. Other toxic effects caused by pesticides are immunosuppression, allergenicity, photosensitivity, estrogenicity, and neurotoxicity. Many of the techniques presently in use for the processing of food give a considerable reduction of pesticide residue levels. Many types of residues can be degraded to harmless products during processing due to heat, steam, light, and acid or alkaline conditions. Furthermore, major reduction of residue levels result from their physical removal by peeling, cleaning, or trimming of foods such as vegetables, fruits, meat, fish, and poultry.

Halogenated aromatic hydrocarbons acting as food contaminants include polychlorinated biphenyls, polychlorinated dibenzodioxins, and polychlorinated dibenzofurans. Polychlorinated biphenyls (PCBs) consist of eight types of compounds, depending on the number of chlorine substituents. They are characterized by their high chemical stability to water, acids, alkalis, and temperatures up to 650°C. Furthermore, they are nonflammable, nonconductors of electricity and have very low vapor pressures, making them well suited for several industrial uses. Some well-known PCBs are 2,4,3',4'-tetra-chlorobiphenyl, 2,3,5,3',4'-penta-chlorobiphenyl, and 2,4,5,2',4',5'-hexachlorobiphenyl. PCBs have been reported to be present in the total diet in many countries, and especially in dairy products, meat, fish, poultry, and cereals. Even though production and importation of PCBs have been terminated in the United States and other countries, their health hazard may remain for a while because of their persistence in the body and the environment. PCB poisoning has been shown to cause chloracne, induction of phase I (i.e., oxidases, reductases) and phase II (i.e., conjugases) xenobiotic-metabolizing enzymes, cancer, teratogenic effects, and neurotoxic effects. The most prominent effect in humans is persistent chloracne on the skin of head and chest. The mechanism of the carcinogenicity of PCBs involves promotion rather than initiation. They stimulate the growth of tumors (induced) in liver, skin, and lungs. Although PCBs have been reported to be carcinogenic in animals, there are only a few reports suggesting that these compounds are also carcinogenic in man. Polychlorinated dibenzodioxins (PCDDs) and polychlorinated dibenzofurans (PCDFs) originate from several sources. PCDD/PCDF emission can result from the incineration of domestic waste containing low-molecular chlorinated hydrocarbons and PCBs. PCDDs and PCDFs are also formed during the production of organochlorine compounds such as polychlorobenzenes, polychlorophenols, and PCBs. The most toxic polyhalogenated aromatic hydrocarbon is 2,3,7,8-tetrachlorodibenzo-p-dioxin (TCDD). Many TCDD-induced effects are similar to those caused by PCBs and other structurally related compounds (e.g., enzyme induction). Other effects of PCDDs and PCDFs include teratogenic effects, immunosuppression, and thymic atrophy.

An important concern of veterinary toxicology is the possible transmission of harmful substances from meat, milk, and other foodstuffs to the human population. This concerns the use of antibiotics as feed additives. These include tetracyclines, nitrofurans, and sulfonamides. Oxytetracycline and furazolidone are suspected of being carcinogens. Oxytetracycline has been reported to react with nitrite to yield (carcinogenic) nitrosamines. In addition, the majority of the antibiotics in use as feed additives pose a serious (indirect) health hazard to humans. Ingestion of these antibiotics may lead to an increased resistance of bacteria, resulting in: (1) transfer of antibiotic-resistant bacteria to humans via food intake, originating from animals treated with antibiotics or infected by resistant bacteria; and (2) transfer of the resistance factor (R-factor) from resistant nonpathogenic bacteria to other bacteria which will lead to widespread resistance.

CONTINUOUS SUBCUTANEOUS INSULIN INFUSION

Provision of insulin 24 hours daily via a small pump worn by an individual that contains a needle attached under the skin.

COPPER

An essential mineral important as an antioxidant, as a component of the cytochromes, and is essential to the use of iron and the synthesis of hemoglobin (see minerals, Table 29).

COPRA, COCONUT OIL

Copra is ground coconut meal from which coconut oil is extracted. Coconut oil is rich in medium chain saturated fatty acids and is one of the group of fats called tropical oils. While solid at 70°F they are liquid at 85°F.

CoQ, COENZYME Q

Also called ubiquinone, serves as an essential component of the respiratory chain and transfers electrons between the flavoproteins and the cytochromes. It is nonpolar and can diffuse through the mitochondrial membrane. It is the only component of the respiratory chain that is not fixed. All the other components are proteins.

CORI CYCLE

A cycle which occurs between the red blood cell, kidneys, muscle, platelets, and the liver and which helps maintain a normal blood glucose level in the face of changes in lactate production. Cori cycle activity is particularly important during exercise as the working muscle is unable to oxidize all the lactate it produces. The muscle does not have gluconeogenic activity. Thus, it must export the accumulating lactate via the blood to the liver which in turn uses it to make glucose. Figure 20 illustrates this cycle.

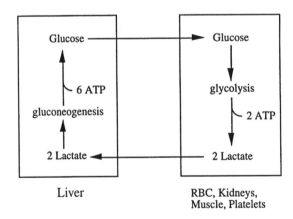

FIGURE 20 The Cori cycle

CORI DISEASE

Glycogen storage disease, Type III, an inherited disease where the mutation has occurred in the gene for the glycogen debranching enzyme. It is characterized by excess stored glycogen having many short branches.

CORONARY ARTERIOGRAPHY

The openness of the coronary vasculature is evaluated using an infused radio-opaque dye and x-ray pictures.

CORONARY ARTERY BYPASS GRAFT (CABG)

A common type of cardiac surgery involving the use of the leg's saphenous vein or the internal mammary artery to bypass blockages in one or more coronary arteries.

CORONARY ARTERY DISEASE

Condition in which one or more coronary arteries are occluded, providing decreased blood supply to the heart and resulting in myocardial damage (see atherosclerosis).

CORTICOSTEROIDS

See adrenocortical steroids.

COUMARIN

A chroman derivative, occurring in many flavoring agents, such as cassie, woodruff, lavender, and lovage. These flavoring agents are extensively used in sweets, liqueurs, and certain wines. Coumarin is a minor constituent of certain edible fruits, e.g., strawberries, cherries, apricots, and a major constituent of tongka beans. Trace quantities of coumarin are also found in citrus oils and carrotseed oil. Coumarin has moderate acute toxicity in animals including man. About 5 g is fatal to sheep; about 4 g produces mild toxic effects in humans; and about 40 g is lethal to horses. Coumarin, which can also be made synthetically, is still allowed for food use in Europe. It is prohibited in the United States, though, as it has been found to cause liver damage in rats.

COUPLED REACTION

Two reactions that have a common intermediate which transfers electrons or reducing equivalents or some other element from one set of reactants to another.

COW'S MILK ALLERGY (CMA)

An immunologic response to milk consumption. Cow's milk contains 30–35 g protein per liter. The main antigens are β-lactoglobulin, casein, α-lactalbumin, serum lactalbumin, and the immunoglobulins. β-lactoglobulin and α-lactalbumin are referred to as the whey proteins. Casein and β-lactoglobulin are the most heat-resistant. Cow's milk allergy is most frequently seen in babies. In 10% of the cases, the symptoms appear in the first week of life, 33% in the second to fourth week, and in 40% during the following months. The main symptoms are eczema and gastrointestinal complaints such as diarrhea, cramps, vomiting, and constipation. Also, rhinitis, asthma, and rash may develop. An often obvious feature is irritability and restlessness. If the diagnosis is cow's milk allergy, a few alternatives for cow's milk are available. Goat's milk and soy milk are sometimes used as are synthetic formulas using purified proteins and/or amino acids.

CREAM

The fat rich layer of nonhomogenized milk that rises to the top of the container.

CREATINE

A metabolite in muscle which is synthesized from glycine and arginine and which can be phosphorylated to form creatine phosphate.

CREATINE KINASE (CREATINE PHOSPHOKINASE)

An enzyme which catalyzes the formation of creatine phosphate.

CREATINE PHOSPHATE

A high energy compound in muscle which has a higher phosphate group transfer potential than ATP. It acts as a reservoir for phosphate so that the muscle can maintain a steady level of ATP to support muscle contraction. It also serves this function in nerve so that a steady supply of ATP for nerve conduction is provided. Creatine phosphate synthesis is shown in Figure 21.

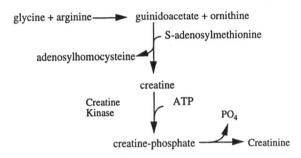

FIGURE 21 Formation of creatine phosphate.

CREATINE PHOSPHOKINASE

Enzyme in skeletal muscle, cardiac muscle, and in brain tissue that catalyzes the transfer of high energy phosphate from phosphocreatine to ADP to make ATP.

CREATININE

The urinary excretion product of creatine breakdown. The conversion of creatine to creatinine is irreversible.

CREATININE CLEARANCE

A test for renal function which measures the degree to which creatinine is cleared from the blood.

CRETINISM

A disease in children which results from too little thyroxine production by the thyroid gland. It is characterized by poor growth and development of children and mental retardation.

CRITICAL CONCENTRATION

The target cell/organ concentration at which adverse (reversible/irreversible) functional changes occur. These changes are called critical effects.

CRITICAL ORGAN

The organ in which the critical concentration is reached first under specified conditions for a given population.

CROHN'S DISEASE

A type of inflammatory bowel disease characterized by diarrhea, malabsorption, and ulcers in the gastrointestinal tract, usually in the terminal ileum and colon. Also known as regional enteritis.

CROSS-SECTIONAL STUDIES

Nonexperimental studies in which data on exposure as well as biological effects are collected at the same time. This kind of study is often used to describe the prevalence of certain exposures or diseases in a population. From an etiological point of view, an essential disadvantage of these studies is the problem of discerning effect from cause.

CRUCIFEROUS VEGETABLES

Vegetables that are members of the cabbage family. Included are various types of cabbage, brussels sprouts, broccoli, kohlrabi, and kale.

CRUDE FIBER

The residue of plant food left after extraction by dilute acid and alkali. Table 16 gives the amounts of crude fiber in many common foods. However, the term crude fiber does not include all the undigested material which may prove to have nutritional value to man. While cellulose, plant fibers, and other so-called nondigestible carbohydrates are not digestible by the enzymes located in the upper portion of the intestine, the intestine contains flora which can partially degrade some of these food components. This degradation provides fatty aids and other useful compounds which are then absorbed by the lower small intestine and colon (see Fiber).

CTP

Cytidine triphosphate. A nucleotide consisting of cytosine (a pyrimidine), ribose, and three high energy phosphate groups.

CURD

The coagulum of milk from which cheese can be made.

CUSHING'S SYNDROME

A disease due to overproduction of glucocorticoids by the adrenal cortex. The syndrome is characterized by abnormal glucose tolerance, excess muscle protein degradation, fatigue, osteoporosis, excess hair growth, excess fat deposition on shoulders and abdomen, and skin discoloration.

CYANOCOBALAMIN

See Vitamin B_{12}.

CYANOGENIC GLYCOSIDES

Glycosides from which cyanide is formed by the activity of hydrolytic enzymes. More than 1000 plant species from 90 families and 250 genera have been reported to be cyanophoric.

The cyanogenic glycoside molecule consists of a monosaccharide (glucose) or disaccharide (vicianose or gentiobiose) and an aglycone in the form of a β-hydroxynitrile. The glycoside

TABLE 16
Fiber Content in Common Foods

Item	Fiber (g/100 g food)
Almonds	2.6
Apples	0.9
Beans, Lima	1.8
Beans, string	1.0
Broccoli	1.5
Carrots	1.0
Flour, whole wheat	2.3
Flour, white wheat	0.3
Noodles, dry	0.4
Oat flakes	1.4
Pears	1.5
Pecans	2.3
Popcorn	2.2
Strawberries	1.3
Walnuts	2.1
Wheat germ	2.5

Source: Adapted from Tables of Food Composition which appeared in *Geigy Scientific Tables*, 7th ed., Diem, K. and Letner, C., Eds., New York: CIBA-Geigy, 1974.

can be hydrolyzed in the presence of β-glucosidase; the nitrile can undergo further degradation by a lyase, generating hydrogen cyanide, an aldehyde, ketone, or in some cases an acid. β-Glucosidase and hydroxynitrile lyase are found in plant cells, possibly in specific organelles. They become available when plant tissue is damaged, an inevitable process when foodstuffs are prepared for consumption. Cyanogenic glycosides in plant foodstuffs can be listed in three categories, based on the sugar moiety: (1) glucosides (sugar: D-glucose); (2) vicianosides (sugar: vicianose); and (3) gentiobiosides (sugar: gentiobiose). Examples of glucosides are dhurrin (aglycone: L-p-hydroxymandelo-nitrile; occurrence: sorghums, kaffir corns), linamarin (aglycone: α-hydroxy-isobutyronitrile; occurrence: lima beans, flax seed, cassava or manioc), lotoaustralian (aglycone: α-hydroxy-α-methylbutyronitrile; occurrence: same as linamarin cassava), prunasin (aglycone: D-mandelonitrile; occurrence: *Prunus* spp. and other Rosaceae), and sambunigrin (aglycone: L-mandelonitrile; occurrence: legumes, elderberry). The cyanogen in the common vetch and similar legumes is a vicianoside (glycoside: vicianin; aglycone: D-mandelonitrile), whereas those of the rose family (*Rosaceae Prunus* spp.: almonds, apple, apricot, cherry, peach, pear, plum, quince) are gentiobiosides (glycoside: amygdalin; aglycone: D-mandelonitrile). Cyanide doses that are lethal to humans can easily be reached or even exceeded after the intake of a variety of cyanogenic foodstuffs. The reported lethal doses in humans are from 0.5 to 3.5 mg/kg body weight. The amounts of HCN produced by lima beans varies from over 200 mg/100 g to less than 20 mg/100 g. Reports of HCN in lima beans include 210 mg/100 g (Burmese, white variety), 300 mg/100 g (Puerto Rican, black variety), 312 mg/100 g (Japanese, colored variety), and less than

20 mg/100 g for most American varieties. Fresh cassava cortex produces HCN in quantities ranging from 1 to 60 mg or more per 100 g, depending on several conditions, such as variety, source, period of harvest, and field conditions. The amount of cyanide produced by cassava varies not only with variety, but also with the manner of preparation. Concerning the different varieties of cassava, cyanide production ranged from 16 to 434 mg/kg, with an average of 158 mg/kg for the whole tuber. Attention should also be directed to the leaves of cassava, which are highly cyanogenic: 78.6 mg HCN/100 g. Cyanide poisoning from cyanogenic glycoside can manifest in one of three forms: (1) acute poisoning, indicative of cytotoxic anoxia; (2) chronic poisoning, indicative of degenerative neuropathy; or (3) chronic poisoning, manifested by goitrogeny. Acute cyanide poisoning has been reported from consumption of lima beans, manioc, unripe sorghum, bitter almonds, apricot kernels, and apple seeds. Characteristic for acute cyanide poisoning are symptoms suggestive of cellular oxygen deprivation. Signs of poisoning begin initially with hyperventilation, headache, nausea, vomiting, general weakness, abdominal distention, and pain. Fatal doses produce, in addition, not only tachypnea and dyspnea, but also paralysis, convulsions, unconsciousness, respiratory arrest, and collapse. Free cyanide is absorbed rapidly in the gastrointestinal tract. Once in the cell, it binds reversibly to cytochrome a_3 in the cytochrome c oxidase complex. Therefore, the enzyme is unable to function in the electron transport chain. The tissues are thus unable to accept oxygen from the blood. Neuronal depression in the medullary centers leads to respiratory arrest and death. This binding can be reversed by hydroxycobalamin, since CN^- has a stronger affinity for cobalt in cyanocobalamin than the iron in cytochrome c oxidase. Concerning the second form of cyanide poisoning, the chronic cyanide poisoning manifested by degenerative neuropathy, two types of neurological degenerative diseases have been reported after increased consumption of cassava. One disease, tropical ataxic neuropathy, is endemic in some parts of Nigeria and Senegal. The disease is believed to be caused in part by the failure of the body to dispose of cyanide owing to cobalamin deficiency. Symptoms of this disease include demyelination and elevated thiocyanate levels in blood plasma and urine. The other disease is called tropical amblyopia, a form of blindness which is common in West African countries. Because this disorder is believed to be the result of secondary cobalamin deficiency, treatment with hydroxycobalamin may cause improvement. Chronic poisoning manifested by goitrogeny is caused by metabolization of cyanide to thiocyanate, in the presence of the enzyme rhodanase. Thus, the high consumption of dry unfermented cassava, containing high levels of cyanogen, has been implicated in the widespread incidence of goiter in eastern Nigeria and other parts of Africa.

CYANOSIS

A dark bluish or purplish skin color due to inadequate oxygenation of the blood in the lungs or to an obstruction to blood flow through the capillaries. The color is due to the accumulation of reduced hemoglobin.

CYCLAMATE

Non-nutritive sweetener; sodium cyclamate. When fed to rats in very high amounts, sodium cyclamate was found to produce bladder tumors. On the basis of this finding, the Delaney Clause of the U.S. Pure Food and Drug Act was exercised and this sweetener withdrawn from use in foods in the United States.

CYCLIC AMP (cAMP)

A second messenger for catabolic hormone effects. The hormone binds to a membrane receptor which in turn stimulates adenyl cyclase which acts on ATP to produce cyclic AMP.

CYCLOPROPENE FATTY ACIDS

Fatty acids occurring in the oils or fat of every plant of the order Malvales, except for cocoa butter from Theobroma cocoa. From a food toxicological point of view, only the acids in the oils of cottonseed and kapok seed are of significance. The most important acids are sterculic and malvalic acids; both are toxic monounsaturated fatty acids. The effects of cyclopropene fatty acids include effects on the reproductive system and carcinogenic effects (by enhancing the activity of aflatoxin B1). Hydrogenation can lead to the disappearance of some of the biological effects.

CYSTATHIONINURIA

A high level of cystathionine in the urine caused by a mutation in the gene for cystathionase which catalyzes the production of cysteine from cystathionine.

CYSTEINE

A nonessential 3 carbon amino acid containing sulfur; can be made from methionine.

CYSTIC FIBROSIS

A genetic disease in which the body fails to conserve the chloride ion.

CYSTINE

A molecule which results when two cysteines are joined through the terminal sulfur atoms.

CYSTINURIA

An inherited disease characterized by excessive amounts of cystine in the urine. The disease is due to a mutation in the gene for the renal carrier of cystine, lysine, and arginine.

CYTIDINE

A nucleotide consisting of cytosine (a pyrimidine) and ribose.

CYTOCHROMES

Electron carriers in the respiratory chain and elsewhere. All cytochromes have a heme prosthetic group which contains iron. The iron fluctuates between the +2 and +3 states.

CYTOPLASM

Cell sap; the medium in which the organelles of the cell are suspended.

CYTOSINE

A pyrimidine base found in the genetic material, DNA and RNA.

CYTOTOXIC AGENTS

Chemicals that destroy specific cells; streptozotocin is an example. This agent destroys the insulin producing β cells of the pancreas.

D

D5W SOLUTION

An isotonic solution containing 50 grams of glucose per liter of solution.

DAILY REFERENCE VALUES (DRVs)

Desirable intakes of specific nutrients.

DARK ADAPTATION

Adaptation of the visual cycle to changes in light intensity. The process is dependent on adequate Vitamin A intake. Failure to adapt to changing light intensity is one of the first symptoms of Vitamin A deficiency.

DAWN PHENOMENON

Early morning hyperglycemia thought to result from decreased sensitivity to insulin.

DE

Digestive energy. The energy of food after the costs (and losses) of digestion are subtracted.

DEAMINASE

An enzyme which catalyzes the removal of an amino group from a carbon chain.

DEAMINATION

The process of amino group removal.

DEBRIDEMENT

Removal of necrotic tissue.

DECARBOXYLASE

An enzyme that catalyzes the removal of a carboxy group from a carbon chain.

DECARBOXYLATION

The reaction in which a carboxy group is removed.

DECIDUOUS TEETH

The first teeth of the young. These teeth are replaced by permanent teeth as the individual matures.

DECUBITUS ULCER

Term previously used to describe a pressure ulcer.

DEEP-FRYING

A processing technique affecting the oxidation of dietary fats and oils. Frying of food under normal conditions may result in the formation of small amounts of stable peroxides. During industrial processing under vacuum, dimers, polymers, and cyclic products may be formed. The products that are formed in cooking oils on heating may be taken up by the fried food products. If oil is used in discontinuous batch-type operations, as in restaurants and at home, it is discarded in time because of either high viscosity or excessive foaming.

DEFIBRILLATION

Ceasing heart fibrillation with drugs or physical means.

DEGRADE

To reduce large molecules to smaller ones.

DEHYDRATASES

Enzymes which catalyze the removal of a molecule of water from a carbon chain. These enzymes frequently require pyridoxine as a coenzyme.

DEHYDRATION

The process of water removal.

DEHYDROASCORBIC ACID

A form of ascorbic acid (Vitamin C) in which two hydrogens have been removed.

DEHYDROGENASES

Enzymes which catalyze the removal of reducing equivalents (hydrogen ions) from carbon chains.

DEHYDROGENATION

Removal of hydrogen ions; catalyzed by a group of enzymes called dehydrogenases.

DELANEY CLAUSE OF THE U.S. FOOD, DRUG AND COSMETIC ACT

Law that prohibits the use of any chemical in foods that can be shown to cause cancer at any level of intake.

DELIRIUM TREMENS

Characterized by agitation, anorexia, hallucinations, and uncontrollable movement during alcohol withdrawal.

DELTA (D)

Change. The Greek symbol is Δ.

ΔG°

Free energy that is available to do work.

$\Delta G^{\circ\prime}$

Standard free energy of biochemical reactions.

DEMENTIA

Condition characterized by a reduction in cognitive function.

DENATURATION

See protein denaturation.

DENSITOMETRY

Measurement of body density.

DENTIN

The major portion of a tooth; about 20% is organic matrix (collagen with some elastin) while 80% is hydroxyapatite containing calcium, phosphorous, magnesium, carbonate, and fluoride.

DEOXYADENOSINE

A nucleoside containing adenine (a purine) and deoxyribose.

DEOXYCYTIDINE

A nucleoside containing cytosine (a pyrimidine) and deoxyribose.

DEOXYGUANINE

A nucleoside containing guanine (a purine) and deoxyribose.

DEOXYRIBONUCLEIC ACID (DNA)

The genetic material in the nucleus and mitochondria (see protein synthesis).

DEPENDENT ACTION

Combination of substances with different sites of action, and interaction between the components. The complexity of the interactions is illustrated with the following example. It has been shown that calcium affords protection against the toxic effects of lead and cadmium. Furthermore, calcium deficiency appears to promote the absorption of both metals. The interaction between calcium on the one hand, and lead and cadmium on the other, is believed to be a competition for binding sites of a carrier protein which is involved in the uptake of the metals from the mucosal wall.

DEPRESSION

Condition characterized by extreme sadness, helplessness, and social isolation.

DERMATITIS

Inflammation of the skin.

DETOXIFICATION

Removal of toxic properties of a substance; metabolic conversion of pharmacologically active compounds to nonactive compounds.

DEUTERIUM

A hydrogen isotope having twice the mass of the common hydrogen atom.

DEUTERIUM OXIDE

Heavy water which contains two molecules of deuterium and one of oxygen.

DEXTRAN

A glucose polymer.

DEXTROSE

Synonymous with glucose.

DHHS

Department of Health and Human Services, United States.

DIABETES INSIPIDUS

A disease of the pituitary which results in excessive urination and thirst due to a lack of ADH.

DIABETES KETOACIDOSIS

Abnormal (greater than 20 mg/l) levels of ketone bodies in blood which cannot be neutralized by the body's buffering system. If untreated can cause coma and death.

DIABETES MELLITUS

A group of diseases characterized by an inappropriate glucose-insulin relationship. These diseases are divided into two major subgroups; insulin-dependent and noninsulin-dependent diabetes, IDDM and NIDDM. Insulin-dependent diabetes mellitus includes juvenile onset diabetes; the term refers primarily to the treatment of the disease by insulin injections and used to be called Type I diabetes. Noninsulin-dependent diabetes mellitus used to be called adult onset or Type II diabetes mellitus. The term refers to the management of the disorder through diet and exercise. The majority of these diseases are genetically determined.

DIABETIC NEPHROPATHY

Renal disease that is a secondary complication of diabetes mellitus and which involves degenerative changes in the glomerulus and thickening of the basement membrane.

DIACYLGLYCEROL

A lipid having two fatty acids esterified to glycerol; also called diglyceride.

DIAGNOSIS RELATED GROUPS (DRGs)

Classes of medical diagnoses in a system devised to control health care costs and used to establish reimbursement for hospital care.

DIALYSIS

Process of removing toxic compounds from blood and body fluid using instrumentation which allows for diffusion and filtration between solutions separated by a semipermeable membrane.

DIAPHORESIS

Excessive perspiration.

DIARRHEA

Abnormal frequent discharge of unformed feces.

DIARRHEIC SHELLFISH POISONING

Characterized by gastrointestinal complaints, including diarrhea, vomiting, nausea, and abdominal spasms. Recently, toxins involved in this poisoning have been chemically identified. They constitute a group of derivatives of a C_{38} fatty acid, okada acid. These shellfish poisons are produced by the dinoflagellate species Dinophysis and Prorocentrum.

DIBASIC AMINO ACID

Amino acids having two amino groups. Lysine and arginine are dibasic amino acids.

DICOUMEROL

Vitamin K antagonist; interferes with normal blood clotting; produced when sweet clover spoils. Other names are dicoumarin, dicumol, dufalone, and melitoxin.

DIET THERAPY

Modification of a normal diet to manage the symptoms of a disease.

DIETARY BEHAVIOR

Includes a multitude of behaviors and can refer to food choice, food preparation, food preservation, and (actual) food consumption.

Attempts have been made to change certain dietary behaviors of the population for reasons of health. These nutritional interventions are aimed at groups of patients, high-risk groups, healthy people, or intermediaries, like people working in the kitchen of a restaurant. The complexity of dietary behavior can also be illustrated by the diversity of the objectives of nutritional interventions such as: increasing the hygienic behavior in the catering industry; reducing the consumption of proteins and sodium by kidney patients to relieve the kidney(s) as much as possible; reducing the total energy intake to prevent or treat obesity; increasing the consumption of food products containing carbohydrates to improve achievements in endurance sports; increasing the knowledge about food preservation to prevent food poisoning, for example, resulting from microbial contamination; and reducing alcohol consumption to decrease the number of alcohol-related traffic accidents. Dietary behavior is determined by many factors, such as availability of food, food policy of the government, social environment, advertising, and experience and opinions people have regarding food safety. In general, three main groups of behavioral determinants can be distinguished: (1) attitude (what do people think of their behavior themselves?); (2) social influence (what is the role of the social environment?); and (3) possibilities (either internal or external to the person) for displaying a behavior. External factors affecting these behavioral determinants are age, education, sex, physiological variables, and habit. An attitude toward a specific behavior reflects whether a person's general feelings are favorable or unfavorable toward that behavior and is determined by the evaluation of all pros and cons of the behavior. To identify the specific pros and cons people may be asked to point out which consequences they believe the behavior is connected with (= beliefs). It is also important to know whether the consequence is considered as an advantage or a disadvantage (= evaluations). Social environment very much affects dietary behavior. There are two kinds of social influence: direct influence (referring to the clear expectations of others as to how someone should behave) and indirect influence (referring to modeling, imitating the behavior of others). The third group of influencing factors are the possibilities or impossibilities for displaying a behavior. Impossibilities for behavior can be external (e.g., unavailability of products, money, or time; noncooperative members of the family) or internal (e.g., lack of information, skills, or perseverance) to the person.

DIETARY FIBER

See Fiber.

DIETARY GUIDELINES FOR AMERICANS

A list of seven general nutrition statements advocating a healthful diet from the U.S. Department of Agriculture and the U.S. Department of Health and Human Services. The specific recommendations vary depending on the agency but in general relate to moderating the intake of fat, total energy, sodium and iron, and including a wide variety of foods in the daily diet.

DIETARY HISTORY METHOD

See interview method.

DIETETIC TECHNICIAN, REGISTERED (DTR)

Individual who has completed a minimum of an associate degree in dietetics or a related areas at a U.S. regionally accredited college or university, completed a supervised clinical experience, and has passed a national examination.

DIETITIAN (RD)

Individual who has completed a minimum of a baccalaureate degree in dietetics or a related area in a U.S. regionally accredited college or university, has completed a supervised clinical experience, and who has passed a national examination. A dietitian is trained in the art of advising clients in the selections of foods appropriate to the age, nutrient needs, and health of the individual. A therapeutic dietitian works closely with a physician to ensure that the food choices are appropriate for the particular medical state the physician wishes to manage. These conditions may include specific nutrient differences, specific nutrient or food intolerances, or metabolic diseases requiring close management of the intake of specific food components, i.e., glucose, saturated fat, specific amino acids, and so forth.

DIFFERENTIAL MISCLASSIFICATION

Errors in the necessary information (e.g., in exposure measurement) which are related to the state of disease. This type of misclassification has more serious consequences than the nondifferential or random misclassification. It can lead to either underestimation or overestimation of the effect.

DIFFUSION

A uniform distribution of solutes on both sides of a permeable membrane.

DIGESTION

See carbohydrate digestion, protein digestion, or lipid digestion.

DIGESTIVE TRACT

That section of the body beginning with the mouth and ending at the anus. Includes the mouth, esophagus, stomach, small intestine (duodenum, jejunum, ileum), cecum, large intestine, rectum, and anus.

DIGITALIS

A drug which assists in the maintenance of a regular heartbeat.

DIGLYCERIDE (DIACYLGLYCEROL)

Two fatty acids esterified to glycerol.

DIHYDROXYCHOLECALCIFEROL

The active form of Vitamin D. Also called 1,25 dihydroxy cholecalciferol (see vitamins Table 49).

DIPEPTIDE

Two amino acids linked together by a peptide bond.

DIRECT CALORIMETRY

The measurement of heat produced by a body through the use of a calorimeter.

DISACCHARIDE

A carbohydrate containing two sugar (saccharide) units. Sucrose, mannose, and lactose are common disaccharides in the human diet.

DISSEMINATED INTRAVASCULAR COAGULATION (DIC)

Acquired clotting disorder occurring simultaneously with another medical condition in which clotting mechanisms become accelerated resulting in occlusion of the microcirculation. Common causes of DIC include obstetric complications, cancer, sepsis, and massive tissue damage.

DISTAL

Away from the center of the body.

DISTENTION

The condition of being expanded or extended beyond normal.

DISULFIDE BRIDGE

A bond containing two sulfur molecules.

DIURESIS

Urine excretion in excess of normal.

DIURETICS

Pharmaceutic agents which increase urinary water loss.

DIURNAL VARIATION

Cyclical changes in one or more features of the body over a 24-hour period.

DIVERTICULITIS

Inflammation of a diverticulum, a small pocket in the wall of the intestine.

DIVERTICULOSIS

The presence of a number of diverticula in the intestine.

DNA

Deoxyribonucleic acid. Dictates all genetically determined characteristics. Each of these characteristics is coded by the sequence of purine and pyrimidine bases that are connected together in a double-stranded helix found in the nucleus of the cell. Some DNA is also found in the mitochondria.

DOPAMINE

A neurotransmitter synthesized from tyrosine in the adrenal medulla and the central nervous system.

DOUBLE-BLIND STUDY

An experiment designed such that neither the subject nor the investigator is aware of the treatment given to the subject.

DRUG-NUTRIENT INTERACTIONS

Drugs that interfere with the action of particular nutrients. In this circumstance the drug becomes an antinutrient.

DUAL ENERGY RADIOGRAPHIC ABSORPTIOMETRY (DRA)

A procedure based on x-rays that measures bone mineralization. Also known as dual x-ray absorptiometry (DXA) and dual energy absorptiometry (DEXA).

DUAL PHOTON ABSORPTIOMETRY

Similar to DEXA but uses photons at two different energy levels to determine bone mineral content.

DUMPING SYNDROME

Characterized by the rapid rate of gastric emptying into the intestine after ingestion of food and frequently resulting in diarrhea, nausea, and weakness.

DUODENUM

The first 12 inches of the small intestine of the human.

DYNAMIC STATE

A state of flux as happens in living cells. Components of the cell are constantly being synthesized and degraded such that there is little net gain except for those products of metabolism which are storage products, i.e., glycogen and triacylglycerides.

DYSGEUSIA

Abnormal taste perception.

DYSPHAGIA

Difficulty with swallowing.

DYSURIA

Painful or difficult urination.

E

EATING DISORDER

Eating behavior that leads to disease or disability including any eating pattern that deviates from the cultural norm. The most common eating disorders include anorexia nervosa, bulimia nervosa, and compulsive overeating.

ECHOCARDIOGRAPHY

Diagnostic procedure which employs ultrasound to inspect the structures of the heart.

ECLAMPSIA

Coma and convulsions that may develop during pregnancy or immediately after partuition. Preceded by hypertension, edema, and proteinuria.

ECOLOGICAL STUDIES

Nonexperimental studies in which the unit of observation is not the individual but a group of people in a particular environment, such as workers in a factory or inhabitants of a city or a country. These studies can be useful if information on individuals is not available; exposure is then an overall measure for the population under investigation. The outcome variable under investigation in ecological studies is often mortality. A well-known phenomenon occurring in this type of study is the so-called ecological fallacy. On comparing countries it may be found that the higher the average level of a risk factor A for a country, the higher the level of mortality due to disease B, while within each country (based on individual measurements of A and B) risk factor A is negatively associated with disease B.

EDEMA

Excess accumulation of water in the body, particularly in the periphery; also called dropsy or hydrops.

EDENTULOUS

Toothless.

EGG ALLERGY

Egg white is the most frequent cause of egg allergy. Egg white contains about 20 allergens, the most important being ovalbumin, ovotransferrine, and ovomucoid. The latter is heat-resistant. Other egg allergens that have been isolated are lysozymes. There is evidence that some cross-reactivity exists between the allergens of the egg white and the egg yolk. Egg allergy is most frequently encountered in children (appearing in the first two years of life).

EICOSANOIDS

A group of compounds synthesized from arachidonic acid. The synthetic pathway is outlined in Figure 22 while the functions of the various compounds are listed in Table 17.

Eicosanoids are 20 carbon molecules having hormone-like activity. In their various forms they are produced and released by many different mammalian cells rather than being produced

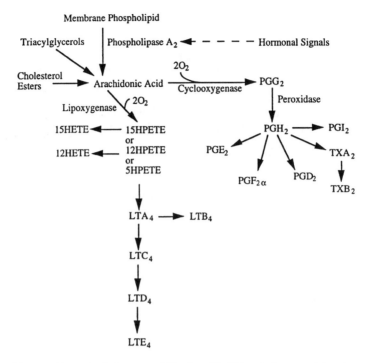

FIGURE 22 Eicosanoid synthesis from arachidonic acid. Abbreviations used for the major classes: PG, prostaglandin; LT, leukotriene; TX, thromboxane; letters and subscripts identify the individual components.

TABLE 17
Functions of Eicosanoids

Eicosanoids	Function
PGG_2	Precursor of PGH_2.
PGH_2	Precursor of PGD_2, PGE_2, PGI_2, and $PGF_{2\alpha}$.
PGD_2	Promotes sleeping behavior.
	Precursor of PGF_2.
PGE_2	Enhances perception of pain when histamine or bradykinin is given. Induces signs of inflammation. Promotes wakefulness. Precursor of $PGF_{2\alpha}$. Reduces gastric acid secretion, induces partuition. Vasoconstrictor in some tissues. Vasodilator in other tissues. Maintains the patency of the ductus arteriosis prior to birth.
$PGF_{2\alpha}$	Bronchial constrictor. Vasoconstrictor especially in coronary vasculature. Increases sperm motility. Induces parturition; stimulates steroidogenesis corpus luteum; induces luteolysis.
PGI_2	Inhibits platelet aggregation.
PGE_1	Inhibits motility of nonpregnant uterus.
	Increases motility of pregnant uterus. Bronchial dilator.
TXA_2	Stimulates platelet aggregation. Potent vasoconstrictor.
TXB_2	Metabolite of TXA_2.
LTA_4	Precursor of LTB_4.
LTB_4	Potent chemotaxic agent.

From Berdanier, C.D., *Advanced Nutrition: Macronutrients*, CRC Press, Boca Raton, FL, 1994, 235.

by highly specialized cells as is the instance of insulin and the β cell in the islets of Langerhans. When each of these compounds is produced, their site of action is local. That is, whereas insulin may be transported from the pancreas to peripheral target cells, the eicosanoids are produced, released, and have as their targets, the surrounding cells. For this reason, the eicosanoids are called local hormones. They have a variety of actions.

The eicosanoids fall into three general groups of compounds: the prostaglandins (compounds of the PG series), the thromboxanes (compounds of the TBX series), and the leukotrienes (compounds of the LKT series). All of these compounds arise from a 20 carbon polyunsaturated fatty acid. This fatty acid is usually arachidonic acid (20 carbons; 4 double bonds at 5, 8, 11, and 14). However, in instances where the diet is rich in omega-3 (n-3) fatty acids, the precursor may be a 20 carbon-5 double bond fatty acid, eicosapentaenoic acid (double bonds at 5, 8, 11, 14, and 17). Other eicosanoids can be synthesized from a 20 carbon fatty acid, dihomo-γ-linoleic acid which has only 3 double bonds at carbons 8, 11, and 14. Each of these precursors yields a particular set of eicosanoids. They are called eicosanoids because they have 20 carbons; during their synthesis they take up oxygen and are cyclized. Dihomo γ-linoleic acid is the precursor of prostaglandin E_1 (PGE$_1$), prostaglandin $E_{1\alpha}$ (PGE$_{1\alpha}$), and subsequent prostaglandins. Arachidonic acid is the precursor of prostaglandins of the 2 series (PGE$_2$, PGF$_{2\alpha}$, etc.) and eicosapentaenoic acid is the precursor of prostaglandins of the 3 series (PGE$_3$, PGF$_{3\alpha}$, etc.).

The cyclization of these 20 carbon fatty acids is accomplished by a complex of enzymes called the prostaglandin synthesis complex. The first step is the cyclooxygenase step which involves the cyclization of C-9. The C-12 of the precursor to form the cyclic 9-11 endoperoxide 15-hydroperoxide (PGG$_2$) is shown in Figure 23.

PGG$_2$ is then used to form prostaglandin H_2 (PGH$_2$) through the removal of one oxygen from the carbonyl group at carbon 15. This reaction is shown in Figure 24. Glutathione peroxidase and prostaglandin H synthase catalyze this reaction. Prostaglandin H synthase is a very unstable, short-lived enzyme with a messenger RNA that is one of the shortest-lived species so far found in mammalian cells. The expression of genes for this enzyme is under the control of polypeptide growth factors such as interleukin 1a and colony stimulating factor 1. Interferon a and b inhibit expression and prostanoid production by the macrophages.

PGH$_2$ is then converted through the action of a variety of isomerases to PGD$_2$, PGE$_2$, prostacylin I_2 (PGI$_2$), or prostaglandin $F_{2\alpha}$ (PGF$_{2\alpha}$). These are the primary precursors of the prostaglandins of the D, E, and F series and PGI or thromboxane. The conversion to subsequent prostaglandins is mediated by enzymes that are specific to a certain cell type and tissue. Not all of these subsequent compounds are formed in all tissues. Thus, PGE$_2$ and PGF$_{2\alpha}$ are

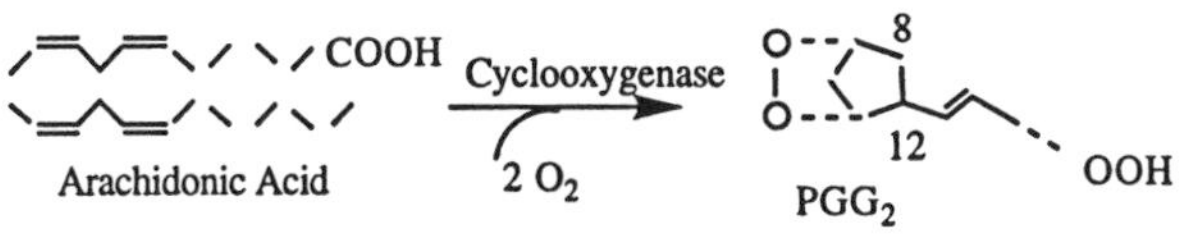

FIGURE 23 Cyclization and oxygenation of arachidonic acid.

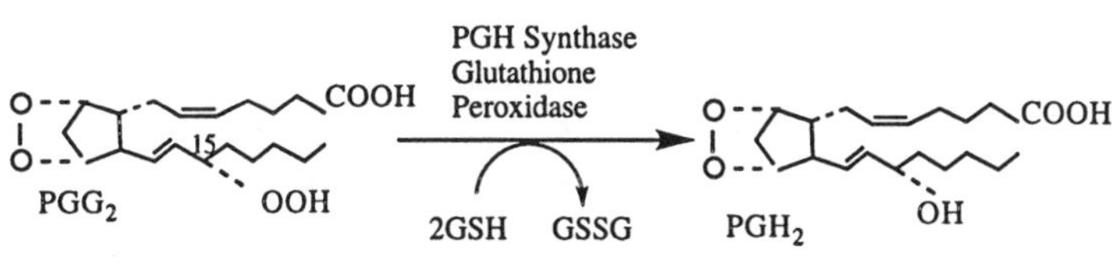

FIGURE 24 Oxygen removal to form PGH$_2$.

produced in the kidney and spleen. Just prior to parturition, $PGF_{2\alpha}$ and PGE are produced in the uterus. PGI_2 is produced by endothelial cells lining the blood vessels. This prostaglandin inhibits platelet aggregation and thus is important to maintaining a blood flow free of clots. It is counteracted by thromboxane A_2 which is produced by the platelets when these cells contact a foreign surface. PGE_2, $PGF_{2\alpha}$, and PGI_2 are formed by the heart in about equal amounts. All of these prostaglandins have a very short half-life. No sooner are they released than they are inactivated.

The thromboxanes are highly active metabolites of the prostaglandins. They are formed when PGH_2 has its cyclopentane ring replaced by a six-membered oxane ring as shown in Figure 25. Imidazole is a potent inhibitor of thromboxane A synthase and is used to block TXA_2 production and platelet aggregation.

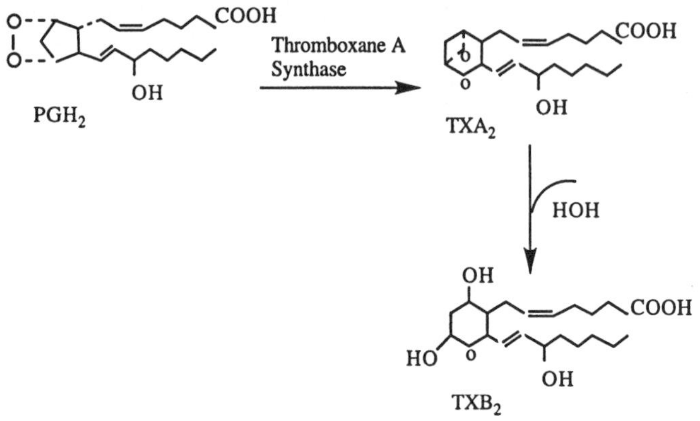

FIGURE 25 Formation of the thromboxanes.

Thromboxane A_2 has a role in clot formation. The half-life of TXA_2 is less than one minute. TXB_2 is its metabolic end-product and has little biological activity. Measuring TXB_2 levels in blood and tissue can give an indication of how much TXA_2 had been produced. PGD_2 and PGE_2 are involved in the regulation of sleep-wake cycles in a variety of species.

The cyclooxygenase reaction illustrated in Figure 23 can be inhibited by certain anti-inflammatory drugs such as aspirin, indomethacin, and phenylbutazone.

When the conversion of arachidonic acid to the prostaglandins is inhibited or when either of the other 20 carbon fatty acids are abundantly available, a different series of prostaglandins and leukotrienes are produced. Eicosapentaenoic acid is not as good a substrate for cyclo-oxygenation as is arachidonic acid. As a result, less of the arachidonic acid-related prostaglandins (even numbered PGs and TBXs) are produced and more of the odd numbered prostaglandins and leukotrienes are produced. Figure 22 shows the overall metabolic pathway for eicosanoid synthesis and degradation.

Although the cyclooxygenase pathway is quite important in the production of prostaglandins, equally important is the lipoxygenase pathway. This pathway is catalyzed by a family of enzymes called the lipoxygenase enzymes. These enzymes differ from the cyclooxygenase enzymes in their catalytic site for oxygen addition to the unsaturated fatty acid. One lipoxygenase is active at the double bond at carbon 5 while a second is active at carbon 11 and a third is active at carbon 15. The products of these reactions are monohydroperoxy-eicosatetraenoic acids (HPETEs) and are numbered according to the location of the double bond to which the oxygen is added. 5HPETE is the major lipoxygenase product in basophils, polymorphonuclear leukocytes, macrophages, mast cells, and any organ undergoing an inflammatory response.

12HPETE is the major product in platelets, pancreatic endocrine cells, vascular smooth muscle, and glomerular cells. 15HPETE predominates in reticulocytes, eosinophils, T-lymphocytes, and tracheal epithelial cells. The HPETEs are not in themselves active hormones; rather, they serve as precursors for the leukotrienes. The leukotrienes are the metabolic end-products of the lipoxygenase reaction. These compounds contain at least three conjugated double bonds. The unstable 5HPETE is converted to either an analogous alcohol (hydroxy fatty acid) or is reduced by a peroxide or converted to leukotriene. The peroxidative reduction of 5'HPETE to the stable 5HETE (5 hydroxyeicosatetraenoic acid) is similar to that of 12HPETE to 12HETE and of 15HPETE to 15HETE. In each instance the carbon-carbon double bonds are unconjugated and the geometry of the double bonds is trans, cis, cis, respectively. In contrast to the active thromboxanes which have very short half-lives, the leukotrienes can persist as long as four hours. These compounds comprise a group of substances known as the slow-acting anaphylaxis substances. They cause slowly evolving but protracted contractions of smooth muscles in the airways and gastrointestinal tract. Leukotriene C_4 is rapidly converted to LTD_4 which in turn is slowly converted to LTE_4. Enzymes in the plasma are responsible for these conversions. The products of the lipoxygenase pathway are potent mediators of the response to allergens, tissue damage (inflammation), hormone secretion, cell movement, cell growth, and calcium flux. The leukotrienes are more potent than histamine in stimulating the contraction of the bronchial nonvascular smooth muscles. In addition, LTD_4 increases the permeability of the microvasculature. The mono HETEs and LTB_4 stimulate the movement of eosinophils and neutrophils making them the first line of defense in injury resulting in inflammation.

When dihomo-γ-linoleic acid or eicosapentaenoic acid serve as substrates for eicosanoid production, the products are either of the 1 series or 3 series. The products they form may be less active than those formed from arachidonic acid, and this decrease in activity can be of therapeutic value. Hence, ingestion of omega 3 fatty acids leads to the decreased production of prostaglandin E_2 and its metabolites; a decrease in the production of thromboxane A_2, a potent platelet aggregator and vasoconstrictor; and a decrease in leukotriene B_4, a potent inflammatory hormone and a powerful inducer of leukocyte hemotaxis and adherence. Counteracting these decreases are an increase in thromboxane A_3 (TXA_3), a weak platelet aggregator and vasoconstrictor; an increase in the production of PGI_3 without an increase in PGI_2 which stimulates vasodilation and inhibits platelet aggregation; and an increase in leukotriene B_5 which is a weak inducer of inflammation and a weak chemotoxic agent.

EJECTION FRACTION

Percentage of the total diastolic volume of blood the heart ejects as it contracts; normal value is 70%.

ELASTIN

A protein found in connective tissue, ligaments, and vascular tissues. Rich in lysine and glycine. It is a very elastic protein.

ELECTROCARDIOGRAM (ECG)

A record of the electrical activity of the heart that provides information about abnormal cardiac rhythm and function.

ELECTROLYTE

An electrically charged particle (anion or cation).

ELECTRON DONOR

In an electron acceptor/donor pair, the electron donor gives or donates electrons to the acceptor. An electron donor is a reducing agent.

ELECTRON TRANSPORT

See respiratory chain.

ELEMENTAL FORMULA

Dietetic formula requiring little digestion.

ELIMINATION DIET

Dietary regimen where foods suspected to cause allergy or intolerance are eliminated from the diet for a period of at least two weeks. If symptoms are reduced or eliminated, foods are reintroduced one at a time and reactions noted to confirm or rule out food involvement in allergy or intolerance.

EMBDEN MEYERHOF PATHWAY

See glycolysis.

EMBOLISM

Obstruction of a blood vessel by blood clot or foreign body.

EMBRYO

The initial stage of development of the fertilized egg; usually the first 12 weeks in human pregnancy.

EMESIS

Vomiting.

EMULSIFIERS

Compounds which facilitate the dispersion of oil in water. Egg yolk serves as an emulsifier in the manufacture of mayonnaise.

EMULSION

A mixture of fat and water held together by an agent which has a lipophilic and a hydrophilic portion of its structure. Bile salts serve as emulsifying agents facilitating lipid digestion and absorption.

ENAMEL

The hard glistening substance covering the crown of the tooth.

ENCEPHALOPATHY

Disease of the encephalus. Dysfunction of the brain associated with advanced liver disease due to excess ammonia and nitrogenous waste product accumulation and characterized by loss of consciousness.

END-STAGE RENAL DISEASE (ESRD)
See Chronic renal failure.

ENDEMIC
Present in a community or population, as in diseases which are localized to a particular group of people.

ENDOCARDITIS
Inflammation of the endocardium, heart valves, or cardiac prosthesis resulting from an infectious agent entering the bloodstream.

ENDOCRINE DISORDERS
Diseases of the endocrine glands which are characterized by either an overproduction or underproduction of the hormone that gland produces.

ENDOCRINE GLANDS
Specialized cells and tissues which release hormones into the blood stream. These hormones have as their targets tissues some distance away from the tissue of origin.

ENDOGENOUS
Coming from within the body

ENDOPLASMIC RETICULUM
See Cell anatomy; Table 15 and Figure 13.

ENDORPHIN
A peptide in the brain which has sedative properties.

ENDOSPERM
That portion of a seed in which the embryotic plant forms.

ENDOTOXIN
A bacterial toxin not freely released into the surrounding medium; may be a component of the bacterial cell wall; is heat stable; may cause symptoms of shock accompanied by diarrhea, fever, and leukocytosis.

ENERGETICS
The physical laws of energy and thermodynamics which apply to all chemical reactions.

ENERGY BALANCE
When energy balance is zero, energy intake equals energy expenditure. When energy balance is positive, intake exceeds expenditure and weight is gained. When energy balance is negative, expenditure exceeds intake and weight is lost.

ENERGY INTAKE
That intake of energy needed to sustain the body and its associated activity. The U.S. recommendations for energy intake are shown in Table 18.

TABLE 18
Recommended Energy Intakes for Infants, Children, and Adults Based on Weight and Height (United States)

Category	Age	Weight (lb.)	Height (in.)	Recommended Energy Intake (kcal)
Infants	0–6 mo	13	24	650
	6–12 mo	20	28	850
Children	1–3 yrs	29	35	1300
	4–6	44	44	1800
	7–10	62	52	2000
Males	11–14	99	62	2500
	15–18	145	69	3000
	19–24	160	70	2900
	25–50	174	70	2900
	51+	170	68	2300
Females	11–14	101	62	2200
	15–18	120	64	2200
	19–24	128	65	2200
	25–50	138	64	2200
	51+	143	63	1900
Pregnant	1st trimester:	No change		
	2nd trimester			+300
	3rd trimester			+300
Lactation	1–6 mo			+500
	7–12 mo			+500

From National Research Council, Food and Nutrition Board, 10th ed., National Academy Press, Washington, D.C., 1989.

ENERGY-PROTEIN MALNUTRITION

Protein-energy malnutrition (PEM or PCM). Starvation is the extreme state of malnutrition that occurs when the individual is provided little or no food to nourish the body. Between starvation and the state of adequate nourishment to meet nutrient needs, there are graded levels of inadequate macronutrient intake. Where the intake of macronutrients is inadequate the syndrome is called protein-calorie malnutrition or more correctly, protein-energy malnutrition.

The needs for these nutrients and energy are determined by the age and health status of the individual. Rapid growth, infection, injury, and chronic debilitating disease can drive up the need for food and the nutrients it contains. It is difficult to segregate symptoms due solely to protein deficiency (Kwashiorkor) from those due solely to energy deficit (Marasmus). In children, one may observe the different symptoms and visualize them all as parts of a continuum called protein-energy malnutrition rather than distinctly different nutritional disorders. The symptoms of protein deficiency intermingle with those of protein and energy deficiency and a clear-cut diagnosis is not possible.

ENGINEERED FOODS

Foods designed by food scientists for specific purposes. These foods have specific properties and functions; they may have more fiber or less salt and/or less fat and/or unusual ingredients that are used as substitutes for usual ingredients.

ENRICHED FOOD

Food product in which micronutrients such as iron or the B vitamins have been added.

ENRICHMENT

Process of adding nutrients back to a food that have been removed during processing.

ENTERAL FEEDING

Feeding by way of a tube inserted through the nose to the stomach.

ENTERAL NUTRITION

Provision of nutrition through a tube that enters the stomach or small intestine through the nasal passage or abdominal area. Used for patients who are unable to consume adequate nutrition by eating sufficient quantities of food.

ENTEROCYTE

Absorptive cells lining the gastrointestinal tract. Usually restricted to the small intestine.

ENTEROHEPATIC CIRCULATION

The path of bile salts and cholesterol from the liver to the gall bladder to the duodenum returning to the liver via the portal circulation upon absorption from the ileum. Some vitamins and minerals also follow this pathway.

ENTHALPY

The thermodynamic function of a system equivalent to the internal energy plus the product of pressure and volume.

ENTROPY

The randomness or disorder of a system.

ENZYMATIC OXIDATION

Enzyme-mediated oxidative degradation of a substance.

ENZYMES

Proteins which serve as catalysts of biological reactions.

EPIDEMIOLOGY

The study of the health status of a population.

EPINEPHRINE

A catecholamine synthesized from tyrosine in the adrenal medulla; a neurotransmitter.

EPITHELIAL CELLS

Cells on the body surface, skin cells; enterocytes are specialized epithelial cells.

EPITHELIUM

The layer of cells that provide the surface covering of the body; the nonvascular cell layer of skin, gastrointestinal tract, and respiratory tract.

ER

Endoplasmic reticulum. See Cell anatomy.

ERGOGENIC, ERGONOMICS

A discipline relating human factors to the design and operation of machines or elements of the physical environment.

ERGOT ALKALOIDS

Mycotoxins which are 3,4-substituted indole alkaloids, produced by the mould *Claviceps purpurea*. There are two types of ergot alkaloids: type I, including ergotamine, ergotaminine, ergocristine, ergocristinine, ergostine, ergostinine, ergosine, α-ergokryptine, α-ergokryptinine, β-ergokryptine, β-ergokryptinine, and ergocornine; type II, including ergine, erginine, ergometrine, ergometrinine, lysergic acid, isolysergic acid methylcarbinolamide, lysergic acid L-valine methyl ester, $\Delta^{8,9}$-lysergic acid, ergosecaline, and ergosecalinine. Most ergot alkaloids are peptides of lysergic acid or isolysergic acid in cyclol form. Lysergic acid alkaloids are levorotatory and highly active pharmacologically. On the other hand, the isolysergic acid alkaloids are dextrorotatory and only weakly active. Thus, the biological activity of *Claviceps purpurea* can be ascribed only to the former type of alkaloids. Ergot alkaloids as a group can result in toxic symptoms of both acute (tachycardia, hypertension, confusion, thirst, abdominal colic, vomiting, diarrhea, hypothermia of the skin) and chronic (disturbances in the gastrointestinal tract, angina pectoris, hypo- or hypertension, and the characteristic symptoms seen in ergotism) nature. Consumption of rye and other cereal grains contaminated by *Claviceps purpurea* causes ergotism. The mould can parasitize the female sex organs of the flowers of grasses, such as rye, wheat, and other grains. This phenomenon is characterized by a black or deep purple, hard, dense mass of cells, or sclerotium, which contains a plethora of compounds that are quite toxic. The sclerotium is capable of germination but may lie dormant in the ground during the winter. In the spring with the alternation of cold (3–4°C) and relatively warm (≥ 14°C) temperatures, the sclerotium germinates. During the harvest the sclerotia may end up between the cereal grains. The consumption by humans of flour contaminated by the sclerotia of *Claviceps purpurea* results in epidemic ergotism. Two types of ergotism have been identified: (1) gangrenous ergotism (general lassitude; pains in the lumbar region, limbs, and calves; mild vomiting; swelling and inflammation of the feet and hands; alternating feeling of hot and cold; numbness; and gangrene); and (2) convulsive ergotism (sudden, painful, convulsive seizures beginning with the fingers or toes and spreading to the arms or legs; coma; drowsiness; giddiness; blindness; deafness; and swollen and edematous hands or feet).

ERUCIC ACID ($CH_3(CH_2)_7CH = CH(CH_2)_{11}COOH$)

A toxic monounsaturated fatty acid, which is found in the plant family Cruciferae, notably in Brassica. The oils from rapeseed and mustardseed are particularly high in erucic acid (20–55%). The toxic effects in animals include fat accumulation in the heart muscle, growth retardation, and liver damage. Because a large intake of erucic acid is necessary to induce myocardial damage in animals, the hazard of erucic acid toxicity in humans is probably minimal. A variety of rapeseed has been developed that produces an erucic acid-free oil. This plant is called canola and its oil is canola oil.

ERYTHROBLAST

An immature red blood cell characterized by the presence of a nucleus and large size. Usually found in the bone marrow.

ERYTHROCYTE

Red blood cell.

ERYTHROCYTEMIA

Abnormal increase in the red blood cells in circulation.

ERYTHROPOIESIS

The process for the synthesis of red blood cells.

ERYTHROPOIETIC PORPHYRIA

Presence of porphyrins in the urine due to excess red blood cell breakdown.

ERYTHROPOIETIN

Substance that stimulates red cell formation.

ESADDI

Estimated safe and adequate daily dietary intakes. Refers to those nutrients for which there are indications of essentiality but for which the database is insufficient to make valid recommendations for intakes.

ESOPHAGEAL VARICIES

Enlarged blood vessels in the collateral circulation of the esophagus.

ESSENTIAL AMINO ACIDS

Amino acids which cannot be synthesized in sufficient quantities in the body to meet the need for protein synthesis (Table 19) (see Amino acids).

TABLE 19
Essential and Nonessential Amino Acids for Adult Mammals

Essential	Nonessential
Valine	Hydroxyproline
Leucine	Cysteine
Isoleucine	Glycine
Threonine	Alanine
Phenylalanine	Serine
Methionine	Proline
Tryptophan	
Lysine	Glutamic Acid
Histidine	Aspartic Acid
Arginine[a]	

[a] Not essential for maintenance of most adult mammals.

ESSENTIAL FATTY ACID DEFICIENCY

Inadequate intake of linoleic and linolenic acids; characterized by dry, scaly skin; weight loss and/or inefficient use of food for weight gain; enlarged heart and kidneys; fatty liver;

disturbed regulation of oxidative phosphorylation; impaired gonadal function; and poor reproduction.

ESSENTIAL FATTY ACIDS

Long chain (18 carbons) unsaturated fatty acids needed by the body but which the body cannot synthesize. These include linoleic and linolenic acids for most species. Members of the cat family cannot synthesize arachidonic acid and therefore require this fatty acid in their diets. Vegetable oils are rich sources of linoleic acid while fish oils, primrose oil, and canola oil are good sources of linolenic acid. The location of the double bonds is indicated as N6 or $\omega6$ counting carbon atoms from the methyl end of the molecule.

$$CH_3CH_2CH_2CH_2CH_2C \overset{H}{=} \overset{H}{C} - CH_2 - \overset{H}{C} = \overset{H}{C}(CH_2)_7COOH$$

18   12   9   1

linoleic acid   (18:2, N-6 or ω-6)

$$CH_3CH_2CH = CHCH_2CH = CHCH_2CH = (CH_2)_7COOH$$

linolenic acid   (18:3, N-3 or ω-3)

$$CH_3(CH_2)_4(CH = CHCH_2)_4(CH_2)_2COOH$$

arachidonic acid   (20:4, N-6 or ω-6)

ESSENTIAL NUTRIENTS

Nutrients needed by the body and which must be provided in the diet. There are species and age differences in the nutrients needed. Some nutrients can be synthesized in the body, but the synthesis may be inadequate to meet the need of the consumer. The essential nutrients for the human include: the amino acids, valine, leucine, isoleucine, threonine, phenylalanine, methionine, tryptophane, lysine, histidine, and arginine. Arginine can be synthesized but not in sufficient quantities in the growing child to meet the need for new tissue growth. Carbohydrate (glucose) can be synthesized. The fatty acids, linoleic, linolenic; the vitamins: retinol and its equivalents, Vitamin D (can be synthesized if body is exposed to ultraviolet light), Vitamin E, Vitamin K, thiamin, riboflavin, niacin, Vitamin B_6, pantothenic acid, folacin, Vitamin B_{12} (cyanocobalamin), biotin, and ascorbic acid (can be synthesized by most species except primates, guinea pig, and fruit bat); the minerals: calcium, phosphorous, iron, copper, selenium, magnesium, zinc, manganese, chloride, sodium, potassium, molybdenum, and fluoride. The needs for some additional minerals are being studied. These are called the trace and ultra-trace minerals, and the need for these is very difficult to establish.

ESTER

A compound containing an oxygen linkage; the product of the condensation of an acid and alcohol with the loss of a molecule of water.

ESTERIFIED CHOLESTEROL

Cholesterol to which a fatty acid is joined.

ESTROGEN

A steroid hormone produced by the ovary in a cyclic fashion and which is an essential hormone for female fertility as well as the development of female characteristics (hair pattern, mammary cell development, etc.)

ESTRUS

That portion or phase of the sexual cycle of female animals characterized by a willingness to accept the male.

ETHANOL

The two-carbon alcohol resulting from the fermentation of glucose.

ETHANOL METABOLISM

Ethanol, once consumed, is rapidly absorbed by simple diffusion. The diffusion is affected by the amount of alcohol consumed, the regional blood flow, the surface area, and the presence of other foods. Absorption is fastest in the duodenum and jejunum; slower in the stomach, ileum, and colon; and slowest in the mouth and esophagus. The rate of absorption by the duodenum depends on gastric emptying time. Complete absorption may vary from two to six hours. The type of beverage can influence ethanol absorption. Ethanol from beer is absorbed slower than that found in whisky which is slower than gin, red wine and, of course, pure ethanol is absorbed the fastest of all. Ethanol is water missible and is rapidly distributed between the intracellular and extracellular compartments. The uptake of ethanol by the fat depots is minimal. Ethanol crosses the plasma membranes but, in so doing, changes them. When ethanol is in contact with a protein, it denatures it. Thus, large and frequent ethanol exposures result in damage to proteins both within and around the cells. The most damaged tissue is the liver since ethanol is carried directly to this tissue via the portal blood. While gut cells are also damaged, these cells have such a rapid turnover time (less than seven days) that damage due to intermittent ethanol consumption is not as long lasting as happens in the liver. Ethanol is metabolized to acetaldehyde (see Figure 26). The acetaldehyde is converted to acetate which can either be joined with a CoA or released to the circulation. If too much acetate is released, acidosis develops. Acetyl CoA can either be used for fatty acid synthesis or be shuttled into the mitochondria via carnitine to be oxidized as through the citric acid cycle. A fatty liver typifies the alcoholic. The fatty liver may progress to alcoholic hepatitis, cirrhosis, liver failure, and death. The fatty liver is due to accelerated hepatic fatty acid synthesis as well as due to an ethanol-induced impairment in hepatic lipid output. If the hepatocyte accumulates too much lipid, the cell will burst and die. Dead tissue within the liver is known as cirrhosis. When too much tissue dies, the liver may cease to function and the alcoholic dies.

ETHNOLOGY

The study of ethnic groups — groups characterized by a common set of customs, beliefs, language, or cultural origin.

ETHOLOGY

A branch of knowledge dealing with human ethos, its evolution, and formation; the study of behavior.

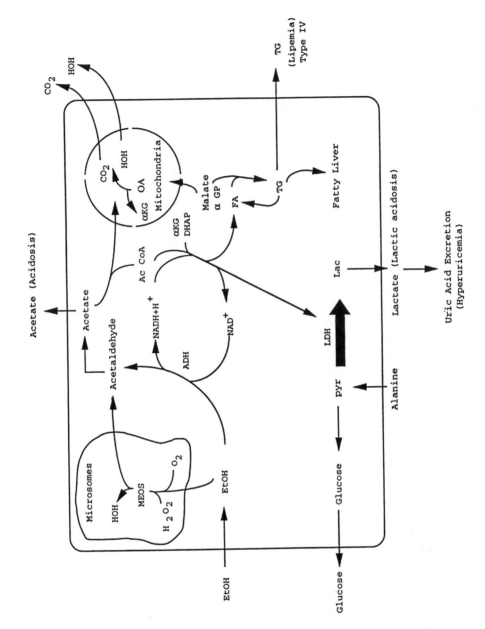

FIGURE 26 Metabolism of ethanol by the liver (From Berdanier, C.D., *Advanced Nutrition: Macronutrients*, CRC Press, Boca Raton, FL, 1994, 205).

ETIOLOGY

The study of the causes and development of a disease.

EUCARYOTES (EUKARYOTES)

Multicelled living beings. Cells are characterized by the presence of a membrane surrounding the nucleus.

EXOCRINE CELLS

Cells that produce secretions into the surrounding environment. Examples are mucous producing cells of the respiratory tract and enzyme producing cells of the intestinal tract.

EXOGENOUS NUTRIENTS

Nutrients in the diet.

EXOPHTHALMIC GOITER

Disease caused by excess thyroxine production. Also called Graves disease, characterized by high metabolic rate; weight loss, particularly muscle and fat loss; bulging eyes; tremor; rapid heart rate; good appetite; and irritability.

EXPANDED FOOD AND NUTRITION EDUCATION PROGRAM (EFNEP)

Nutrition education program available in the United States to low income mothers of young children.

EXPERIMENTAL STUDIES

Studies in which the exposure conditions are chosen by the investigator. For ethical reasons, exposure restrictions exist. The most important one is that examining potentially toxic substances in humans is prohibited. This implies that potentially adverse effects of food components can only be investigated in animal studies. In experimental studies, two groups of subjects are compared with regard to the outcome variable — subjects exposed to the substance under investigation (treatment group) and subjects not exposed (control group). An essential condition of this type of study is that the exposure is randomly distributed over the subjects. Maintaining all conditions constant except for the exposure has to be achieved by randomization of the study subjects, as life-style and genetic background differ greatly from one person to another. If possible, the study should be double-blind. This means that the investigator as well as the study subjects do not know whether they are in the treatment group or the control group. In this way, the observations are not influenced by the investigator or the respondent.

EXTERNAL VALIDITY

Determines whether the results can be generalized beyond the study population. Internal validity is a prerequisite for external validity. If an association is not validly assessed for the population under investigation, it cannot be generalized to other populations. For external validity, a judgment must be made as to the plausibility that the effect observed in the study population can be generalized.

EXTRACELLULAR

Outside of the cell, as in serum which surrounds the blood cells.

EXTRACELLULAR WATER

The fluid compartment which surrounds cells, tissues, and organs. It is distributed into several subcompartments (plasma, interstitial, and lymph fluids; fluids around connective tissue, cartilage, and bone; and transcellular fluids) which are not clearly defined. About 45% of the total body water is found in the extracellular compartments.

EXTRAVASCULAR

Outside the vascular system as the fluids which are between the cells in the tissues or between the capillaries and the cells they supply.

EXTRINSIC FACTOR

Vitamin B_{12}.

EXUDATE

Fluid that has left blood vessels and deposited in or on tissues.

F

FACILITATED TRANSPORT

Transport against a concentration gradient using a carrier but which is not energy or sodium dependent.

FAD, FMN-FLAVIN ADENINE DINUCLEOTIDE, FLAVIN MONONUCLEOTIDE

Coenzymes that carry reducing equivalents (H$^+$) in reactions of intermediary metabolism. Riboflavin is an essential component of these nucleotides.

FAILURE TO THRIVE

Term usually referring to infants and children who fail to grow and develop in the normal way but in whom no definitive cause for this failure can be identified. The term can also be used to refer to the elderly who appear ill for no apparent cause.

FANCONI'S SYNDROME

A genetic disease associated with abnormal metabolism of cystine. Characterized by abnormal renal function, glycosuria, phosphaturia, amino aciduria, and bicarbonate wasting.

FASTING BLOOD GLUCOSE

The level of glucose in the blood after 12–16 hours without food, usually between 80–100 mg/dl or 4–5 mmol/l (see hypoglycemia; hyperglycemia).

FAT SOLUBLE VITAMINS

Vitamins that are soluble in fat solvents (alcohol, ether, chloroform, etc.). Includes retinol and its equivalents (Vitamin A), Vitamin D, Vitamin E, and Vitamin K (see Vitamins, Table 49).

FAT SUBSTITUTES

Synthetic compounds designed to provide the food characteristics of fat without the energy value (see simplesse, olestra).

FATTY ACID DESATURATION

Saturated fatty acids can be converted to unsaturated fatty acids in the body. Desaturation occurs in the endoplasmic reticulum and in the microsomes. The pathway is shown in Figure 27. The enzymes that catalyze desaturation are the Δ9, Δ6, or Δ3 desaturases. They are sometimes called mixed function oxidases because two substrates (fatty acid and NADPH) are oxidized simultaneously. Desaturation of stearic acid to form oleic acid results in the formation of a double bond at the ω-6 or Δ9 position. This is the first committed step of the desaturation pathway. Fatty acid desaturation can be followed by elongation and repeated such that a variety of mono- and polyunsaturated fatty acids can be formed. These fatty acids contribute fluidity to membranes because of their lower melting point. An increase in the activity of the desaturation pathway is a characteristic response of rats fed a diet high in saturated fatty acids. The body can convert the dietary saturated fatty acids to unsaturated fatty acids thus maintaining an optimal P:S ratio in the tissues.

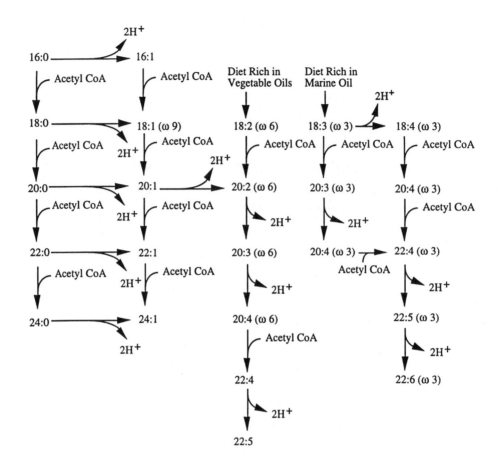

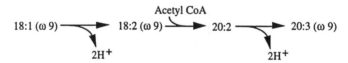

FIGURE 27 Pathways for the synthesis of long chain polyunsaturated fatty acids. The reaction sequences show both elongation and desaturation with the initial substrate being palmitate (From Berdanier, C.D., *Advanced Nutrition: Macronutrients*, CRC Press, Boca Raton, FL, 1994, 229).

The activity of the desaturases can be increased through feeding saturated fat and/or high sugar diets. Both dietary maneuvers increase the need to synthesize unsaturated fatty acids. Desaturase activity is stimulated by insulin, triiodothyronine, and glucocorticoid. Desaturase activity is decreased when high polyunsaturated fats are fed.

FATTY ACID ELONGATION

The lengthening of fatty acids by the addition of two carbon units (acetyl groups). Elongation occurs in either the endoplasmic reticulum or the mitochondria. The reaction differs depending on where it occurs. In the endoplasmic reticulum, the reaction sequence is similar to that described for the cytosolic fatty acid synthase complex. The source of the two carbon unit is malonyl CoA, and NADPH provides the reducing power. The intermediates are CoA esters not the acyl carrier protein 4′ phosphopantetheine. The reaction sequence (Figure 27) produces stearic acid (18:0) in all tissues that make fatty acids except the brain. In the brain, elongation can proceed further producing fatty acids containing up to 24 carbons. In the mitochondria, elongation uses acetyl CoA rather than malonyl CoA as the source of the two carbon unit. It uses either NADH⁺H⁺ or NADPH⁺H⁺ as the source of reducing equivalents and uses, as substrate, carbon chains of less than 16 carbons. Mitochondrial elongation is the reversal of fatty acid oxidation which also occurs in this organelle.

FATTY ACID ESTERIFICATION

Fatty acids are joined to glycerol via an esterification reaction shown in Figure 28. The resultant product is a monoglyceride, diglyceride, or triglyceride (triacylglyceride). Triacylglycerides are formed in a stepwise fashion. First, a fatty acid (usually a saturated fatty acid) is attached at carbon 1 of the glycerophosphate. The phosphate group at carbon 3 is electronegative and because it pulls electrons toward it, it leaves carbon 1 more reactive than carbon 2. The fatty acid (as acyl CoA) is transferred to carbon 1 through the action of a transferase. The attachment uses the carboxy end of the fatty acid chain and makes an ester linkage releasing the CoA. Now the molecule has electronegative forces at each end — the phosphate group on carbon 3 and the oxygen plus carbon chain at carbon 1. Now carbon 2 is vulnerable and reactive and another carbon chain can be attached. In this instance the fatty acid is usually an unsaturated fatty acid. At this point, the 1,2 diacylglyceride-phosphate loses its phosphate group so that carbon 3 is now reactive. The 1,2 diacylglyceride can either be esterified with another fatty acid to make triacylglyceride or can be used to make the membrane phospholipids, phosphatidylcholine, phosphatidylethanolamine, phosphatidylinositol, cardiolipin, and phosphatidylserine.

FATTY ACID OXIDATION

A process which occurs after the glycerides are hydrolyzed to glycerol and fatty acids. The oxidation is shown in Figure 29. This oxidation is called β oxidation and occurs in the mitochondria.

Prior to oxidation, the fatty acids must be transported into the mitochondria via the acyl carnitine transport system (see Figure 10). The fatty acids are activated by conversion to their CoA thioesters. This activation requires ATP and the enzyme, acyl CoA synthase or thiokinase. There are several thiokinases which differ with respect to their specificity for the different fatty acids. The activation step is dependent on the release of energy from ATP. Once the fatty acid is activated it is bound to carnitine with the release of CoA. The acyl carnitine is then translocated through the mitochondrial membranes into the mitochondrial matrix via the carnitine acylcarnitine translocase. As one molecule of acylcarnitine is passed into the matrix, one molecule of carnitine is translocated back to the cytosol and the acylcarnitine is converted back to acyl CoA. The acyl CoA can then enter the β oxidation pathway shown in Figure 29. Without carnitine, the oxidation of fatty acids, especially the long chain fatty acids, cannot proceed. Acyl CoA cannot traverse the membrane into the mitochondria and thus requires a translocase for its entry. The translocase requires carnitine. While most of the fatty acids that enter the β oxidation pathway are completely oxidized via the citric acid cycle and respiratory chain to CO_2 and HOH, some of the acetyl CoA is converted to the ketones, acetoacetate, and β hydroxybutyrate. The condensation of two molecules of acetyl CoA to acetoacetyl CoA occurs in the mitochondria via the enzyme β-ketothiolase. Acetoacetyl CoA then condenses with another acetyl CoA to form HMG CoA. At last, the HMG CoA is cleaved into acetoacetic acid and acetyl CoA. The acetoacetic acid is reduced to β hydroxybutyrate, and this reduction is dependent on the ratio of NAD⁺ to NADH⁺H⁺. The enzyme for this reduction, β hydroxybutyrate dehydrogenase is tightly bound to the inner

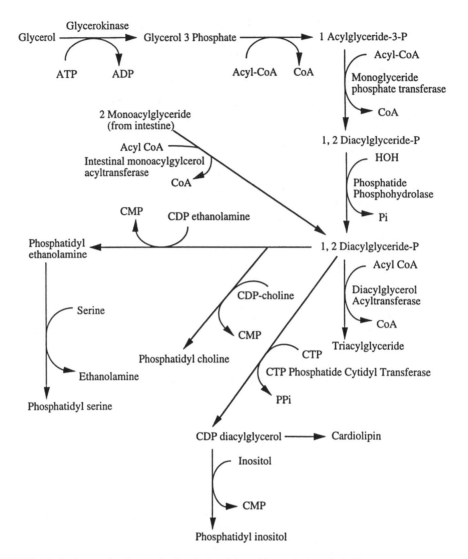

FIGURE 28 Pathways for the synthesis of triacylglycerides and phospholipids.

aspect of the mitochondrial membrane. Because of its high activity, the product (β hydroxy-butyrate) and substrate (acetoacetate) are in equilibrium.

HMG CoA is also synthesized in the cytosol, however, because this compartment lacks the HMG CoA lyase, the ketones are formed only in the mitochondria. In the cytosol, HMG CoA is the beginning substrate for cholesterol synthesis. The ketones can ultimately be used as fuel but may appear in the blood, liver, and other tissues at a level of less than 0.2 mM. In starving individuals or in people consuming a high fat diet, blood and tissue ketone levels may rise above normal (3–5 mM). However, unless these levels greatly exceed the body's capacity to use them as fuel (as is the case in uncontrolled diabetes mellitus with levels up to 20 mM) a rise in ketone levels is not a cause for concern. Ketones are choice metabolic fuels for muscle and brain. Although both tissues may prefer to use glucose, the ketones can be used when glucose is in short supply. Ketones are used to spare glucose wherever possible under these conditions.

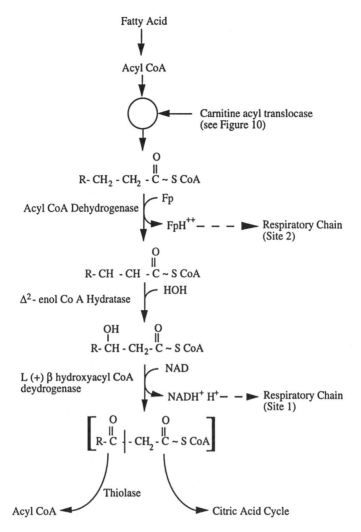

FIGURE 29 β oxidation of fatty acids.

The oxidation of unsaturated fatty acids follows the same pathway as the saturated fatty acids until the double bonded carbons are reached. At this point, a few side steps must be taken that involve a few additional enzymes. The pathway is shown in Figure 30.

Linoleate has two double bonds in the cis configuration. β oxidation removes three acetyl units leaving a CoA attached to the terminal carbon just before the first cis double bond. At this point an isomerase enzyme, Δ^3 cis Δ^6 trans enoyl CoA isomerase, acts to convert the first cis bond to a trans bond. Now this part of the molecule can once again enter the β oxidation sequence and two more acetyl CoA units are released. The second double bond is then opened and a hydroxyl group is inserted. In turn, this hydroxyl group is rotated to the L position and the remaining product can then re-enter the β oxidation pathway. Other unsaturated fatty acids can be similarly oxidized. Each time the double bond is approached, the isomerization and hydroxyl group addition takes place until all of the fatty acid is oxidized.

While β oxidation is the main pathway for the oxidation of fatty acids some fatty acids undergo α oxidation so as to provide the substrates for the synthesis of sphingolipids. These reactions occur in the endoplasmic reticulum and mitochondria and involve the mixed function

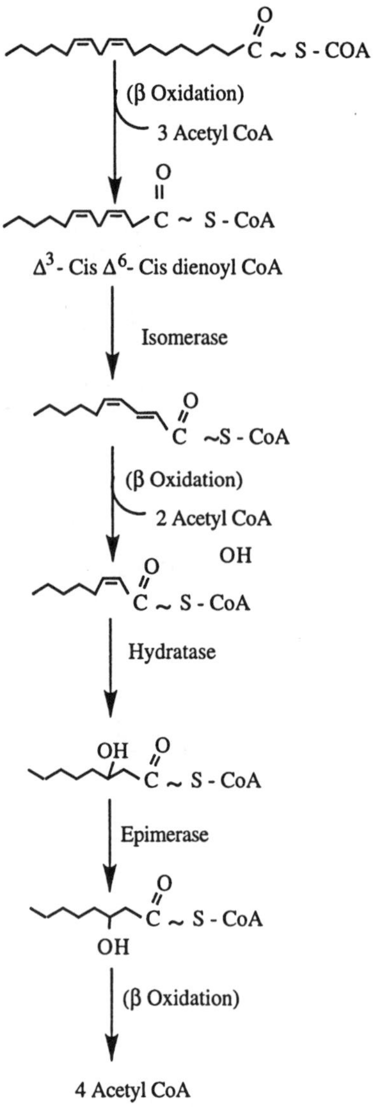

FIGURE 30 Modification of β oxidation for unsaturated fatty acid.

oxidases because they require molecular oxygen, reduced NAD, and specific cytochromes. The fatty acid oxidation that occurs in organelles other than the mitochondria are energy wasteful reactions because these other organelles do not have the citric acid cycle nor do they have the respiratory chain which takes the reducing equivalents released by the oxidative steps and combine them with oxygen to make water releasing energy that is then trapped in the high energy bonds of the ATP. Peroxisomal oxidation in the kidney and liver is an important aspect of drug metabolism. The peroxisomes are a class of subcellular organelles that are important in the protection against oxygen toxicity. They have a high level of catalase activity which suggests their importance in the antioxidant system. The peroxisomal fatty acid oxidation pathway differs in three important ways from the mitochondrial pathway. First, the initial dehydrogenation is accomplished by a cyanide insensitive oxidase which produces H_2O_2. This H_2O_2 is rapidly extinguished by catalase. Second, the enzymes of the pathway prefer long chain fatty acids and are slightly different in structure from those (with the same function) of the mitochondrial pathway. Third, β oxidation in the peroxisomes stops at eight carbons rather than proceeding all the way to acetyl CoA. The peroxisomes also serve in the conversion of cholesterol to bile acids and in the formation of ether lipids (plasmalogens).

FATTY ACID SYNTHESIS

Fatty acid synthesis occurs in the cytosol of the living cell using two carbon units (acetyl units) that are the result of glucose oxidation or amino acid degradation.

Fatty acid synthesis (Figure 31) begins with acetyl CoA. Acetyl CoA arises from the oxidation of glucose or the carbon skeletons of deaminated amino acids. Acetyl CoA is converted to malonyl CoA (Figure 32) with the addition of one carbon (from bicarbonate)

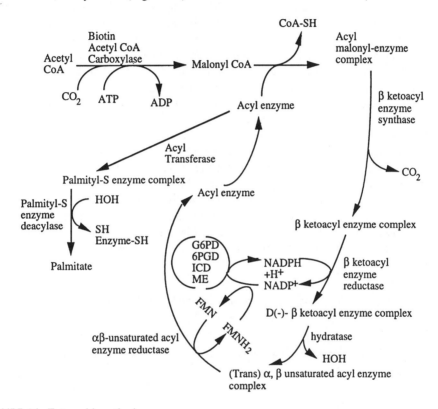

FIGURE 31 Fatty acid synthesis.

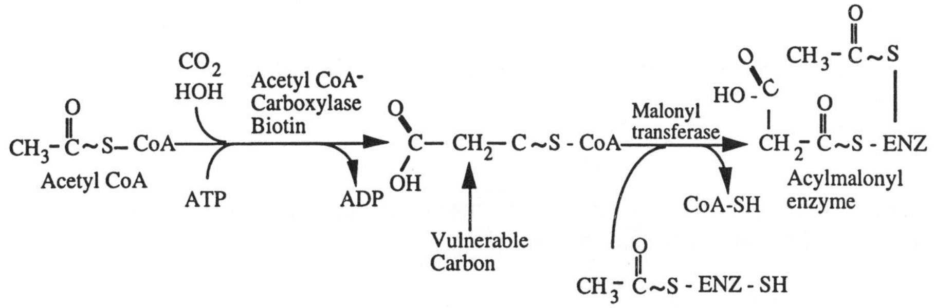

FIGURE 32 Details of the initial steps in fatty acid synthesis.

in the presence of the enzyme acetyl CoA carboxylase. The reaction uses the energy from one molecule of ATP and biotin as a coenzyme. This reaction is the first committed step in the reaction sequence that results in the synthesis of a fatty acid. The activated carbon dioxide attached to the biotin-enzyme complex is transferred to the methyl end of the substrate. Although most fatty acids synthesized in mammalian cells have an even number of carbons, this first committed step yields a three carbon product. This results in an asymmetric molecule which becomes vulnerable to attack (addition) at the center of the molecule with the subsequent loss of the terminal carbon. The vulnerability is conferred by the fact that both the

$$\overset{O}{\overset{\|}{}}$$

carboxyl group at one end and the $-C \sim S - CoA$ group at the other end are both powerful attractants of electrons from the hydrogen of the middle carbon. This leaves the carbon in a very reactive state, and a second acetyl group carried by a carrier protein with the help of phosphopantethine which has a sulfur group connection can be joined to it through the action of the enzyme, malonyl transferase. Subsequently, the "extra" carbon is released via the enzyme β ketoacyl enzyme synthase leaving a four carbon chain still connected to an SH group at the carboxyl end. This SH group is the docking end for all the enzymes that comprise the fatty acid synthase complex. These enzymes catalyze the addition of two carbon acetyl groups in sequence to the methyl end of the carbon chain until the final product palmityl CoA and then palmitic acid is produced. Members of this fatty acid synthase complex include the aforementioned malonyl transferase and β ketoacyl synthase, β ketoacyl reductase which catalyzes the addition of reducing equivalents carried by FMN, and an acyl transferase. Upon completion of these six steps, the process is repeated until the chain length is 16 carbons long. At this point, the SH-acyl carrier protein is removed through the action of the enzyme palmityl-S-enzyme deacylase and the palmitic acid is available for esterification to glycerol to form a mono-, di-, or triacylglyceride (see Fatty acid esterification).

FATTY ACIDS

Carbon chains having a carboxyl group at one end and a methyl group at the other end.

FATTY FOODS

Foods having a high percentage of their energy content as fat. The fat content of some common foods is shown in Table 20.

FAVISM

A condition which develops after consuming certain species (vicia faba) of beans, characterized by fever, headache, abdominal pain, severe anemia, prostration, coma, and sometimes death.

FDA

Food and Drug Administration. A subunit of the U.S. Department of Health and Human Services.

FECES

Excrement discharged from the bowel, contains undigested food, intestinal secretions, intestinal flora, and desquamated intestinal cells.

FERMENTATION

A processing technique affecting the oxidation of dietary carbohydrates, fats, and oils. Some types of fermentation are used for the production of substances that are undesirable in other

TABLE 20
Fat Content of Some Common Foods

Food[a]	% Fat (g/100 g food)	% Cholesterol (g/100 g food)
Codfish	0.67	0.043
Halibut	2.94	0.041
Mackerel	6.30	0.076
Salmon	3.45	0.052
Beef steak, cooked	31.8	0.36
Hamburger, cooked	12.8	0.10
Stew meat	18.8	1.0
Roast lamb	19.0	
Lamb chops, cooked	36.0	1.11
Pork chops, cooked	21.1	1.03
Pork sausage	46.2	1.35
Bacon	53.0	
Bologna	28.6	1.04
Chicken, white meat	3.5	0.64
Eggs, whole	12	4.2
Egg white	<3.0	—
Whole milk	3.3	0.32
Skim milk	Trace	Trace
Cheddar cheese	32.0	1.0
Cottage cheese (4%)	4.29	0.21
Mozzarella cheese, skim milk	17.9	4.5
Ice cream	10.0	
Butter	81.4	2.4
Margarine	81.4	—
Walnuts	60.0	
Fruits, all kinds	<1.0	—
Avocado	13.0	—
Leafy vegetables	<1.0	—
Legumes (except peanuts)	1.0	—
Peanut butter	50.0	
Root vegetables	<1.0	—
Cereals and grains	1.0–2.0	0
Crackers	1.0	0
Bread, whole wheat	2.6	
Bread, white, enriched	3.3	<0.1

[a] These foods were selected from the vast array of foods presented in Handbooks 8–15, United States Department of Agriculture, Human Nutrition Information Service, U.S. Government Printing Office, Superintendent of Documents, Washington, D.C. 20402.

products. Examples are the formation of short-chain fatty acids and carbonyl compounds in cheeses and the high rancidity of a number of traditional Asian fermented fish and soy products.

FERRITIN

An iron binding protein which transports this mineral from the absorption site in the intestine to the site where it is used.

FETAL ALCOHOL SYNDROME

Malformed infants whose malformations can be traced to the alcohol consumed by their mothers during pregnancy. Characterized by abnormal eye placement, nose, and mouth development, and failure of the infant to grow and develop normally with full intellectual capacity. Various learning disabilities have also been associated with this condition.

FETUS

An unborn child; stage of development of a human from embryo to birth or from about 12 weeks post fertilization to full gestational age (approximately 40 weeks).

FIBER

Dietary fiber refers to those carbohydrates that are indigestible and unabsorbed.

The component glucose moieties are joined by β linkages rather than α linkages. They may also contain additional substituents but their chief characteristic is that of nondigestibility by the α amylases of the mammalian gastrointestinal system. These nondigestible carbohydrates are plant products and fall into five major categories: celluloses, hemicelluloses, lignins, pectins, and gums. The celluloses, hemicelluloses, and lignins provide bulk to the gastrointestinal contents due to their property of absorbing water. The increased bulkiness of the gut contents stimulates peristalsis and results in shorter passage time and more frequent defecation. In addition to its water holding property, fibers of the lignin type adsorb cholesterol and noxious agents in the gut contents aiding in their excretion in the feces. Pectins and gums also influence gastric emptying but in the opposite direction. These fiber types form gels that slow gastric emptying and slow the digestion and absorption of sugars, starches, and also fats. Fruits are good sources of pectin, while cereal grains and the woody parts of vegetables are good sources of the celluloses, hemicelluloses, and lignins. Dried beans and oats are good sources of gums. The fiber content of several common foods is given in Table 16 (page 86).

FIBRINOGEN

The precursor of fibrin which provides a network of fibers that forms the structural element in clot formation.

FIBROUS PLAQUE

Lipids that collect on a fibrous network within or on the arterial walls during the atherogenic process creating a projection into the lumen of the vessel and impeding flow.

FISH ALLERGY

Allergic reactions to fish are often serious. The cod-fish allergen is heat stable and resistant to proteolytic enzymes. In addition to symptoms such as rhinitis, dyspnea, eczema, urticaria, nausea, and vomiting following digestion of food, urticaria may occur after skin contact with fish. Also, shellfish can cause strong allergic reactions. Probably, fish families have a species-specific antigen as well as cross-reactive antigens. Antibodies and allergic reactions may be directed against a specific fish or multiple fish families.

FISH OILS

Marine oils, rich in omega-3 (N-3) unsaturated fatty acids, affect (decrease) platelet aggregation because they stimulate the synthesis of thromboxane A_3. Thromboxane A_3 does not have the platelet aggregating property of the other eicosanoids. In addition, eicosapentaenoic acid is used to make the anti-aggregating prostaglandin, PGI_3. Animals fed omega-3 rich oils produce significantly more of the eicosanoids of the LTB_5 series. LTB_4 is an important inflammatory mediator whereas LTB_5 is not. Fish oil consumption results in an increased neutrophil LTB_5 production with a concomitant decrease in LTB_4 production. This diet influenced change in LTB_4 and LTB_5 production seems to be related to a reduced incidence of autoimmune-inflammatory disorders such as asthma, psoriasis, and rheumatoid arthritis in populations consuming omega-3 fatty acids routinely. Thus, eicosanoid synthesis can be used as an explanation of the beneficial effects of fish oil ingestion on rheumatoid arthritis. In arthritics, the joints are inflamed and painful. The prostaglandins PGE_2 and leukotriene are both produced from arachidonate. PGE_2 induces the signs of inflammation which include redness and heat due to arteriolar vasodilation, swelling, and localized edema resulting from increased capillary permeability. Leukotriene prevents platelet aggregation. If there is less arachidonate available for the synthesis of these prostaglandins, then the inflammation is inhibited.

Tumorigenesis likewise can be influenced by the relative amounts of the various eicosanoids. Prostaglandin G of the 2-series acts as a tumor promoter. It down regulates macrophage tumoricidal activities and inhibits interleukin 2 production. Increased PGE_2 levels (from omega-6 fatty acids) have been associated with aggressive growth patterns of both basal and squamous cell skin carcinomas in humans. Vegetable oils are rich in these fatty acids. Products of the lipooxygenase pathway (stimulated by the omega-3 fatty acids) have the reverse effect.

FLATULENCE

Release from the anus of gases (methane, sulfur dioxide, etc.) produced in the large intestine through the action of intestinal flora on food residue. If the gas is not released, intestinal distention and discomfort result.

FLAVONOIDS

A class of plant pigments that are widely present in human food. These pigments are polyhydroxy-2-phenylbenzo-γ-pyrone derivatives, occurring as aglycones, glycosides, and methyl ethers. They are divided into six main subgroups: (1) flavanone, 3-OH: flavanol; (2) flavone, 3-OH: flavonol; (3) anthocyanidin, 3-OH: catechin, 3-OH: condensed tannins; (4) isoflavanone; (5) chalcone; and (6) aurone.

FLUORIDATION

The addition of fluoride to water; as a treatment of teeth to prevent decay.

FLUORIDE

Present in low but varying concentrations in drinking water (1 mg/ l), plants (e.g., tea) and animals (fish, 50–100 mg per 100 g). It accumulates in human bone tissue and dental enamel. Its beneficial effects on dental health have clearly been demonstrated. If consumed in excessive amounts, fluoride is toxic. The normal daily intake is 1–2 mg. Daily ingestion of

20–80 mg of fluoride leads to fluorosis, which is characterized by calcification resulting in effects on kidney function and possibly muscle and nerve function.

FLUOROSIS

A condition of excess fluoride intake chiefly characterized by a mottled appearance of the tooth enamel.

FMN

Flavin mononucleotide. A nucleotide coenzyme containing riboflavin.

FOLACIN

An essential B vitamin which particiates in one carbon transfer. Its structure is shown in Figure 33.

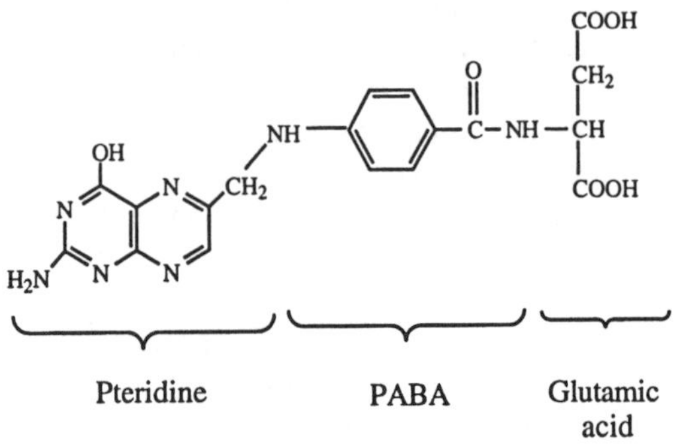

FIGURE 33 Structure of folacin.

FOLATE DEFICIENCY

A state which develops when an inadequate intake of folacin occurs. The main characteristic is macrocytic anemia. Green leafy vegetables, liver, and yeast are good sources of folacin. Inadequate intake of folacin by pregnant women has been linked to neurotube defects in the child. Folacin has para-aminobenzoic acid, glutamate, and pteridine in its structure (see Vitamins, Table 49).

FOLLICULOSIS

Presence of lymph follicles in large numbers.

FOLLOW-UP STUDIES (COHORT STUDIES)

Population studies in which the subjects (also referred to as the cohort) are followed for some time (follow-up period). At the start of the study (also called the baseline), the cohort consists of people who are free of the disease under investigation and differ in exposure conditions. All persons are examined and information on variables of interest is collected. During the course of the study, the occurrence of disease is recorded. From this, the incidence of the disease in the study population can be calculated. Based on these data, inferences on the association between exposure and occurrence of disease can be drawn. An important advantage of a follow-up study is that exposure is measured before the disease has developed. The appropriate follow-up period depends on the associations which are studied. Because the majority of follow-up studies concern chronic diseases, the follow-up period is usually long.

Consequently, results are only available after many years. Furthermore, for the assessment of associations between exposure and disease, it is necessary for the number of cases which manifest themselves during the follow-up period to be sufficiently large. This means that the cohort approach is not suitable for studying rare diseases. Another advantage of follow-up studies is that a large number of both exposures and outcomes can be studied. At baseline, a large number of parameters are measured in all study subjects. For a cohort study on a chronic disease, for example, these parameters may include lifestyle factors such as diet, physical activity, and smoking habits, and biological variables such as blood pressure, serum cholesterol concentration, height, and weight. Recent developments in the design of cohort studies include storage of biological material such as serum and white or red blood cells. This can be very useful if during the follow-up period new hypotheses arise about the role of variables which have not been measured at baseline. In this way additional baseline information on the study subjects can still be obtained even after the study is complete. There are two special types of cohort studies. For a study on a particular effect of an industrial chemical, a cohort can be selected from groups of industrial workers who have been exposed to the chemical. Such cohorts are referred to as special cohorts. The prevalence of adverse health effects in such a cohort can then be compared with that among workers in the same industry who have not been exposed or with that in the general population. Because a cohort has to be followed for many years after exposure has been measured, a retrospective cohort study is sometimes carried out. This means that a cohort is selected that has been exposed in the past. The investigator then has to establish the appearance of adverse health effects for all individuals of that cohort at the time of the actual study.

FONTANEL

One of several membranous intervals at the angles of the cranial bones in the head of an infant.

FOOD ADDITIVES

See Additives.

FOOD ALLERGY

Immunological reaction to food or a food product. There are many foods which may cause allergic reactions, but in only a few have the allergens been isolated and identified. The most common foods are cow's milk, soy, fish, egg, nuts, peanut, and wheat. The clinical symptoms of allergic food reactions can be characterized as: (1) skin symptoms (itching, erythema, angioedema, urticaria, increase of eczema); (2) respiratory symptoms (itching of eyes, nose, throat; tearing, redness of the eyes; sneezing, nasal obstruction; swelling of the throat; shortness of breath; cough); (3) gastrointestinal symptoms (nausea, vomiting, abdominal cramps, diarrhea); (4) systemic symptoms (hypotension, shock); and (5) controversial symptoms (arthritis, migraine, glue ear, irritable bowel syndrome). Sometimes, the allergic reaction only develops if the food intake is followed by exercise. This is referred to as exercise-induced food allergy.

FOOD AND AGRICULTURAL ORGANIZATION (FAO)

An international organization dedicated to improving the health of third world nations through improvement of agricultural practices.

FOOD AVERSION

A psychogenic reaction to a food (product).

FOOD-BORNE DISEASES

Diseases that develop as a result of consuming contaminated food.

Bacterial infection and poisoning which result from ingestion of bacteria-contaminated food. Food-borne diseases can be divided into food-borne infections or food-borne intoxications, depending on whether the pathogen itself or its toxic product (a microbial toxin or toxic metabolite, produced in the food or in the human body) is the causal agent. The most important bacterial food-borne pathogens causing infections include Salmonella (incubation time: 6–36 hours; duration of disease: 1–7 days), Shigella (incubation time: 6–12 hours; duration of disease: 2–3 days), *Escherichia coli* (incubation time: 12–72 hours; duration of disease: 1–7 days), *Yersinia enterocolitica* (incubation time: 24–36 hours; duration of disease: 3–5 days), *Campylobacter jejuni* (incubation time: 3–5 days; duration of disease: 5–7 days), *Vibrio parahemolyticus* (incubation time: 2–48 hours; duration of disease: 2–5 days), and *Aeromonas hydrophila* (incubation time: 2–48 hours; duration of disease: 2–7 days). Examples of pathogens causing food–borne intoxications are *Staphylococcus aureus* (in food; incubation time: 2–6 hours; duration of disease: 1 day or less), *Clostridium botulinum* (in food; incubation time: 12–96 hours; duration of disease: 1–8 days), *Clostridium perfringens* (in intestine; incubation time: 8–22 hours; duration of disease: 1–2 days), and *Bacillus cereus* (emetic type — in food; incubation time: 1–5 hours; duration of disease: 1 day or less; diarrheal type — in intestine; incubation time: 8–16 hours; duration of disease: > 1 day). Other microbial agents causing food-borne intoxications include toxins produced by fungi (mycotoxins), and by algae, and toxic metabolites such as biogenic amines and ethyl carbamate produced by bacteria in yeasts. In general, five sources of bacteria are recognized in causing food-borne diseases: (1) fecal matter and/or urine of infected humans or animals; (2) nasal and throat discharges of sick individuals or asymptomatic carriers; (3) infections on body surfaces of food handlers (hands and arms); (4) infected soils, mud, surface waters, and dust; and (5) sea water, marine materials, and marine life (see also Botulism; Ciguatera poisoning; Salmonella; Contamination of food with plant toxins, metals, organic chemicals; Ergot alkaloids; Glycoalkaloids; Immuno-active endotoxins; Lesion-causing bacterial toxins; Membrane affecting bacterial toxins; Mycotoxins).

FOOD CONTAMINANTS

Substances that are included unintentionally in foods.

FOOD DIARY

A record kept by an individual of food and beverages consumed, their quantity, and method of preparation.

FOOD EXCHANGE LISTS

Lists of food developed by dietitians which allow patients to exchange one food for another in planning their day's food intake. Lists of fruits, vegetables, meats, etc., have been developed for the control of fat intake, or sodium intake, or total energy, or balancing the intake of carbohydrates, fats, and proteins as is needed to manage a diabetic condition. The American Dietetic Association Food Exchange System is widely used and can be obtained through correspondence with their headquarters (ADA, P.O. Box 97215, Chicago, IL 60678-7215).

FOOD FADS

Instances where certain foods are consumed frequently for reasons other than for providing needed nutrients.

FOOD FAT

See fat content of common foods (Table 20); fatty foods.

FOOD FREQUENCY METHOD

A method for recording and estimating food intake. It is a relatively quick and simple method to obtain dietary information from study subjects in a large-scale study. Food frequency questionnaires ask about the usual intake frequency (and sometimes also the quantities) of a limited number of food products. Only products which contribute substantially to the intake of the nutrients of interest are selected. A disadvantage of this method is that no information on total food consumption is obtained. Since food consumption patterns differ widely from one population to another, a new food frequency list has to be designed and validated for every study.

FOOD GUIDE PYRAMID

Graphic representation of the United States Department of Agriculture's (USDA) Dietary Guidelines that displays complex carbohydrates at the base to emphasize their contribution to the daily diet and fats and sweets at the top.

FOOD INTAKE REGULATION

Control (both external and internal) of the amount and kind of foods consumed.

Most animals other than man eat primarily to satisfy their nutritional needs; man's motivation for eating (or not eating) frequently is to satisfy both non-nutritonal and nutritional needs. His food selection is based on a combination of forces arising from his culture, his family, his educational level, his economic circumstances, and his individual needs and idiosyncrasies.

In addition to the social, cultural, and economic influences on food intake, the selection of foods involves a complex interaction between the special senses: reactions of the eye, ear, nose, mouth, and the sensations of pain and touch are all involved. The appearance, texture, smell, and taste of food, which, in many ways, are inextricably bound to one's cultural heritage, as well as the sensation of hunger, determine whether and when food is consumed. The appearance of food, its color, its consistency, and its temperature are perceived by the sensory system which includes vision, the sense of touch, the sense of temperature, and the sense of smell. Temperature, taste, texture, and smell are perceived via sensory receptor systems located in the nose and mouth.

Neuronal signals for hunger and satiety

Internal cues regulate food intake through a number of signals and responses which ultimately result in the initiation or cessation of feeding. These cues are in addition to those described above which involve the cerebrum. Both short- and long-term controls are exerted which, over time, serve to regulate the food intake of normal individuals so that they neither gain nor lose weight. Food intake control rests, in part, with the integration of a variety of hormonal and nonhormonal signals which are generated both peripherally and centrally. The hypothalamus is thought to be the main integrator of these signals. Other discrete areas are also involved. The paraventricular nucleus located slightly in front of the dorsomedial nucleus is involved in glucose homeostasis and also senses body size. A number of hormones, diet ingredients, metabolites, and drugs have been shown to influence food intake and feeding behavior. Some of the more important ones are shown in Table 21. Hormones that can enhance food intake at one level can suppress it at another level.

Within this framework are a number of afferent and efferent systems which influence food intake by providing information to the brain and relaying instructions via neuronal signals (usually peptides) from the brain to the rest of the body. Food intake can be increased or

TABLE 21
Factors That Affect Food Intake

Enhances		Suppresses
Insulin	Cachectin (Tumor necrosis factor)	Anorectin
Testosterone	Estrogen	Corticotropin-releasing hormone
Glucocorticoids	Phenylethylamines[a]	(CRH)
Thyroxine	Mazindol	Neurotensin
Low serotonin levels	Substance P	Bombesin
Dynorphin	Glucagon	Cyclo-his-pro
β endorphin	"Satietin" (a blood borne factor)	High protein diets
Neuropeptide Y	High fat diet	High blood glucose
Galanin	Serotonin	Enterostatin
	Leptin	
		Calcitonin
Opioid peptides	Fluoxetine	Thyrotropin releasing factor
Growth hormone-releasing	Pain	
hormone	Histidine (precursor of histamine)	
Desacetyl-melanocyte	Amino acid imbalance in diet	
stimulating hormone	Tryptophan (precursor of serotonin)	
Antidepressants[b]	Cholecystokinin (CCK)	
	Somatostatin	
	Thyrotropin releasing hormone	

[a] These are drugs and except for the drug phenylpropanolamine are controlled substances. Many have serious side effects. They are structurally related to the catecholamines. Most are active as short-term appetite suppressants and act through their effects on the central nervous system, particularly through the β adrenergic and/or dopaminergic receptors. This group includes amphetamine, methamphetamine, phenmetrazine, phentermine, diethylpropion, fenfluramine, and phenylpropanolamine. Phenylpropanolamine-induced anorexia is not reversed by the dopamine antagonist haloperidol.

[b] All of these drugs are controlled substances and their use must be carefully monitored. This group includes amitriptyline, buspirone, chlordiazepoxide, chlorpromazine, cisplatin, clozapine, ergotamine, fluphenazine, impramine, iprindole, and others that block 5-HT receptors.

Adapted from Berdanier, C.D., *Advanced Nutrition: Macronutrients*, CRC Press, Boca Raton, FL, 1994, 89.

decreased with reciprocal effects on the central nervous system when these peptides are administered. Galanin, neuropeptide Y, opioid peptides, growth hormone-releasing hormone, and desacetyl-melanocyte stimulating hormone increase food intake, whereas glucagon, cholecystokinen, anorectin, corticotropin-releasing hormone, neurotensin, bombesin, cyclo-his-pro, and thyrotropin-releasing hormone reduce food intake. Several of these hormones or peptides have specific actions with respect to the intake of specific food components. For example, increases in neuropeptide Y result in increased carbohydrate intake while increases in the level of galanin and opioid peptides increase fat intake. Fat intake is suppressed when the blood level of enterostatin rises. Rising blood levels of glucagon suppresses protein intake. All of the above are short-term signals that appear to regulate food selection as well as the amount of food consumed. Although most of these studies have been done in carefully prepared experimental animals (usually rats) there is sufficient indirect evidence to suggest that short-term food intake is similarly regulated in man. In humans, serotoninergic agents are being developed for use as treatments for obesity and eating disorders. These agents either block the binding of serotonin (5-hydroxytryptamine, 5-HT) to its receptor, or upregulate the receptors' binding affinity. 5-HT receptors are widespread throughout the cerebral cortex, the limbic system, the striatum, the brain stem, the choroid plexus, and almost every other region of the central nervous system. Because serotonin suppresses feeding if the receptor is blocked, feeding is enhanced. Thus, drugs that block these receptors are useful in treating anorexia (decreased desire to eat) especially the anorexia that accompanies anxiety, depression, obsessive-compulsive disorders, panic disorders, migraine, and chemotherapy emesis. In contrast, drugs that potentiate the binding of 5-HT to its receptor will result in a suppression of appetite and may be useful in treating the hyperphagia of Prader Willi syndrome and that associated with genetic obesity.

Drugs, particularly those used in cancer chemotherapy, frequently have as a side effect, appetite suppression. In part, this reduction in food intake may be due to disease and/or drug-induced changes in taste and aroma perception and in part, due to the effects of the disease and/or drugs on the central nervous system, particularly the adrenergic and serotonergic receptors. Several of the drugs listed in Table 22 are appetite suppressants and are chemically related to the catecholamines. As indicated, some of these drugs can be addictive and are therefore controlled substances. It appears that none of the drugs listed in Table 22 are free of side effects.

Some steroids affect food intake. Adrenalectomized animals or humans with Addison's disease (glucocorticoid deficient states) do not perceive normal hunger signals. If without food for extended periods of time, these individuals are difficult to realiment. However, once eating commences, a normal feeding pattern will be maintained. In excess, glucocorticoid stimulates feeding and patients with Cushing's disease (excess glucocorticoid production) or patients who are receiving long-term glucocorticoid treatment will report increased hunger and food intake. Patients with Cushing's disease are often characterized by large fat depots across the shoulders and in the abdomen. In addition, obese patients are frequently characterized by excess blood levels of both glucocorticoids and insulin. As noted above, these hormones stimulate the appetite and feeding.

Within the normal range, doses of testosterone and estrogen, although also steroids, have opposite effects with respect to food intake. In experimental animals, day to day variations in food intake by females will follow the same pattern as their day to day variation in estrogen level. When estrogen is high, food intake is suppressed and vice versa. Women who are

TABLE 22
Some Drugs That Affect Nutrient Intakes and Use

Drug	Effect
Phenethylamine and related compounds	Anorexia
Amphetamine	Anorexia
Ethanol	Inhibits intestinal absorption of folate, B_{12} increases need for niacin, riboflavin, thiamin and pyridoxine
Diphenylhydantoin (Dilantin)	Impairs use of folate
Oral contraceptives	Increased folate turnover
Azulfidine	Decreases folate absorption, B_{12} and fat-soluble vitamins
Neomycin	Decreases lipid absorption
P-aminosalicylic acid	Promotes diarrhea and results in decreased absorption of almost all nutrients
Colchicine	Promotes diarrhea and results in decreased absorption of almost all nutrients
Biguanides (Penformin, metformin)	Decreased absorption of B_{12}
Bile salt sequestrants	Decreased fat and fat soluble vitamin absorption

Adapted from Berdanier, C.D., *Advanced Nutrition: Macronutrients*, CRC Press, Boca Raton, FL, 1994, 90.

anestrus due to ovariectomy or who are postmenopausal frequently lose their day to day estrogen-mediated food intake pattern. With this loss is a more even (and somewhat increased) food intake and subsequent body fat gain. This has been found as well in castrated female rats.

The gain in body weight as fat is explained by the loss in food intake control exerted by the estrogens rather than by an estrogen inhibiting effect on lipogenesis. Testosterone increases food intake marginally but it also stimulates protein synthesis and spontaneous physical activity. As a result, body fat does not increase. As testosterone levels decline in males with age, protein synthesis declines and the body tends to sustain its fat synthetic activity. This results in a change in body composition with an increase in body fat stores. The age-related decline in testosterone production may not be accompanied by a decline in food intake.

Although food intake can vary from day to day in response to minor day to day variations in food supply, activity, and hormonal status, body weight is relatively constant. The mechanisms that control body weight are very complex, and the fine details of this regulation are far from clear. However, suffice it to say, major long-term deviations in either food intake or physiological state can affect body weight or energy balance. If food intake (energy intake) is curtailed for days to months, body weight will fall; similarly, if food intake is dramatically increased, body weight will increase.

FOOD INTOLERANCE

General term describing an abnormal physiological response to food or food additives that does not appear to be immunological in nature.

FOOD JAGS

Periods of time when one or more foods are consumed in large amounts or in amounts relatively greater than usual.

FOOD-ORIENTED CHEMICALS

Chemicals with no nutritional value which are primarily associated with food. They include food additives (preservatives such as benzoic acid; antioxidants such as butylated hydroxyanisole, BHA; sweeteners, such as sorbitol; food contaminants such as nitrate, lead, cadmium, polycyclic aromatic hydrocarbons); and natural toxins (aflatoxins).

FOOD POISONING

See food-borne illness.

FOREMILK

The early milk of the lactating mother; also called the colostrum.

FORTIFICATION

The addition of nutrients to food products as they are manufactured.

FREE ENERGY

Energy not trapped or used further; usually dissipated as heat.

FREE RADICALS

Very reactive products of the auto-oxidation of unsaturated fatty acids. Some amino acids also may be radicalized.

FREEZE-DRYING

A processing technique that results in dehydration of the food at temperatures below freezing.

FRUCTOSE

A six carbon sugar having a 5-membered ring and a ketone group instead of an aldehyde group at its terminus.

FRUCTOSE INTOLERANCE

Inability to use dietary fructose; a genetic disease of fructose metabolism. Three hereditary diseases resulting from a mutation in one of three key enzymes of fructose metabolism: fructokinase, aldolase B, and fructose 1,6-bisphosphatase (see Figure 34). A mutation in the gene for fructokinase is characterized by elevated blood and urine levels of fructose. A second mutation has been identified in the gene for aldolase B. This is the enzyme which catalyzes the splitting of fructose 1 phosphate to glyceraldehyde phosphate and dihydroxyacetone phosphate. Aldolase B is located in the liver only. The mutation is such that the enzyme has a reduced affinity for its substrate, fructose 1 phosphate. The results of this reduced affinity include hypoglycemia due to an inhibition of glycogenolysis by fructose 1 phosphate. This hypoglycemia is not responsive to glucagon stimulation. In addition to the disturbance in glycogenolysis, patients with this disorder vomit after a fructose load, have elevated levels of urine and blood fructose, grow poorly with evidence of jaundice, hyperbilirubinemia (high levels of bilirubin in the blood), albuminuria (albumin in the urine), and amino aciduria (amino acids in the urine), and some patients may have damaged renal proximal convoluted tubules.

The third mutation involves only the liver enzyme fructose 1,6-bisphosphatase. The muscle enzyme is normal in activity. This enzyme is a key enzyme in the hepatic gluconeogenic pathway so, as one might expect, hypoglycemia is one of the characteristics of a mutation in this enzyme. Other characteristics include an enlarged liver, poor muscle tone, and increased blood lactate levels. All of these mutations are uncommon and all are autosomal recessive traits. Heterozygotes are not detectable.

FRUCTOSE METABOLISM

Fructose is converted to glucose after phosphorylation as shown in Figure 34. Although two enzymes are available for the phosphorylation of fructose one of these, the fructokinase, is present only in the liver. Hexokinase can catalyze the phosphorylation of fructose. However, fructokinase is a much more active enzyme. Its activity is so high that, in fact, most of the dietary fructose whether as the free sugar **or** as a component of sucrose is metabolized in the liver. This is in contrast to glucose which is metabolized by all the cells in the body. As a result, fructose- or sucrose-rich diets fed to rats or mice will result in a fatty liver. This occurs because the dietary overload of fructose or sucrose exceeds the capacity of the liver to oxidize it so it uses the sugar metabolites as substrate for fatty acid and triacylglyceride synthesis. Until the hepatic lipid export system increases sufficiently to transport this lipid to the storage depots, the lipid accumulates, hence, the fatty liver. Adaptation to a high fructose intake can and does occur in normal individuals.

FULL LIQUID DIET

Diet containing foods and beverages that are liquid at room temperature.

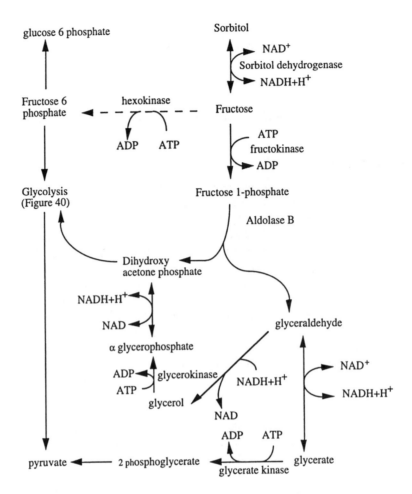

FIGURE 34 Metabolism of fructose.

G

GABA

Gamma amino butyric acid. A neurotransmitter formed through the decarboxylation of glutamic acid.

GALACTOSE

A monosaccharide which, with glucose, forms the dissaccharide, lactose, or milk sugar. Galactose is converted to glucose and eventually enters the glycolytic sequence as glucose 6-phosphate. The entire pathway is shown in Figure 35. Galactose is phosphorylated at carbon 1 in the first step of its conversion to glucose. It can be isomerized to glucose 1-phosphate or converted to UDP-galactose by exchanging its phosphate group for a UDP group. This UDP-galactose can be joined with glucose to form lactose in the adult mammary tissue under the influence of the hormone prolactin. However, usually the UDP-galactose is converted to UDP-glucose and thence used to form glycogen.

GALACTOSEMIA

An inability to use galactose; a genetic disease of galactose metabolism. Abnormally high blood levels of galactose. Three autosomal recessive mutations in the genes for enzymes involved in galactose conversion to glucose have been described. Galactosemia results in each instance. Two of these mutations involve the gene for galactose 1-phosphate uridyl transferase. Two variants have been described. One is fairly innocuous in that the mutation occurs only in the enzymes found in the red cell. This variant is called the Duarte variant, and affected individuals have 50% less red cell galactose 1-phosphate uridyl transferase activity than normal individuals. These people have no other discernible characteristics. The second variant is far more severe in its effects on the patient. The enzyme in the liver is abnormal and does not function to convert galactose 1-phosphate to UDP galactose. As a result, galactose 1-phosphate accumulates and some is converted to the sugar alcohol galactitol via NADH aldose reductase action. Cataracts in the eye form in this disease accompanied by mental retardation and increased tissue levels of galactose 1-phosphate, galactitol, and galactonic acid. These last metabolites are excreted in the urine. Also characteristic of this mutation in galactose 1-phosphate uridyl transferase are decreased blood glucose levels, decreased glycogenesis, decreased mutase activity, and decreased pyrophosphorylase activity. Since UDP-galactose is necessary for the formation of the galactoyl lipids, chondroitin sulfate formation is decreased. A mutation in the gene for galactokinase also results in accumulations of galactose and galactitol and cataracts. The galactitol accumulation was found to be the causative agent in the formation of cataracts. Except for cataract formation due to galactitol accumulation, no other symptoms have been described for this form of galactosemia.

GALL STONES

Gall stones develop when the bile salts and cholesterol accumulate in the gall bladder. With time, the cholesterol precipitates out providing a crystalline structure for the stone. Since the bile also contains a variety of minerals, these minerals form salts with the bile acids and are deposited within and around the cholesterol matrix. Eventually these stones irritate the lining of the gall bladder or may lodge themselves in the duct connecting the bladder to the

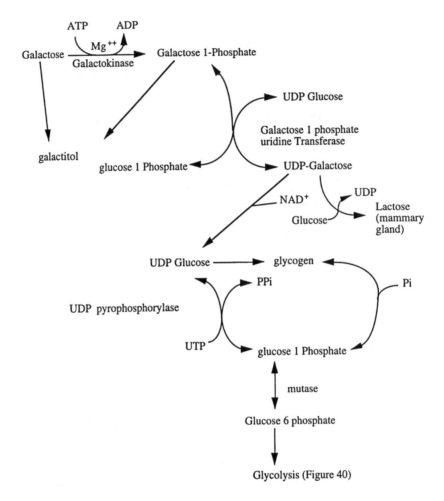

FIGURE 35 Conversion of galactose to glucose.

duodenum. When this happens, the bladder becomes inflamed, the duct may be blocked, and the patient becomes unable to tolerate food. In some cases, treatment consists of reducing the irritation and inflammation through drugs, but often the patient has the gall bladder and its offending stones removed.

GAMMA AMINO BUTYRATE (GABA)

A metabolite produced when glutamic acid is decarboxylated. It is an inhibitory neurotransmitter which quiets excited neurons. Low levels of GABA are associated with convulsions.

GANGLIOSIDE

A cerebroside containing glucose and/or galactose and neurominic acid (an amino uronic acid).

GASTRIC ACID

Hydrochloric acid.

GASTRIN

A small peptide hormone produced by gastric cells. Gastrin stimulates the parietal cells to release hydrochloric acid.

GASTRITIS

Inflammation of the stomach.

GASTROENTERITIS

Inflammation of the stomach and intestines.

GASTROESOPHAGEAL REFLUX

Condition characterized by the return of gastric contents up the esophagus resulting in a "burning sensation" under the sternum.

GASTROINTESTINAL TRACT

Flexible muscular tube from the mouth, through the esophagus, stomach, small intestine, large intestine, and rectum to the anus.

GASTROINTESTINAL TRANSIT TIME

The time which elapses between food entry and fecal excretion of the residual nondigested food components.

GASTROJEJUNOSTOMY

Known as the Billroth II procedure in which an opening between the stomach and jejunum is surgically created.

GASTROPARESIS

Condition in which the stomach is slower than normal in emptying.

GASTROPLASTY

Reduction of the stomach size via surgery.

GAUCHER'S DISEASE

A genetic disease due to a mutation in the gene for the synthesis of the enzyme glucocerebrosidase. This enzyme catalyzes the cleavage of the sphingolipid, glucocerebroside. Characterized by accumulation of cerebrosides in the brain and other tissues.

GDP

Guanosine diphosphate. A dephosphorylated form of GTP important in the activation of substances participating in the biosynthesis of proteins.

GENE

Carrier of specific genetic code for a specific characteristic of the organism.

GENERALLY RECOGNIZED AS SAFE (GRAS)

See additives.

GENETIC CODE

The sequence of purine and pyrimidine bases which are in a specific order and which dictate the amino acid sequence of all proteins synthesized by cells.

GENETIC DISEASES

Diseases due to mutations in the gene codes for specific proteins.

GENOTOXIC CARCINOGENS

Chemicals that attack DNA causing mutated cells to develop and reproduce in an uncontrolled manner.

GENOTYPE

The inherited character of the individual.

GEOPHAGIA

The eating of dirt; an abnormal appetite.

GERIATRICS

A medical subspecialty relating to the care and treatment of elderly people.

GERM

Pathogenic microorganism.

GERMPLASM

The heart of a plant seed from which a new plant grows.

GERONTOLOGY

The study of senescence (old age).

GESTATION

The period of growth initiated at conception and terminated by partuition.

GESTATIONAL DIABETES

Carbohydrate intolerance, in variable severity, with onset first recognized during pregnancy. Detected during screening between 24 and 28 weeks gestation with a 50 g oral glucose test. If results at 1 hour post-prandial are ≥140 mg/dl, the oral glucose tolerance test is used to confirm diagnosis.

GI TRACT

Gastrointestinal tract.

GIP

Gastric inhibitory peptide. A peptide hormone inhibiting gastric motility and acid secretion.

GLOBULIN

A protein in blood that is globular in shape. Gamma globulin is a protein which carries antibodies to a variety of antigens especially those related to communicable diseases.

Hemoglobin is a globular protein in red blood cells which contains heme iron which in turn carries oxygen.

GLOMERULAR FILTRATION RATE

Test used as an indicator of renal function that reflects the ability of the kidney to filter and reabsorb fluids.

GLOMERULONEPHRITIS

Occurs when the nephrons of the kidney become inflamed. Glomerulonephritis occurs most often one to two weeks after a streptococcal throat or skin infection and generally affects children.

GLOSSITIS

A shiny red appearance of the tongue.

GLUCAGON

A polypeptide synthesized and released by α cells of the Islets of Langerhans in the pancreas. Serves as an anti-insulin with respect to glucose homeostasis. Glucagon stimulates gluco-neogenesis and glycogenolysis.

GLUCOGENIC AMINO ACIDS

Amino acids whose carbon skeletons can be used for glucose synthesis. These are listed in Table 23.

TABLE 23
Amino Acids that Contribute a Carbon
Chain for the Synthesis of Glucose

Amino Acid	Enters As:
Alanine	Pyruvate
Tryptophane → Alanine	Pyruvate
Hydroxyproline	Pyruvate
Serine	Pyruvate
Cysteine	Pyruvate
Threonine	Pyruvate
Glycine	Pyruvate
Tyrosine	Fumarate
Isoleucine	Succinyl CoA
Methionine	Succinyl CoA
Valine	Succinyl CoA
Histidine → Glutamate	α ketoglutarate
Proline → Glutamate	α ketoglutarate
Glutamine → Glutamate	α ketoglutarate
Arginine → Glutamate	α ketoglutarate

GLUCONEOGENESIS

The synthesis of glucose from noncarbohydrate precursors.

Gluconeogenesis occurs primarily in the liver and kidney. Except under conditions of prolonged starvation, the kidneys do not contribute appreciable amounts of glucose to the circulation. Most tissues lack the full complement of enzymes needed to run this pathway. In particular, the rate-limiting enzyme phosphoenolpyruvate carboxykinase is not found to be active in tissues other than liver and kidney. The enzymes that are unique to gluconeogenesis are shown in Figure 36. The other reactions shown use the same enzymes as glycolysis and do not have control properties with respect to gluconeogenesis. The rate-limiting enzymes are glucose 6-phosphatase, fructose 1,6 biphosphatase, and phosphoenolpyruvate carboxykinase (PEPCK). Pyruvate kinase and pyruvate carboxylase are also of interest because their control is a coordinated one with respect to the regulation of PEPCK.

Oxalacetate is essential to gluconeogenesis because it is the substrate for PEPCK which catalyzes its conversion to phosphoenolpyruvate (PEP). This is an energy-dependent conversion which overcomes the irreversible final glycolytic reaction catalyzed by pyruvate kinase. The activity of PEPCK is closely coupled with that of pyruvate carboxylase. Whereas the pyruvate kinase reaction produces one ATP, the formation of PEP uses two ATPs — one in the mitochondria for the pyruvate carboxylase reaction and one in the cytosol for the PEPCK reaction. PEPCK requires GTP provided via the nucleoside diphosphate kinase reaction which uses ATP. ATP transfers one high-energy bond to GDP to form ADP and GTP.

In starvation or uncontrolled diabetes, PEPCK activity is elevated as is gluconeogenesis. Starvation elicits a number of catabolic hormones that serve to mobilize tissue energy stores as well as precursors for glucose synthesis. Uncontrolled diabetes elicits similar hormonal responses. In both instances, the synthesis of the PEPCK enzyme protein is increased. Unlike other rate limiting enzymes, PEPCK is not regulated allosterically or by phosphorylation-dephosphorylation mechanisms. Instead, it is regulated by changes in gene transcription of its single copy gene from a single promoter site. This regulation is unique because all of the known factors (hormones, vitamins, metabolites) act in the same place. They either turn on the synthesis of the messenger RNA for PEPCK, or they turn it off. What is also unique is the fact that liver and kidney cells translate this message into sufficient active enzyme protein which catalyzes PEP formation. Other cells and tissues have the code for PEPCK in their nuclear DNA but do not usually synthesize the enzyme. Instead, these cell types synthesize the enzyme which catalyzes glycerol synthesis. In effect then, only the kidney and liver have active gluconeogenic processes.

The next few steps in gluconeogenesis are identical to those of glycolysis but are in the reverse direction. When the step for the dephosphorylation of fructose 1,6 bisphosphate occurs, there is another energy barrier and instead of a bidirectional reaction catalyzed by a single enzyme, there are separate forward and reverse reactions. In the synthesis of glucose, this reaction is catalyzed by fructose 1,6-bisphosphatase and yields fructose 6-phosphate. No ATP is involved, but a molecule of water and an inorganic phosphate are produced. Rising levels of fructose 2,6-bisphosphatase allosterically inhibits gluconeogenesis while it stimulates glycolysis. AMP likewise inhibits gluconeogenesis at this step.

Lastly, the removal of the phosphate from glucose 6-phosphate via the enzyme complex glucose 6-phosphatase completes the pathway to yield free glucose. This is an irreversible reaction which does not involve ATP. The glucose 6-phosphate moves to the endoplasmic reticulum where the phosphatase is located and glucose is released for use.

GLUCOSE

A six carbon monosaccharide. The preferred metabolic fuel for most cell types particularly those of the central nervous system (CNS).

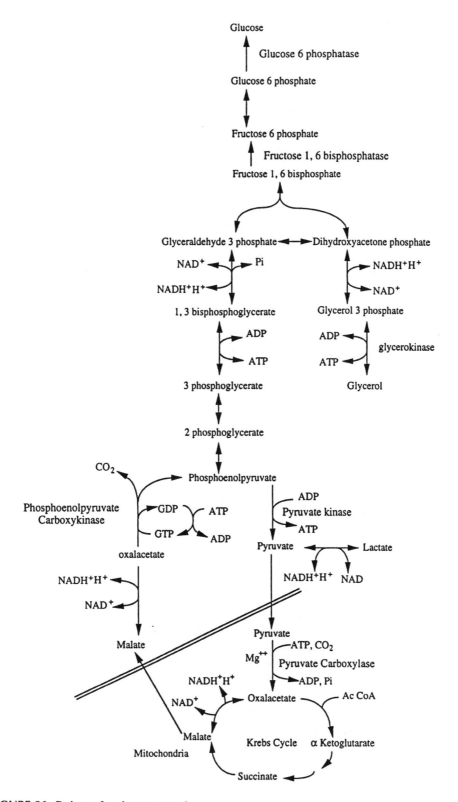

FIGURE 36 Pathway for gluconeogenesis.

GLUCOSE TOLERANCE TEST

Test performed on an individual that has fasted at least 12 hours and then provided 75–100 grams of glucose. Blood glucose levels are monitored at hourly intervals and compared to established norms to confirm the diagnosis of diabetes mellitus.

GLUCOSE TRANSPORTERS (GLUT 1, 2, 3, 4, 5)

A group of special proteins that transport glucose into the cell. There are five glucose transporters called GLUT 1, 2, 3, 4, and 5. Some cell types have only one of these while others have more than one. The transporters differ slightly in their structure and function with respect to the function of the tissues which contain them. Table 24 lists the transporters and their location. The glucose transporter is referred to as a mobile transporter because when it is not in use, it is sequestered in an intracellular pool. When needed, it leaves its storage site, moves to the interior aspect of the plasma membrane, forms a loose bond with the membrane, picks up the glucose molecule, and moves it through the membrane into the cytosol whereupon the glucose can be phosphorylated and metabolized.

Aberrations in the mobile glucose transporters affect glucose use. The consequences of such mutations are listed in Table 25.

TABLE 24
Location of the Mobile Glucose Transporters

Transporter	Location
GLUT 1	Ubiquitous but found mainly in brain, placenta, and cultured cells; is not particularly responsive to insulin regulation
GLUT 2	Liver, β cells of pancreas, kidney
GLUT 3	Ubiquitous in human tissue
GLUT 4	Adipose tissue, heart, skeletal muscle
GLUT 5	Small intestine

TABLE 25
Consequences of Aberrations in the Mobile Glucose Transporters

Protein	Consequences of an Error
GLUT 1	Minimal changes in glucose uptake by all tissues that use glucose
GLUT 2	Liver. Glucose metabolic pathways suppressed; increased gluconeogenic activity β cell. Pancreas unresponsive to glucose stimulation Kidney. Increased gluconeogenic activity
GLUT 3	Minimal changes in glucose uptake and metabolism
GLUT 4	Adipose tissue. Decreased glucose use by fat cell; compensatory increased in hepatic glucose use; increased hepatic lipogenesis and lipid output; increase hepatic glycogen store Heart, muscle. Decreased glucose use by muscle could be lethal if compensatory use of fatty acids and ketones is insufficient.
GLUT 5	Small intestine. Glucose uptake by intestinal cells is impaired. If diet is high in carbohydrates, osmotic diarrhea might result.

From Berdanier, C.D., *Advanced Nutrition: Macronutrients*, CRC Press, Boca Raton, FL, 1994, 206.

GLUCOSINOLATES

See type B antinutritives.

GLUCOSURIA

Glucose in the urine.

GLUTAMIC ACID

A five carbon amino acid with two carboxyl groups (see Table 5). Glutamate is the precursor of the neurotransmitter gamma amino butyric acid (GABA).

GLUTAMINE

The amine of glutamic acid; the two carboxyl groups of glutamic acid are replaced by two amino groups. Plays a key role in transporting amino groups to the urea cycle.

GLUTATHIONE

A tripeptide with a free sulfhydryl group that, in a reduced state, helps maintain iron in its appropriate oxidized state (ferrous) in hemoglobin.

GLUTEN-SENSITIVE ENTEROPATHY

Characterized by the gastrointestinal intolerance to the protein in wheat, rye, oats, and barley. Also known as nontropical sprue, celiac disease, and idiopathic steatorrhea.

GLYCEMIC INDEX

An index for the glucose contribution of a food to the blood glucose level.

GLYCEROL

A three carbon monosaccharide which, when phosphorylated, provides the backbone for the synthesis of triglycerides.

GLYCEROPHOSPHATE SHUTTLE

A shuttle for the transfer of reducing equivalents into the mitochondria from the cytosol. Shown in Figure 37. Is a rate limiting step for glycolysis.

GLYCINE

A two carbon nonessential amino acid (see Table 5).

GLYCOALKALOIDS

Minor components of potatoes and tomatoes that if consumed in large quantities are toxic. Steroidal alkaloids are mainly present as glycosides in the family of the Solanaceae, including the potato and the tomato. The major glycoalkaloids in potatoes are α-solanine and α-chaconine, both glycosides of solanidine. Solanine and chaconine are potent irritants of the intestinal mucosa and cholinesterase inhibitors, the first being the most active. Poisoning with either substance can result in gastrointestinal symptoms of vomiting and diarrhea, and neurological symptoms such as irritability, confusion, delirium, and respiratory failure, which may ultimately result in death. Furthermore, poisoning is often accompanied by high fever. In general, the glycoalkaloid contents of potato tubers do not pose harmful effects in humans. Serious poisonings have been reported following the consumption of large amounts of potatoes with high glycoalkaloid contents (≥200 mg per kg). Potatoes that have been exposed to

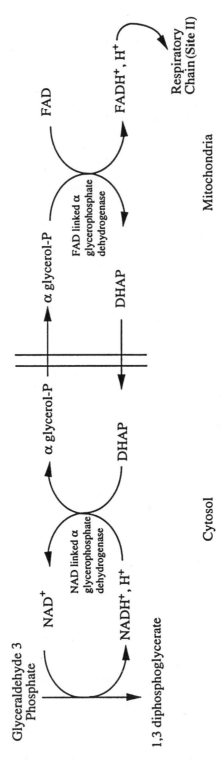

142

FIGURE 37 Glycerophosphate shuttle.

light and those that are diseased by fungal infection or mechanically bruised may contain toxic levels of glycoalkaloids. The major glycoalkaloid in tomatoes is α-tomatidine, with tomatidenol as the aglycon. It is present in all parts of the plant. In the fruit the concentration decreases during ripening. Poisonings in humans due to the consumption of tomatoes have not been reported.

GLYCOCHOLATE

Bile salt required for fat digestion and absorption.

GLYCOGEN

Glucose polymer formed in mammalian liver and muscle. A storage form of glucose.

Glycogen, when stimulated to release its glucose by the catabolic hormones, glucagon, epinephrine, the glucocorticoids, and thyroxine, and/or by the absence of food in the digestive tract, provides glucose to the body. Because the glycogen molecule has molecules of water as part of its structure, it is a very large molecule and cumbersome to store in large amounts. The average 70 kg man has only an 18 hour fuel supply stored as glycogen while that same individual might have up to a 2 month supply of fuel stored as fat. Muscle and liver glycogen stores have very different functions. Muscle glycogen is used to synthesize ATP for muscle contraction whereas hepatic glycogen is the glucose reserve for the entire body particularly the central nervous system. The amount of glycogen in the muscle is dependent upon the physical activity of the individual. After bouts of strenuous exercise, the glycogen store will be depleted only to be rebuilt during the resting period following exercise. Hepatic glycogen stores are dependent on nutritional status. They are virtually absent in the 24-hour starved animal while being replenished within hours of ad libitum feeding. Clusters of glycogen molecules with an average molecular weight of 2×10^7 form quickly when an abundance of glucose is provided to the liver. The amount of glycogen in the liver is diet dependent. There is a 24-hour rhythmic change in hepatic glycogen that corresponds to the feeding pattern of the animal. In nocturnal animals such as the rat, the peak hepatic glycogen store will be found in the early morning hours while the nadir will be found in the evening hours just before the nocturnal feeding begins. In humans accustomed to eating during the day, the reverse pattern will be observed.

GLYCOGEN STORAGE DISEASES

Genetic diseases which are characterized by excess glycogen stores. One very rare autosomal recessive disease is due to a mutation in the gene for the branching enzyme. This results in an accumulation of straight chain glycogen which, because it is less compact than the normally branched chain glycogen, results in an enlarged liver. This disorder is called amylopectinosis and is usually grouped with the other disorders characterized by enlarged glycogen stores. However, this disorder affects synthesis rather than degradation (which is normal) and there is not an excess in glycogen. People with this disorder do not have a problem with the synthesis of α glycogen in the muscle, only with the branching of the straight chain. They have poor muscle tone and are exercise intolerant. Poor weight gain and early death are also characteristic of the disorder.

Five mutations in the genes which code for the enzymes of glycogenolysis have been described. These include a mutation in the lysomal α 1,4 glucosidase (also called acid maltase) which results in a generalized excess of glycogen not only in the liver and muscle but also in the viscera and central nervous system. This disorder is called Pompe's Disease and is characterized by an enlarged liver and heart and extreme muscular weakness.

A mutation in the gene for the debranching enzyme (amylo-1,6-glucosidase) results in the accumulation of highly branched short chain glycogen in the muscles and liver. The usual glycogen has a branch point at every fourth glucosyl residue in the interior of the molecule and further apart on the outer regions. The glycogen stored in people lacking the debranching enzyme have their branch points very close together. This occurs when glucose is mobilized from glycogen and only the outer limbs of the molecule are used. Without a functioning debranching enzyme, the remaining inner core is untouched. These cores accumulate and are responsible for the enlarged liver and heart. Because the glycogen gives up only a small amount of its glucose, the muscle which needs it for ATP synthesis is very weak. This condition is called Forbes disease.

McArdle's disease affects only the muscle, and the enzyme lacking is the muscle phosphorylase. Patients with this disorder are intolerant to exercise and accumulate glycogen in the muscle but not the liver. This disorder was discovered in military recruits during World War II when in a few isolated instances, young men were found who could not endure the rigorous physical training of boot camp. Unfortunately, the first few were thought to be malingerers and were forced to exercise to death by their drill instructors. When their deaths were investigated, the reason for their exercise intolerance was understood. The mutation in the muscle phosphorylase gene might not have been discovered otherwise.

In the liver, a mutation in phosphorylase is far more serious. This disorder, known as Her's Disease, results in growth retardation, an enlarged liver due to glycogen accumulation, and elevated serum lipids. In both McArdle's Disease and Her's Disease, glycogen is not phosphorylated because of a mutation in the enzyme which catalyzes the initial step in glycogenolysis. This is also the case for another glycogen storage disease but instead of a mutation in the gene for phosphorylase, the mutation is in the gene for the phosphorylase kinase, the enzyme that is responsible for the activation of glycogen phosphorylase b to glycogen phosphorylase a. Without the addition of energy through the hydrolysis of ATP, the glycogen phosphorylase cannot transfer this phosphate to the glycogen molecule and produce a molecule of glucose 1-phosphate. People with this disorder have the same symptoms as those with Her's Disease and, in addition, have increased rates of gluconeogenesis and hypoglycemia when without food for long periods of time. They also have decreased phosphorylase activity in hepatocytes and leukocytes.

All of these disorders in glycogen synthesis and degradation are rare and all appear as autosomal recessive traits. Their long-term outlook is not very good. Nutritional manipulations include a continual nasogastric drip of a starch suspension which is directed toward reducing hypoglycemia episodes. Because the hypoglycemia is due to an inability to normally mobilize the glycogen-glucose, care must be given to avoid prolonged periods without food. The glucose that is needed by all the body's cells must be provided either by the diet or through an active gluconeogenic process.

GLYCOGEN SYNTHESIS

Shown in Figure 38. Glycogen synthesis begins with glucose 1-phosphate formation from glucose 6-phosphate through the action of phosphoglucomutase. Glucose 1-phosphate then is converted to uridine diphosphate glucose (UDP-glucose) which can then be added to the glycogen already in storage (the glycogen primer). UDP-glucose can be added through α 1,6 linkage or α 1,4 linkage. Two high energy bonds are used to incorporate each molecule of glucose into the glycogen. The straight chain glucose polymer is comprised of glucoses joined through the 1,4 linkage and is less compact than the branched chain glycogen which has both 1,4 and 1,6 linkages. The addition of glucose to the primer glycogen with α 1,4 linkage is catalyzed by the glycogen synthase enzyme while the 1,6 addition is catalyzed by the so-called glycogen branching enzyme, Amylo $(1 \rightarrow 4, 1 \rightarrow 6)$ transglucosidase. Once the liver and muscle cell achieve their full storage capacity, these enzymes are product inhibited and glycogenesis is "turned off." Glycogen synthase is inactivated by a cAMP-dependent kinase and activated by a synthase phosphatase enzyme that is stimulated by changes in the ratio of ATP to ADP. Glycogen synthesis is stimulated by the hormone insulin and suppressed by the catabolic hormones. The process does not fully cease but operates at a very low level. Glycogen does not accumulate appreciably in cells other than liver and muscle although all cells contain a small amount of glycogen. Note in Figure 38 that a glycogen primer is required for glycogen synthesis to proceed. This primer is carefully guarded so that some is **always** available when glycogen is synthesized. This means that glycogenolysis **never** fully depletes the cell of its glycogen content.

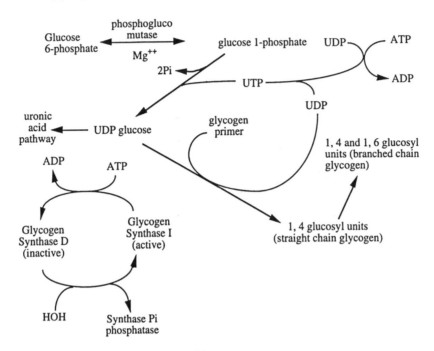

FIGURE 38 Glycogen synthesis (glycogenesis).

GLYCOGENOLYSIS

The process of releasing glucose from glycogen shown in Figure 39. Glycogenolysis is a carefully controlled series of reactions referred to as the glycogen cascade. It is called a cascade because of the stepwise changes in activation states of the enzymes involved. To release glucose for oxidation by the glycogenolytic pathway, the glycogen must be phosphorylated. This is accomplished by the enzyme glycogen phosphorylase. Glycogen phosphorylase exists in the cell in an inactive form (glycogen phosphorylase b) and is activated to its active form (glycogen phosphorylase a) by the enzyme phosphorylase b kinase. In turn, this kinase also exists in an inactive form which is activated by the calcium-dependent enzyme, protein kinase, and active cAMP-dependent protein kinase. These activations each require a molecule of ATP. Lastly, the cAMP-dependent protein kinase must have cAMP for its activation. This cAMP is generated from ATP by the enzyme adenylate cyclase which, in itself, is inactive unless stimulated by a hormone such as epinephrine, thyroxine, or glucagon. As can be seen, this cascade of activation is energy dependent with three molecules of ATP needed to get the process started. Once started, the glycolytic pathway will replenish the ATP needed initially as well as provide a further supply of ATP to provide needed energy. As mentioned, the liver and muscle differ in the use of glycogen. This also affects how ATP is generated within the glycogen containing cell and how much is generated by cells that do not store glycogen.

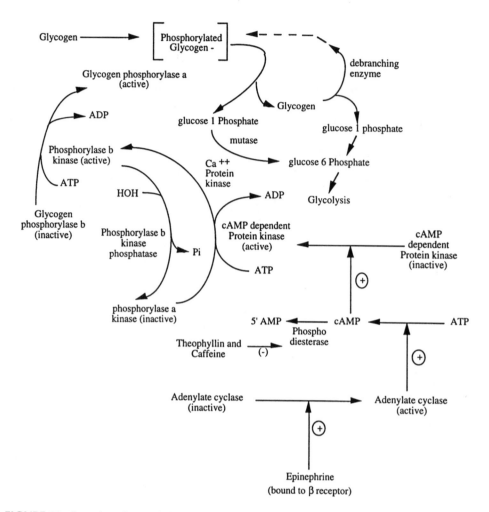

FIGURE 39 Stepwise release of glucose molecules from the glycogen molecule (glycogenolysis).

GLYCOLIPID

A complex lipid containing a carbohydrate moiety.

GLYCOLYSIS

The oxidation of glucose is shown in Figure 40. The glycolytic pathway for the anaerobic catabolism of glucose can be found in all cells in the body. The pathway begins with glucose, a 6 carbon unit, and through a series of reactions produces 2 molecules of ATP and 2 molecules of pyruvate. The control of glycolysis is vested in several key steps. The first step is the activation of glucose through the formation of glucose 6-phosphate. In the liver and pancreatic β cell this step is catalyzed by the enzyme glucokinase. A molecule of ATP is used and magnesium is required. Glucose 6-phosphate is a key metabolite. It can proceed down the glycolytic pathway or move through the hexose monophosphate shunt (see hexose mono-phosphate shunt), or be used to make glycogen. How much glucose 6-phosphate is oxidized directly to pyruvate depends on the nutritional state of the animal, the type of cells, the genetics of the animal, and its hormonal state. Some cell types, the brain cell for example, do not make glycogen. Some people do not have shunt activity in the red cell because the code for glucose-6-phosphate dehydrogenase has mutated such that the enzyme is not func-tional. Insulin deficient animals likewise have little shunt activity due to the lack of insulin's effect on the synthesis of its enzymes. All these factors determine how much glucose-6-phosphate goes in which direction.

Two enzymes are used for the activation of glucose: glucokinase and hexokinase. In the liver both enzymes are present. While hexokinase activity is product inhibited, glucokinase is not. The hexokinase in the nonhepatic tissues must be product inhibited to prevent the hexokinase from tying up all the Pi in the cells as glucose-6-phosphate. The Km for glucokinase is greater than that for hexokinase so the former is the main enzyme for the conversion of glucose to glucose-6-phosphate in the liver. The other enzyme will phosphorylate not only glucose but six other carbon sugars such as fructose. However, the amount of fructose phosphorylated to fructose-6-phosphate is small in comparison to the phosphorylation of fructose at the carbon 1 position catalyzed by fructokinase. The metabolism of fructose is shown in Figure 34.

Glucose-6-phosphate is isomerized to fructose-6-phosphate and then is phosphorylated once again to form fructose-1,6-bisphosphate. Another molecule of ATP is used, and again magnesium is an important cofactor. Both kinase reactions are rate-controlling reactions in that their activity determines the rate at which subsequent reactions proceed. The phosphofructokinase reaction is unique to the glycolytic sequence while the glucokinase or hexokinase step is not. Thus, one could argue that the formation of fructose-1,6-bisphosphate is the first **committed** step in glycolysis. Glycolysis is inhibited when phosphofructokinase is inhibited. This occurs when levels of fatty acids in the cytosol rise as in the instance of high rates of lipolysis and fatty acid oxidation. Phosphofructokinase activity is increased when levels of fructose-6-phosphate rise or when cAMP levels rise. Stimulation occurs also when fructose-2,6-bisphosphate levels rise. In any event, glycolysis then proceeds with the splitting of fructose-1,6-bisphosphate to dihydroxyacetone phosphate (DHAP) and glyceraldehyde-3-phosphate. At this point another rate-controlling step occurs. This step is one which shuttles reducing equivalents into the mitochondria for use by the respiratory chain. This is the α-glycerophosphate shuttle (see Figure 37). This shuttle carries reducing equivalents from the cytosol to the mitochondria. DHAP picks up reducing equivalents when it is converted to α-glycerol phosphate. These reducing equivalents are produced when glyceraldehyde-3-phosphate is oxidized in the process of being phosphorylated to 1,3-diphosphate glycerate. The α-glycerophosphate enters the inner mitochondrial membrane whereupon it is converted back to DHAP, releasing its reducing equivalents to FAD that in turn transfers the reducing equivalents to the mitochondrial respiratory chain. The reason why this shuttle is rate limiting is due to the need to regenerate NAD^+. Without NAD^+ the glycolytic pathway ceases. $NADH^+$ is produced during glycolysis when reducing equivalents are accepted by NAD^+. $NADH^+$ itself cannot pass through the mitochondrial membrane so substrate shuttles are necessary. Another means of producing NAD^+ is by converting pyruvate to lactate. This is a nonmitochondrial reaction catalyzed by lactate dehydrogenase. It occurs when an oxygen debt is developed as happens in exercising muscle. In these muscles more oxygen is consumed than can be provided. Glycolysis is occurring at a rate faster than can be accommodated by the respiratory chain that joins the reducing equivalents transferred to it by the shuttles to molecular oxygen making water. If more reducing equivalents are generated than can be used to make water, the excess are added to pyruvate to make lactate. Thus, rising lactate levels are indicative of oxygen debt.

There are other shuttles which also serve to transfer reducing equivalents into the mitosol. These are the malate-aspartate shuttle and the malate-citrate shuttle. Neither of these are rate limiting with respect to glycolysis. The malate-aspartate shuttle has rate controlling properties with respect to gluconeogenesis while the malate-citrate shuttle is important to lipogenesis.

Once 1,3-bisphosphate glycerate is formed it is converted to 3-phosphoglycerate with the formation of one ATP. The 3-phosphoglycerate then goes to 2-phosphoglycerate and then to phosphoenolpyruvate. These are all bidirectional reactions that are also used in gluconeogenesis.

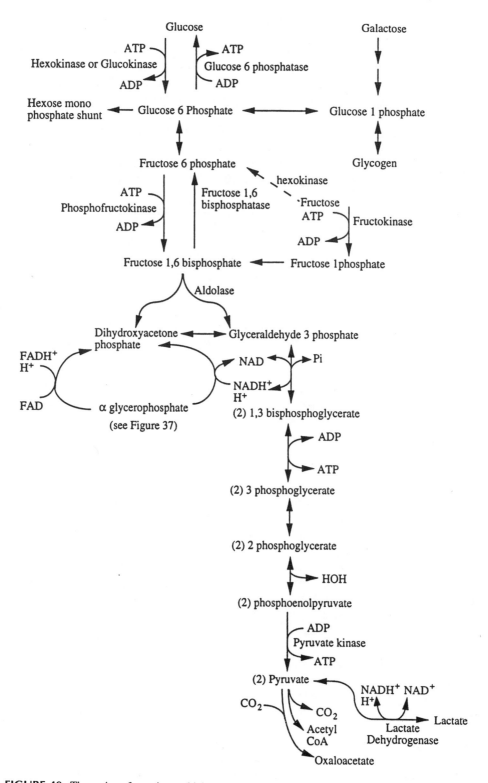

FIGURE 40 The series of reactions which comprise glycolysis.

The phosphoenolpyruvate is dephosphorylated to pyruvate with the formation of another ATP. Because of the great energy loss to ATP formation at this step, this reaction is not reversible. Gluconeogenesis uses another enzyme, phosphoenolpyruvate carboxykinase to reverse this step. Glycolysis uses pyruvate kinase to catalyze the reaction. At any rate, pyruvate can now be converted to acetyl CoA via pyruvate dehydrogenase or carboxylated to oxalacetate via pyruvate carboxylase.

The glycolytic pathway is dependent upon both ATP for the initial steps of the pathway, the formation of glucose-6-phosphate and fructose-1,6-bisphosphate, and on the ratio of ATP to ADP and inorganic phosphate, Pi. In working muscle the continuance of work and the continuance of glycolysis depends on the cycling of the adenine nucleotides and the export of lactate to the liver. ATP must be provided at the beginning of the pathway, and ADP as well as Pi must be provided in the latter steps. If the tissue runs out of ATP, ADP, or Pi, or accumulates lactate and H^+, glycolysis will come to a halt and work cannot continue. This is what happens to the working skeletal muscle. Exhaustion sets in when glycolytic rate is down regulated by an accumulation of lactate.

GLYCOPROTEIN

A complex protein containing a carbohydrate moiety. Glycoproteins play a role in antigen recognition.

GMP

Guanosine monophosphate. A nucleotide containing guanine (a purine), ribose, and a high energy phosphate group.

GOITER

Enlargement of the thyroid gland usually due to an inadequate intake of iodine (see minerals, Table 28).

GOITROGEN

A compound which interferes with the normal production of thyroxine by the thyroid gland.

GOSSYPOL

A toxic yellow pigment found in cotton seeds.

GOUT

Condition in which excess uric acid in the blood is deposited in tissues and joints.

GRAVES DISEASE

Disease characterized by hyperplasia of the thyroid gland, excessive secretion of its hormones, and increased metabolic rate.

GRAVIDA

A pregnant woman.

GROWTH

A well-orchestrated series of processes which result in an increase in size of individual tissues, organs, and whole animals.

GRP

Gastrin releasing peptide. A neuroactive peptide originating in nerves of the gut and stimulating the release of gastrin from gastric cells.

GSH

Glutathione, reduced.

GSSG

Glutathionine, oxidized. A tripeptide containing glutamic acid, cysteine, and glycine. Its sulfhydryl group can undergo reversible oxidation and reduction allowing the peptide to serve as a buffer. Its chief function is to serve as a reductant of toxic peroxides.

GTP

Guanosine triphosphate. A high-energy, phosphate-containing compound needed for protein synthesis.

GUANINE

A purine base.

GUANOSINE

A nucleoside containing guanine and ribose.

GUT-ASSOCIATED LYMPHOID TISSUE (GALT)

See immunological defense mechanism.

GUT HORMONES

Hormones produced by the endocrine cells of the gastrointestinal tract. Includes gastrin, cholecystokinin, bombesin, somatostatin, and others. At least 20 have been identified. Most are small peptides.

GYNOID OBESITY

Excess body fat deposited mainly on hips and thighs.

H

HALF-LIFE

The time required for half of the amount of a given substance to disappear or be degraded.

HALOGENATED AROMATIC HYDROCARBONS

Organic cyclic compounds containing a fluorine, chlorine, iodine, or bromide substituent. Thyroxine is an example.

HANES (NHANES I, II, III, or HHANES)

Health and Nutrition Examination Survey sponsored by the U.S. Centers for Disease Control, a unit of the U.S. Public Health Service.

HARRIS-BENEDICT EQUATION

Equation used to estimate basal energy expenditure (see Table 2).

HEARTBURN

Burning sensation in the lower esophagus resulting from gastric acid reflux.

HEAT OF COMBUSTION

The heat produced when a food substance is oxidized in a bomb calorimeter.

HEAT PRODUCTION

The heat produced by the body in the course of its metabolism.

HEIGHT-WEIGHT INDICES

Various ratios or indices used to express weight in terms of height. Body mass index is one such expression and is used to indicate relative body fatness.

HELPER T CELLS

Component of the immune system which serves to direct antibody production by B cells in response to an antigen presented to the B cells by the macrophages.

HEMATOCRIT

Volume of erythrocytes packed by centrifugation in a given volume of blood.

HEME

The protein portion of hemoglobin which holds iron and is responsible for the carriage and release of oxygen by red blood cells.

HEME IRON

Iron held by heme.

HEMOCHROMATOSIS

A disease of iron metabolism in which iron accumulates in liver, under the skin, and in other tissues. Heart failure is a common consequence in this disorder.

HEMODIALYSIS

Process of removing toxic substances from blood with the aid of a synthetic semipermeable membrane.

HEMODILUTION

Dilution of the volume of red blood cells by an expansion of the extracellular water compartment.

HEMOGLOBIN

The iron-containing protein in the red blood cell responsible for carrying oxygen to the cells.

HEMOLYSIS

Rupture of the red blood cell.

HEMORRHAGIC DISEASE OF THE NEWBORN

Failure of the blood of the newborn to clot normally.

HEMORRHOIDS

Enlarged veins in the mucous membrane of the anus.

HEMOSIDERIN

An iron-containing compound which results from the breakdown of hemoglobin.

HEPARIN

A mucopolysaccharide; used in the prevention and treatment of thrombosis and embolism; an anticoagulant.

HEPATITIS

Inflammation of the liver. Can be caused by pathogens or may be the result of exposure (either chronic or acute) to a toxin.

HEPATOMEGALY

Enlargement of the liver.

HERS DISEASE

Genetic disease characterized by excess hepatic glycogen due to a mutation in the gene for hepatic phosphorylase.

HETEROGEUSIA

Altered taste perception; may be due to specific drugs or toxins or nutrient deficiencies. Zinc deficiency is an example.

HETEROZYGOTE

An individual having unlike copies of a gene coding for a given characteristic.

HEXOSE

A six carbon sugar.

HEXOSE MONOPHOSPHATE SHUNT

An alternative pathway for the metabolism of glucose as shown in Figure 41. The shunt provides an alternative pathway for the use of glucose-6-phosphate and generates phosphorylated ribose for use in nucleotide synthesis. It is estimated that approximately 10% of the glucose-6-phosphate generated from glucose is metabolized by the shunt.

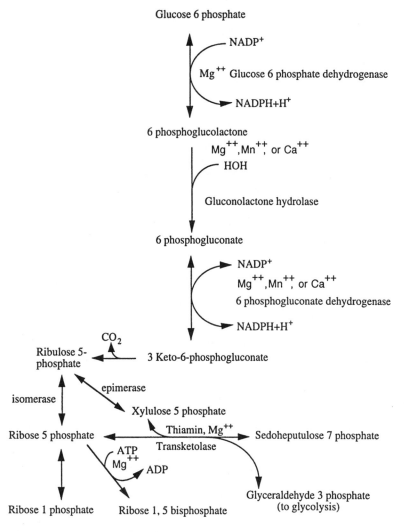

FIGURE 41 Reaction sequence of the hexose monophosphate shunt commonly referred to as the "shunt."

The shunt contains two NADP-linked dehydrogenases, glucose-6-phosphate dehydrogenase and 6 phosphogluconate dehydrogenase. These two enzymes comprise the rate limiting steps in the reaction sequence. In the instance where there is an active lipogenic state, these reactions provide about 50% of the reducing equivalents needed by the lipogenic process. There is an excellent correlation between this dehydrogenase activity and lipogenesis. The microsomal P450 enzymes also use the reducing equivants carried by $NADP^+$ as does the red blood cell in the maintenance of glutathione in the reduced state. The glutathione system in the red cell maintains the redox state and integrity of the cell membrane. If sufficient reducing equivalents are not produced by the shunt dehydrogenase reactions to reduce glutathione, the red cell membrane integrity is lost and hemolytic anemia results. This is important to the red blood cell function of carrying oxygen and exchanging it for carbon dioxide. There are a number of genetic mutations in the code for red cell glucose-6-phosphate dehydrogenase. The code is carried as a recessive trait on the X chromosome and thus only males are affected. These mutations are usually silent. That is, the male, having a defective red cell glucose-6-phosphate dehydrogenase, does not know he has the problem unless his cells are tested **or** unless he is given a drug such as quinine or one of the sulfur antibiotics that increases the oxidation of $NADPH^+H^+$. When this happens $NADPH^+H^+$ is depleted and is not available to reduce oxidized glutathione. In turn, the red cell ruptures. In almost all cases the affected male has sufficient enzyme activity to meet the normal demands for $NADPH^+H^+$. It is only when stressed by these drugs that a problem develops.

In any event as shown in Figure 41, glucose-6-phosphate proceeds to 6-phosphogluconolactone, a very unstable metabolite which is in turn reduced to 6-phosphogluconate. 6-phosphogluconate is decarboxylated and dehydrogenated to form Ribulose 5-phosphate with an unstable intermediate (keto-6-phosphogluconate) forming between the 6-phosphogluconate and ribulase 5-phosphate. Ribulose 5-phosphate can be isomerized to ribose 5-phosphate or epimerized to Xylulose 5-phosphate. Xylulose and ribose 5-phosphate can reversibly form sedoheptulose 7-phosphate with release of glyceraldehyde 3-phosphate.

HIATAL HERNIA

Protrusion of the stomach through the esophageal opening into the chest cavity.

HIGH DENSITY LIPOPROTEINS (HDL)

A protein-lipid complex responsible for the transport of lipids (triacylglycerides and cholesterol) in the blood from/to the liver to/from storage sites in the periphery. The complex is very dense and contains phospholipids as well as glycerides and sterols. Elevated HDL is associated with a reduction in risk for cardiovascular disease.

HIGH ENERGY COMPOUND

A compound having high energy phosphate bonds. When these bonds are broken a large amount of energy is released.

HIGH FIBER DIET

Diet characterized by significantly more fiber containing foods than the norm; most high fiber diets contain at least 20–35 grams of mixed fiber daily.

HINDMILK

Milk produced by the mammary gland at or near the end of the lactation period.

HISTAMINE

A vasoactive amine, which is normally present in food products such as cheese, wine, cream, fish (especially sardine), sauerkraut, and sausages. Excessive intake of histamine can cause headache, abdominal cramps, tachycardia, urticaria and, in severe cases, hypotension, bronchoconstriction, chills and muscle pain. These symptoms appear within one hour after ingestion and may last for several hours. Histamine can also be produced by bacteria in the gut. It is metabolized very quickly by enzymes in the gut mucosa and liver.

HISTAMINE RELEASERS

Biologically active substances, which can be involved in the pharmacological reactions of food intolerance. Known histamine releasers are lectins, present in certain legumes, fruits, and oat. Furthermore, foodstuffs like chocolate, strawberries, tomato, fish, eggs, pineapple, ethanol, and meat have been reported to cause histamine release. Symptoms following non-immunoglobulin E-mediated histamine release resemble real allergic symptoms.

HISTIDINE

An amino acid that is essential for growth (see Table 5).

HISTIDINEMIA

A genetic disease characterized by an excess amount of histidine in the blood.

HMG CoA

3-hydroxy-3-methylglutaryl coenzyme A. A metabolic intermediate in cholesterol synthesis.

HNIS

Human Nutrition Information Service of the U.S. Department of Agriculture.

HOLOENZYME

The complete active enzyme.

HOMEOSTASIS

A state of physiological equilibrium where anabolic and catabolic processes are in balance.

HOMOCYSTINURIA

A genetic disease characterized by a high level of homocystine in the urine. Due to an error in the gene for the Vitamin B6-dependent enzyme cystathionine synthetase.

HOMOGENTISIC ACID

A metabolite in the pathway for the conversion of phenylalanine and tyrosine to fumarate and acetoacetate (see Figure 6).

HOMOZYGOTE

An individual who has two identical genes coding for a given characteristic.

HORMONE

A substance synthesized and released by an endocrine cell, carried by the blood and having its site of action distal to its site of origin. Hormones can be peptides, proteins, or steroids. Some of these are listed in Table 26.

HOSPICE CARE

Nonhospital comfort care offered to people with terminal diseases.

24-HOUR RECALL METHOD

See interview method.

HUMAN IMMUNODEFICIENCY VIRUS (HIV)

Virus which attacks the body's immune system; the virus is thought to cause acquired immunodeficiency syndrome (AIDS).

HUNGER

Physiologic drive to eat.

HYDROGENATED FATS

Fats whose double bonds have been converted to single bonds with the resultant change in physical state (oil or liquid state to a solid state).

HYDROGENATION

The addition of hydrogen atoms to a compound; the conversion of unsaturated fats to saturated fats.

HYDROLASE

An enzyme which catalyzes the addition of water and thereby serves to split the compound into two fragments.

HYDROLYSIS

The process whereby a molecule is fragmented when water is added.

HYDROLYTIC RANCIDITY

A process resulting from the hydrolysis of glycerides to fatty acids and glycerol. It can be catalyzed by lipases (enzymes present in foods or originating from microorganisms), alkali, or acids. From a food safety point of view, hydrolytic rancidity has no important direct implication. Indirectly, however, it may be involved in combined actions. On the other hand, it can be considered desirable, for instance in strong tasting cheeses. Hydrolytic rancidity can be minimized by cold storage, proper transportation, careful packaging, and sterilization.

HYDROPHILIC

A compound that will dissolve in water.

HYDROPHOBIC

A compound that will not dissolve in water.

TABLE 26
Some Protein and Peptide Hormones and their Functions

Hormone	Source	Type	Function
Thyroid	Thyroid gland	Dipeptide of tyrosine	Regulates oxygen consumption by tissues
Thyroid stimulating hormone (TSH)	Pituitary	Polypeptide	Stimulates synthesis and release of thyroid hormone by thyroid gland
Thyroid releasing factor	Hypothalamus	Tripeptide	Stimulates pituitary to release thyroid stimulating hormone
Calcitonin	Thyroid gland	Polypeptide	Stimulates bone uptake of calcium
Parathyroid hormone	Parathyroid glands	Polypeptide	Raises serum calcium levels, lowers serum phosphorus levels; increases urinary phosphorus excretion, decreases urinary calcium excretion; activates Vitamin D in renal tissue
Insulin	β cells of islets of langerhans (pancreas)	Protein	Regulates glucose utilization; stimulates glucose uptake; influences lipid and protein synthesis
Glucagon	α cells of islets of langerhans (pancreas)	Polypeptide	Rapid mobilization of hepatic glucose from glycogen; mobilizes fatty acids from adipose tissue stores; enhances hepatic glucose production from amino acids and glycerol
Somatostatin	D cells of islets of langerhans (pancreas)	Polypeptide	Inhibits food passage along gastrointestinal system, decreases gall bladder release of bile, slows uptake of nutrients from intestinal lumen; inhibits growth hormone release
Epinephrine	Adrenal medulla	Tyrosine derivative	Stimulates lipolysis, stimulates glycogen breakdown; increases vasodilation of arterioles of skeletal muscles, vasoconstriction of arterioles in skin and viscera
Norepinephrine	Adrenal medulla	Tyrosine derivative	Exerts an overall vasoconstriction effect on the vascular system
ACTH	Pituitary	Polypeptide	Stimulates production and release of adrenal corticoid hormones
Antidiuretic hormone (ADH) (Vasopressin)	Pituitary	Polypeptide	Promotes water conservation; controls water resorption by kidney; raises blood pressure
Follical stimulating hormone (FSH)	Anterior pituitary	Peptide	Controls testicular function; spermatogenesis; stimulates ovum production; enhances release of estrogen
Luteotropic hormone (LH) (Prolactin)	Anterior pituitary	Small protein	Controls testicular function and spermatogenesis; stimulates ovum production; enhances release of estrogen
Growth hormone	Anterior pituitary	Small protein	Stimulates growth of long bones and muscles; stimulates production of somatomedin
Gastrin	Gastric glands	Polypeptide	Stimulates acid and pepsin secretion; stimulates growth of gastric mucosa
Cholecystokinin	Intestine, pancreas	Polypeptide	Stimulates gall bladder contraction; stimulates pancreatic enzyme release
Secretin	Intestine, pancreas	Polypeptide	Stimulates pancreatic secretion; augments action of cholecystokinin

From Berdanier, C.D., *Advanced Nutrition: Macronutrients*, CRC Press, Boca Raton, FL, 1994, 124.

HYDROSTATIC PRESSURE

The pressure of fluids against their container.

HYDROSTATIC WEIGHING

Reliable method for determining body fat known as underwater weighing.

HYDROXYACID ANALOGUES

Used in the treatment of chronic renal failure; produced by the replacement of an amino group with a hydroxy group to decrease the nitrogen load in the body.

HYDROXYAPPETITE

The mineral complex that is deposited in the ground substance and which provides hardness to bones and teeth.

HYDROXYLATION

The addition of a hydroxyl (–OH) group to a compound.

HYDROXYLYSINE

An amino acid in collagen. A special form of lysine which is made after the lysine is incorporated into the collagen protein.

HYDROXYPROLINE

A ring structured nonessential amino acid (see Table 5).

HYPERALIMENTATION

Early term for parenteral nutrition; nutrition support provided when a hypertonic solution of nutrients is infused via the subclavian or umbilical vein.

HYPERAMMONEMIA

Excess (>40 μmol/l) levels of ammonia in blood.

HYPERBILIRUBINEMIA

Excess (>7 μmol/l) levels of bilirubin in blood.

HYPERCALCEMIA

Excess (>2.5 μmol/l) levels of calcium in blood.

HYPERCHOLESTEROLEMIA

Above normal levels of cholesterol in blood. Normal levels are <180 mg/dl or between 4 and 7 mmol/l.

HYPERCORTISOLISM (CUSHING'S DISEASE)

See Cushing's Syndrome.

HYPEREMESIS

Excessive vomiting.

HYPERGLYCEMIA

Levels of glucose >120 mg/dl (6 mmol/l) blood.

HYPERKALEMIA

Excessive levels of potassium (>5 mmol/l) in blood.

HYPERKINESIS (HYPERACTIVITY)

Excessive motor activity.

HYPERLIPEMIA (HYPERLIPIDEMIA)

Levels of lipids in excess of normal (5–6 g/l).

HYPERMAGNESEMIA

Excessive (>1.25 mmol/l) levels of magnesium in blood.

HYPERMETABOLISM

Above normal metabolic rate.

HYPERNATREMIA

Excessive (>145 mmol/l) levels of sodium in blood.

HYPERPHAGIA

Excess food intake.

HYPERPLASIA

Increase in the number of cells.

HYPERPLASTIC ANEMIA

An increase in the size of the red blood cell with a reduction in its oxygen carrying capacity (see anemia).

HYPERPLASTIC OBESITY

Obesity characterized by an increase (above normal) in the number of adipocytes.

HYPERSENSITIVITY

See allergy.

HYPERTENSION

Blood pressure that exceeds 120/80 by 20%.

HYPERTHYROIDISM (GRAVES DISEASE)

Excess thyroid hormone production.

HYPERTONIC SOLUTIONS

Solution with a greater osmolality than plasma; >290 to 300 mOsm/kg of water.

HYPERTROPHY
Increased cell size.

HYPERTROPHIC OBESITY
Obesity characterized by increase in adipocyte size.

HYPERURICEMIA
Excess (>0.29 mmol/l) level of uric acid in the blood; a key symptom of gout.

HYPERVITAMINOSIS
A toxic syndrome resulting from intake of Vitamins A and D in great excess of the required amounts.

HYPERVOLEMIA
Increased circulating blood volume.

HYPOCHLORHYDRIA
Decreased production of hydrochloric acid in the stomach.

HYPOCHROMIC MICROCYTIC ANEMIA
Red blood cells that are fewer in number and size and lacking the normal amount of hemoglobin (see anemia).

HYPODIPSIA
Decreased thirst.

HYPOGEUSIA
Abnormal taste perception; loss of taste perception.

HYPOGLYCEMIA
Lower than normal blood glucose level (<80 mg/dl blood or 4 mmol/l).

HYPOKALEMIA
Below normal blood levels of potassium (<2.5 mmol/l).

HYPONATREMIA
Below normal blood level of sodium (<136 mmol/l).

HYPOPROTEINEMIA
Decreased protein in the blood.

HYPOSMIA
Diminished sense of smell.

HYPOTHALAMUS
A part of the central nervous system which consists of a group of nuclei at the base of the brain in relation to the floor and walls of the third ventricle.

HYPOTHYROIDISM

Below normal activity of the thyroid gland resulting in low levels of thyroxine in the blood.

HYPOTONIC SOLUTION

Solution with a lower osmolality than plasma; <290 to 300 mOsm/kg of water.

HYPOTONY

Decreased tone of the gastrointestinal tract that impedes transit time.

HYPOVITAMINOSIS

Below normal intakes of vitamins.

HYPOVOLEMIA

Diminished circulating blood volume.

HYPOXIA

Subnormal content of oxygen in arterial blood.

IJK

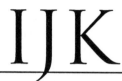

IATROGENIC

An abnormal state in a patient induced by inappropriate or erroneous treatment.

IBW

Ideal body weight.

IDIOPATHIC DISEASE

A disease of no known cause.

IDIOPATHIC STEATORRHEA

See gluten-sensitive enteropathy.

IDIOSYNCRATIC REACTION

An individual intolerance of a certain food or additive. The underlying mechanism is unknown.

ILEOSTOMY

Procedure in which a part of the ileum is brought through the abdominal wall for defecation.

ILEUM

The last third of the small intestine.

ILIAC CREST

The crest or top of the ilium or the longest of the three bones comprising the pelvis. Sometimes called the top of the hip bone.

ILEOCECAL VALVE

The valve at the junction between the large and small intestine.

IMMUNITY

The process whereby antibodies are developed to specific antigens.

IMMUNO-ACTIVE BACTERIAL ENDOTOXINS

Toxic substances produced by food-borne microorganisms.

An example of a bacteria producing immuno-active endotoxin is *Escherichia coli. E. coli* are motile, gram-negative, rod-shaped, aerobic bacteria. There are several serotypes of *E. coli*, characterized by the antigens they produce. These are somatic (O), capsular or surface (K; three types: A, B, and L), and flagellar (H).

The enteropathogenic strains of *E. coli* (EEC) can be listed into 5 groups — group A: classic enteropathogenic *E. coli*; group B: enterotoxigenic *E. coli*; group C: enteroinvasive *E. coli*; group D: facultative enteropathogenic *E. coli*; and group E: enterocytoxic *E. coli*. The serotypes of group A (CEEC) have been associated with outbreaks of infantile and childhood diarrhea. In general, they do not produce the heat-stable and heat-labile toxins. The serotypes of group B (ETEC) have been reported to cause cholera-like diarrhea, infantile diarrhea (in developing countries), and travelers' diarrhea. Unlike the serotypes of group A, they produce the heat-stable and heat-labile toxins. The heat-stable toxin, which survives heating at 100°C for 15 minutes, is a very potent toxin with a molecular weight between 1000 and 10,000. The heat-labile toxin, which is inactivated at 60°C for 30 min, is a larger molecule (molecular weight 91,000) and has been shown to possess antigenic characteristics similar to cholera toxin. The serotypes of group C (EIEC) behave like shigellae by being able to invade the epithelial cells of the colon, resulting in dysenterylike symptoms, i.e., bloody diarrhea with mucus, tenesmus, urgency, high fever, hypotension, cramps, chills, vomiting, and nausea. A lipopolysaccharide with a specific structure appears to be required in causing the disease. The invasion is followed by death of adjacent cells, inflammation, ulceration, and hemorrhage. The serotypes of group D (FEEC) are pathogens from the intestines, causing sporadic cases of diarrhea and other forms of infection. Many of them are characterized by mannose-resistant hemaglutination of human red blood cells. The only serotype of group E (ECEC) has been associated with hemorrhagic colitis, a syndrome characterized by symptoms like bloody diarrhea, abdominal cramps, and the presence or absence of low-grade fever. The strain does not produce heat-stable or heat-labile toxins or invade the enterocytes.

The minimum infective dose for enteropathogenic *E. coli* may vary from 1 million to 10 billion organisms, depending on the host and the strain. The incubation period varies with the dose, ranging between 5 to 72 hours in adults and between 18 hours and 6 days in infants. Symptoms include diarrhea, abdominal pain, nausea, pain in the limbs and head, vomiting, and fever.

Sources of contamination with enteropathogenic *E. coli* are human feces and infected foods. Food types involved in this food-borne infection include milk, cheese, red meat, poultry meat and substitute coffee drink. Furthermore, outbreaks can be the result of contaminated water, especially since enteropathogenic *E. coli* survives in water for a prolonged period of time.

IMMUNOGLOBULINS

Proteins that develop in response to antigens.

IMMUNOLOGICAL DEFENSE MECHANISM

One of the defense mechanisms in the digestive tract, protecting the body against unwanted effects of food, like allergic reactions. The immunological defense is formed by the gut-associated lymphoid tissue (GALT). The GALT consists of lymphoid organs (follicles, appendix, tonsils, and Peyer's patches) and solitary lymphocytes. Lymphoid organs contain B and T lymphocytes as well as antigen-presenting cells (APCs), mast cells, eosinophils, and basophils. Peyer's patches, which can be found in the small intestine, are situated just beneath the mucous membrane and are covered by epithelial cells. Between the latter the so-called M cells (microfold cells) are found, which transport the antigens from the gut lumen to the dome area by pinocytosis. The dome area consists of B cells, plasma cells, T cells, and APCs. The APCs present the antigen to the B and T cells. The T cells produce cytokines which stimulate the B cells to switch from immunoglobulin M (IgM) production to immunoglobulin A (IgA) production, and activate the B cells to proliferate. The B cells migrate to other parts of the body, such as the respiratory mucosa. Meanwhile, they can receive other T-cell signals which stimulate differentiation to Ig-producing plasma cells. After this a number of these plasma cells return to the GALT. Most of the plasma cells produce IgA (70–90%), some of them IgM (20%), and only a few immunoglobulin G (IgG) or immunoglobulin E (IgE). The IgA binds not only to antigens, but also to microorganisms, to prevent infection. A small number of antigens, bound to IgA, is taken up and transported by the portal system to the Kupffer cells in the liver and eliminated. Also, in healthy individuals, these immune complexes circulate in the blood shortly after a meal.

IMMUNOSUPPRESSION

Decreased ability to fight infection; decreased antibody response to antigens.

IMMUNOTHERAPY

Treatment with antibodies to enhance the response of the body to harmful substances. Treatment with very low doses of antigens to stimulate the body's production of antibodies to that antigen. The latter treatment is the basis for immunization against communicable disease.

IMPEDENCE

The opposition to an alternating current composed of two elements: resistance and reactance.

IN UTERO

In the uterus.

INBORN ERRORS OF METABOLISM

Genetic diseases of metabolism caused by a mutation in specific genes for specific enzymes, carriers, receptors, protein hormones, or cytokines.

INCIDENCE

The number of new events or cases of a disease in a population within a specified time period.

INDEPENDENT ACTION

Combination of substances with different sites of action, and no interaction between the components. However, different mechanisms can underlie the same effect and this may mean that the effects of some components of a mixture consisting of a large number of substances are similar and are integrated into an overall effect (effect integration).

INDIGENOUS

Native to a particular geographic area.

INDIRECT CALORIMETRY

Determination of energy expenditure using the measurement of oxygen consumption.

INDISPENSIBLE NITROGEN

Nitrogenous compounds that must be sustained for good health.

INFARCT

Death of local tissue fed by an obstructed artery or occluded vein.

INFECTIOUS DISEASE

Any disease caused by the invasion and multiplication of an invading pathogen.

INFLAMMATORY BOWEL DISEASE

See Crohn's Disease.

INFORMATION BIAS

Errors in the necessary information, leading to errors in the classification of subjects. The misclassification can be characterized as random (or nondifferential) or differential.

INORGANIC

Compounds that are not carbon compounds but are minerals and mineral salts.

INOSITOL

A carbohydrate (six carbon monosaccharide) that is an essential ingredient of the inositol phosphate second messenger system.

INOSITOL PHOSPHATE

A phospholipid in the plasma membrane which releases phosphoinositol when stimulated by phospholipase C.

INOSITOL PHOSPHATE CYCLE

See PIP cycle.

INSENSIBLE WATER LOSS

Water lost through the skin and through the lungs that is not noticed by the individual.

INSULIN

The hormone synthesized and released by the β cells of the Islets of Langerhans in response to rising levels of blood glucose.

INSULIN-DEPENDENT DIABETES MELLITUS (IDDM)

A disease caused by failure of the pancreas to produce and release sufficient insulin to regulate glucose homeostasis. It is characterized by defective glucose utilization.

In its most severe form, the symptoms of excessive thirst, excessive urination, rapid weight loss, and perhaps coma and death are observed. The body fat stores are raided, but because insulin is needed to complete fatty acid oxidation, this oxidation is incomplete. As a result, acetone, β hydroxybutyrate, and acetoacetate, products of incomplete fatty acid oxidation, accumulate. These are the ketone bodies. Elevated blood levels of these ketones (ketonemia) are observed as is an elevated urinary excretion (ketonuria). Rising levels of ketones increase the need for buffering power since they tend to lower pH. Acidosis is a characteristic feature of diabetes. Not only are the fat stores raided but so too is the body protein. Proteolysis (body protein breakdown) is enhanced, and amino acids thus liberated are used for energy or as substrates for intracellular glucose synthesis. The ammonia released as a product of the deamination of these amino acids assists in the buffering of the accumulating ketones. However, this ammonia is in itself cytotoxic so the body must increase its capacity to convert it to urea. Humans with uncontrolled diabetes thus are characterized by a loss in body protein, an increase in blood and urine levels of ammonia, an increase in urea synthesis, a negative nitrogen balance, a loss in fat store, elevated blood and urine levels of glucose, and elevated levels of fatty acid oxidation products. Some of these metabolic products are also excreted via the lungs in the expired air. The breath of an uncontrolled diabetic has the aroma of the ketones, somewhat like the aroma of fingernail polish remover.

Pancreatic β islet cell failure

Several explanations for pancreatic insulin production failure have been offered. The two most generally accepted are: (1) failure due to autoimmune disease and (2) failure due to viral destruction of the islet β cells. In each of these instances, the genetic heritage of the individual plays a role. In both, the immune system is involved. In the former, the autoimmune disease, the insulin producing pancreatic islet cell is destroyed because the immune system has sensed the presence of an antigen which it recognizes, not as a self-made protein, but as a foreign protein. What this self antigen might be is not known, but as a result of the antigen-antibody reaction, the insulin-producing β cells of the pancreatic islets are destroyed and with this destruction, the clinical symptoms of severe diabetes of the insulin-dependent type develop.

Diabetes secondary to viral infections

Studies of the incidence of IDDM in human populations indicate that major increases in new cases have followed outbreaks of communicable viral diseases. Certain strains of mice likewise have been found to develop IDDM following exposure to two closely related viruses, the encephalomyocarditis virus and the Coxsackie B virus. Not all rodents however will respond to these viruses by developing IDDM. Some strains are responsive while others are not. This is true in humans as well. This suggests a genetic determination of susceptibility to these infections that probably involves genes that code for the various components of the immune system. Such variability in the human population is also likely and explains why some humans may develop IDDM secondary to a viral infection while others do not. Viruses work by inserting their DNA into normal cells, converting them to an abnormal cell or causing the normal cell to destroy itself. If the person is susceptible, he/she would not be able to repel the virus and prevent its entry into the β cell. Fluorescein labeling of viral antibody has confirmed the entry of such viruses into the β cell. Evidence of virus-induced IDDM in man has been gathered through post mortem studies of pancreatic tissue excised from children with fatal viral infections caused by a variety of viruses.

INSULIN PUMP

Small instrument that senses changes in blood glucose and delivers insulin subcutaneously so as to maintain an optimal insulin-glucose relationship.

INTERCELLULAR COMPARTMENT

The water that surrounds cells and is contained in the intracellular space. Plasma is part of this compartment and surrounds the red blood cells in the blood.

INTERMEDIATE-DENSITY LIPOPROTEIN

Lipoprotein resulting from removal of triglycerides from very low density lipoproteins and chylomicrons.

INTERNAL VALIDITY

The validity of the inferences drawn for the population under investigation. In general, internal validity can be influenced by three types of bias: (1) selection bias; (2) information bias; and (3) confounding bias. However, the distinction between these three is not always strict.

INTERSTITIAL FLUID

Fluid located between cells and in some body cavities such as joints, pleura, and the gastrointestinal tract.

INTERSTITIAL SPACES

Space between tissues.

INTERVENTION STUDIES

See experimental studies.

INTERVIEW METHOD

A method for estimating food intake. Two frequently used interview methods are the 24-hour recall method and the dietary history method. In the 24-hour recall method, a complete description of the total food intake during the 24-hours preceding the interview is requested. As with the two-day record method, a single 24-hour recall does not give a good estimate of food consumption by individuals, because of the large day-to-day variation in food intake. With the dietary history method, respondents are asked about their usual food intake during a specific period of time, usually the 2–4 weeks preceding the interview. This method gives a better indication of the usual dietary intake by individuals. Since a dietary history interview takes about 1-2 hours, this method cannot be applied in studies in which many thousands of people participate.

INTESTINAL BYPASS

A surgical procedure wherein part or all of the small intestine is removed and the remaining fragments connected. The gastrointestinal tract is thus reduced in length.

INTRACELLULAR COMPARTMENT

Body water compartment consisting of fluids within the cells.

INTRAVASCULAR

Within the vascular tree. An intravascular (i.v.) injection is one where the substance is injected into a vein.

INTRAVENOUS THERAPY

Provision of fluids and/or nutrients or drugs into a vein.

INTRINSIC FACTOR

A protein secreted by the gastric cells and which is needed for the absorption of Vitamin B_{12}.

INVERT SUGAR

A mixture of glucose and fructose that results from the hydrolysis of sucrose.

INVERTASE (SUCRASE)

Enzyme that catalyzes the hydrolysis of sucrose to glucose and fructose.

IODIDE

The ion of iodine, an essential nutrient required primarily for the synthesis of thyroxine. The deficiency disorder is called goiter and is characterized by thyroid gland enlargement (see minerals, Table 29).

ION

An element with either a positive or negative charge.

IRON

An essential mineral nutrient which serves as a component of hemoglobin and the cytochromes (see minerals, Table 29).

IRRADIATION OF FOOD

Preservation technique based on the irradiation of food with x-rays.

IRRITABLE BOWEL SYNDROME

Chronic condition, characterized by diarrhea and with abdominal pain.

ISCHEMIA

Impaired blood flow causing oxygen and nutrient deprivation resulting in pain and, if severe, death of some or all parts of the tissue.

ISF (INTERSTITIAL FLUID)

Fluid surrounding the extravascular cells providing a medium for passage of nutrients to and from cells.

ISLETS OF LANGERHANS

The particular segments of the pancreas having an endocrine function. These islets consist of several cell types, one of which is the β cell that produces the hormone insulin. Another is the α cell which produces glucagon, and a third, the D cell, produces somatostatin.

ISOELECTRIC POINT

The pH of a protein in solution at which there are equal numbers of positive and negative charged groups.

ISOENERGETIC (ISOCALORIC)

State where the energy consumed is equal to the energy expended.

ISOLEUCINE

An essential amino acid (see Table 5).

ISOPRENE

A five carbon unit used in the synthesis of sterols.

ISOTONIC SOLUTION

Solution with an osmolality similar to plasma; 290–300 mOsm/kg of water.

ISOTOPIC DILUTION TECHNIQUE

A technique using very small amounts of isotopically labelled substrate to measure the volume of and amount of a large pool of that substrate. The technique is based on the Fick principle where the volume and concentration of the infused labelled substrate is known. It is infused, and at a set time later a known volume is withdrawn and the concentration determined. This allows the computation of the volume of distribution of the substrate in the larger volume of the body. The equation for this computation is $C_1/V_2 = V_1/C_2$.

IU (INTERNATIONAL UNIT)

An amount defined by the International Conference for Unification of Formulae.

JAUNDICE

A yellow color of the skin which arises when bilirubin accumulates in the subcutaneous layer of cells and in the blood. Can be a symptom of hepatitis.

JEJUNUM

The middle third of the small intestine.

JEJUNOSTOMY

Surgical opening in the jejunum.

JELLY

A colloidal suspension of fruit juice. The suspension is created by the hydration of pectin.

JOULE

A unit of work or energy in the metric system. The amount of work done by a force of 1 newton acting over the distance of 1 meter.

KELP

Seaweed.

KERATIN

A scleroprotein found primarily in fingernails, hair, horns, etc.; contains a large amount of sulfur.

KERNICTERUS

Jaundice of newborn with degenerative lesions in parts of the brain.

KESHAN DISEASE

Selenium deficiency disease resulting in cardiomyopathy (see minerals, Table 30).

KETO ACID

Used in the treatment of chronic renal failure; produced by the replacement of an amino group with a keto group to decrease the nitrogen load in the body.

KETOGENIC AMINO ACIDS

Amino acids which, when catabolized, yield ketones. These include leucine, phenylalanine, tyrosine, lysine, threonine, and tryptophan.

KETONEMIA

Excess levels of ketones in blood (levels greater than 20 mg/l).

KETONES

Carbon compounds having a double bond oxygen substituent. Typical ketones are acetone and β hydroxybutyrate.

KETONURIA

Excess ketones in urine.

KETOSIS

State where excess ketones are being produced.

KIBBLED

Coarsely ground meal or grain.

KIDNEY FAILURE

See Chronic renal failure.

KIDNEY STONES

Precipitates of calcium phosphate or oxalate. These stones vary in size from the size of coarse gravel to pea size. Also called calculi; condition is called urolithiasis or nephrolithiasis.

KILOCALORIE (kcal)

The amount of energy required to raise the temperature of 1 kg water 1°C. 1 kilojoule = 4.189 kcal.

KINETIC ENERGY

Mechanical energy.

KJELDAHL

Chemical method for determining the nitrogen content of foods and animal tissues. The quantity of nitrogen is multiplied by 6.25 to obtain the proximate protein content of the sample (6.25 is an average conversion factor). Specific foods and specific tissues may have different conversion factors.

K_m

Michaelis constant. The substrate concentration that produces half maximal velocity of the reaction. The affinity of the enzyme for its substrate determines K_m. If the affinity is high, the reaction will proceed very quickly. If two enzymes work on the same substrate, the one with the greater affinity will be more active and have a higher K_m.

KREBS CYCLE

See Citric acid cycle.

KWASHIORKOR

Protein-deficiency disorder. Kwashiorkor usually affects the young child after he/she is weaned from his/her mother's breast. The child is usually between 1 and 3 years old; he/she is weaned because his/her mother has given birth to another child or is pregnant and cannot support both children. If the child has no teeth, he/she is given a thin gruel. This may be a fruit, vegetable, or cereal product mixed with water; it is not usually a good protein source. Cultural food practices or taboos may further limit the kinds and amounts of protein given to the child. Concurrent infections, parasites, seasonal food shortages, and poor distribution of food amongst the family members may also contribute to the development of kwashiorkor. The deficiency develops not only because of inadequate intake but also because at this age the growth demands for protein and energy are high. **Growth failure** is the single most outstanding feature of protein malnutrition. The child's height and weight for his/her age will be less than that of his/her well-nourished peer. **Tissue wastage** is present but may not be apparent if edema is present. The **edema** begins with the feet and legs and gradually presents itself in the hands, face, and body. If edema is advanced, the child may not appear underweight but many appear "plump." The edema is thought to result from insufficient ADH production and a deficient supply of serum and tissue proteins needed to maintain water balance. The protein-deficient child is usually **apathetic**, has little interest in his/her surroundings, and is listless and dull. This child is usually "fussy" and irritable when moved. Mental retardation may or may not result. **Hair changes** are frequently observed. Texture, color, and strength are affected. Black, curly hair may become thin, lusterless, and brown or reddish-brown in color. **Lesions of the skin** are not always present, but if present, they give the appearance of old flaky paint. Depigmentation or darkly pigmented areas may develop with a tendency for these areas to appear in places of body friction such as the backs of legs, groins, and elbows. **Diarrhea** is almost always present. The diarrhea may be a result of the inability of the body to synthesize the needed digestive enzymes so that the food that is consumed can be utilized, and/or it may be the result of concurrent infections and parasites. **Anemia** due to an inability to synthesize hemoglobin as well as red blood cells is invariably present. **Hepatomegaly** (enlarged liver) is usually observed.

In children consuming energy sufficient-protein insufficient diets, the enlarged liver is usually fatty because the child is unable to synthesize the lipid transport proteins which are needed to transport the lipids out of the liver.

L

LABILE

Easily degraded; unstable.

LACTALBUMIN

One of the whey proteins in milk.

LACTATE

End product of glycolysis.

LACTATE DEHYDROGENASE

Enzyme which catalyzes the removal of reducing equivalents from lactate to produce pyruvate.

LACTATION

Milk production and release by the mammary gland. The process is under the control of the hormone prolactin and can be diminished in the poorly nourished mother. Lactation increases the mother's need for most nutrients (see RDA, Table 45)

LACTIC ACIDOSIS

Condition where lactate levels are elevated above normal; occurs in muscles of exercising animals; occurs in uncontrolled diabetes mellitus.

LACTOFLAVIN

An outdated name for riboflavin (Vitamin B_2).

LACTOSE

A disaccharide present in milk; when hydrolyzed by lactase, glucose and galactose result.

LACTOSE INTOLERANCE

Inability to digest lactose due to decreased (or absence) of lactose activity. In the absence of lactase, lactose is not hydrolyzed (digested) and acts as an osmotic agent stimulating peristalsis with the clinical symptoms of flatulence, bloating, cramps, and diarrhea. Whether lactase deficiency is a genetic disease is subject to much discussion. Lactase deficiency has been reported in 55% of Mexican-American males, 73.8% of adult Mexicans from rural Mexico, 44.7% of Greeks, 56% of Cretans, 66% of Greek Cypriots, 68.8% of North American Jews, 50% of Indian adults, 20% of Indian children, 45% of Negro children in the United States, 80% of Alaskan Eskimos, and greater in Oriental adults compared with Caucasian adults. Current evidence indicates that lactose intolerance is more common than lactose tolerance. Notable exceptions to these observations are Caucasians of Scandinavian or Northern European background. These populations have less than 5% with lactose intolerance and traditionally consume diets containing large amounts of milk and milk products.

Lactose intolerance is age related. Prevalence of lactose intolerance is greater in adult populations than in populations of children, suggesting that if there is a genetic tendency toward lactase deficiency, this tendency may be modified by such environmental factors as milk availability, sanitation, adequacy of diet with respect to essential nutrients, and the presence of parasites. That lactose intolerance does not appear until after weaning and is related to milk drinking or avoidance, suggests that high milk consumption may be a stimulus for prolonging lactase activity in the mucosal brush border during the postweaning period. Genetic studies of lactose intolerant families suggest that true lactase deficiency is an autosomal recessive trait. Therapy for lactose intolerant individuals consists simply of restricting lactose intakes. Some individuals tolerate fermented products such as yogurt and cheese fairly well, while varying amounts of milk or ice cream induce the typical symptoms of diarrhea and flatulence.

LAETRILE
A nitritoside having questionable nutritional value.

LARD
Pig fat.

LDL RECEPTOR
A protein on the surface of the cell which has a particular affinity for low density lipoprotein (LDL). When aberrant, lipids transported to the adipose tissue are not transported into the cell and stored. This results in an increase in LDL in the blood.

LEAD
A mineral which is toxic to the neuromuscular system.

LEAN BODY MASS
That fraction of the body exclusive of stored fat. This fraction is considered to be the active metabolic fraction.

LECITHIN
The trivial name for the phospholipid, phosphatidyl choline.

LECTINS
See type A antinutritives.

LEEK
A member of the onion family.

LEGUMES
A large family of plants that have nodules on their roots containing nitrogen fixing bacteria. Peas and beans are legumes. Some legumes contain substances that interfere with vitamins or have other antinutrient effects. These are listed in Table 27.

LEPTIN
A cytokine produced by the adipocyte. Leptin signals the brain that the fat store is full and that satiety has been attained. Mutation of either the gene for its production or the gene for its receptor has been associated with the development of obesity.

TABLE 27
Antinutritional and/or Toxic Factors Which May be Present in Certain Legumes

Type of Factor(s)	Effect of Factor(s)	Legumes Containing the Factor(s)
Antivitamin Factors:	Interfere with the actions of certain vitamins.	
Antivitamin A	Lipoxidase oxidizes and destroys carotene (provitamin A).	Soybeans
Antivitamin B-12	Increases requirement for Vitamin B-12.	Soybeans
Antivitamin D	Causes rickets unless extra vitamin D is provided.	Soybeans
Antivitamin E	Damage to the liver and muscles.	Alfalfa, Common beans (*Phaseolus vulgaris*), Peas (*Pisum sativum*).
Cyanide-Releasing Glucosides	Releases hydrocyanic acid. The poison may also be released by an enzyme in *E. coli*, a normal inhabitant of the human intestine.	All legumes contain at least small amounts of these factors. However, certain varieties of lima beans (*Phaseolus lunatus*) may contain much larger amounts.
Favism Factor	Causes the breakdown of red blood cells in susceptible individuals.	Fava beans (*Vicia faba*).
Gas-Generating Carbohydrates	Certain indigestible carbohydrates are acted upon by gas-producing bacteria in the lower intestine.	Many species of mature dry legume seeds, but not peanuts. The immature (green) seeds contain much lower amounts.
Goitrogens	Interfere with the utilization of iodine by the thyroid gland.	Peanuts and soybeans.
Inhibitors of Trypsin	The inhibitor(s) binds with the digestive enzyme trypsin.	All legumes contain trypsin inhibitors. These inhibitors are destroyed by heat.
Lathyrogenic Neurotoxins	Consumption of large quantities of lathyrogenic legumes for long periods (several months) results in severe neurological disorders.	Lathyrus pea (*L. sativus*) which is grown mainly in India. Common vetch (*Vicia sativa*) may also be lathyrogenic.
Metal Binders	Bind copper, iron, manganese, and zinc.	Soybeans, Peas (*Pisum sativum*).
Red Blood Cell Clumping Agents (Hemagglutinins)	The agents cause the red blood cells to clump together.	Occurs in all legumes to some extent.

Adapted from Ensminger et al., *Foods and Nutrition Encyclopedia*, 2nd ed., CRC Press, Boca Raton, FL, 1994, pp. 1284–1285.

LESCH NYHAN SYNDROME

A genetic disease affecting only males that is due to a mutation in the gene for hypoxanthine-guanine phosphoribosyl transferase, an enzyme that is essential in making guanosine from the purine, guanine. The disorder is characterized by mental retardation, self mutilation, and renal failure.

LESION-CAUSING BACTERIAL TOXINS

Bacteria-producing, lesion-causing toxins include *Bacillus cereus*. *Bacillus cereus* are gram-positive, rod-shaped, spore-forming, aerobic bacteria, which produce enterotoxins (type I and II) as well as several enzymes of pathogenic relevance (e.g., hemolysin and lecithinase).

Type I (diarrheal type) is a proteinous enterotoxin (molecular weight 50,000), which is formed in the intestine. This enterotoxin is heat-sensitive and can be degraded by trypsin.

Type II (emetic type) is an enterotoxin (molecular weight ≤5000), which is formed in the food during the logarithmic phase of bacterial growth. Type II is stable at pH 10 and heat-resistant.

It has been reported that cereus counts ranging from 36,000 to 950 million cells/g of food result in enteritis. Type I enterotoxin occurs most frequently and is mildly toxic. After an incubation period of 8–16 hours, 50–80% of the consumers develop abdominal cramps and diarrhea which may last for 24 hours. Type II enterotoxin is less common. After a short incubation period of 1–5 hour(s), violent vomiting occurs. Symptoms may last for 8–10 hours. The sudden onset of symptoms, short duration of illness, characteristic lack of fever, requirement for large numbers of organisms to produce response, and variability of fecal isolation of the organism are all suggestive of the noninfective nature of the disease and indicate that cereus food-borne poisoning is an intoxication.

Factors affecting growth and survival of Bacillus cereus are:

1. temperature (growth of *Bacillus cereus*: 7–50°C (optimum: 30–35°C); germination of spores: –1 to 59°C (optimum: 30°C));
2. acidity (growth of *Bacillus cereus*: pH 4.9–9.3);
3. type of substrates and nutritional factors (growth of *Bacillus cereus*: affected by the amino acid composition of the medium, especially by arginine, cysteine, glutamic acid, histidine, isoleucine, leucine, methionine, phenylalanine, serine, threonine, and valine; enterotoxin production: further enhanced by adding glycine, lysine, aspartic acid, and tyrosine);
4. presence of other microorganisms (*Streptococcus lactis* produces an antibiotic, nisin, that suppresses growth of *Bacillus cereus* in milk at low temperatures (≤5°C) of storage. The antibiotic has no effect at 15°C or higher, whereas the spores of *Bacillus cereus* appear to be resistant to nisin);
5. NaCl (tolerance: 5%);
6. time (generation time: 27 min).

Sources contributing to *Bacillus cereus* contamination are soil and dust; principal food types involved include custards, cereal products, puddings, sauces, and meat-loaf. There is no evidence that human factors are involved in the contamination. Type I enterotoxin is mainly associated with sauces, pastries, etc., type II enterotoxin with cooked or fried rice. The main prevention measure is adequate and immediate cooling after cooking. This should be carried out in shallow layers enabling fast heat transfer; storage should be at ≤10°C.

LESIONS
A wound or injury; an abnormality of a cell or tissue that is indicative of disease.

LETHARGY
Lack of energy; drowsiness.

LEUCINE
An essential amino acid (see Table 2).

LEUKEMIA
Cancer; white blood cell production is uncontrolled.

LEUKOCYTES
White blood cells.

LEUKOTRIENES

Eicosanoids synthesized from arachidonic acid (see eicosanoids).

LEVULOSE

Fructose.

LHA

Lateral hypothalamus.

LIFE EXPECTANCY

The number of years a human can expect to live; can vary depending on nutritional status, genetics, environment, and physical activity.

LIGNIN

A complex indigestible fiber that provides structure to very mature vegetables.

LIMITING AMINO ACIDS

A food that is poor in one or more essential amino acids is said to have these amino acids as limiting.

LINGUAL LIPASE

A lipase found in the saliva that initiates the digestion of triacylglycerides (see lipid digestion).

LINOLEIC ACID

An essential fatty acid of the n-6 or ω6 family of fatty acids.

LINOLENIC ACID

An essential fatty acid of the n-3 or ω3 family of fatty acids.

LIPASE

An enzyme responsible for the hydrolysis of the ester bond which links a fatty acid to its glycerol backbone.

LIPID DIGESTION

The digestion of food lipids consists of a series of enzyme-catalyzed steps resulting in absorbable components.

Food lipids (fats and oils) are digested initially in the mouth then in the stomach and intestine. The digestion of lipid is begun in the mouth with the mastication of food and its mixing with the acid stable lingual lipase. Digestion can proceed only when the large particles of the food are made smaller through chewing. The action of the tongue and later the churning action of the stomach mix the food particles with the various digestive juices and in the stomach with hydrochloric acid. These actions separate the lipid particles exposing more surface area for enzyme action and providing the opportunity for emulsion formation. These changes in physical state are essential steps that precede absorption. In the stomach the proteins of lipid-protein complexes are denatured by gastric hydrochloric acid and attacked by the proteases (pepsin, parapepsin I, and parapepsin II) of the gastric juice with the resultant release of lipid. Little degradation of fat occurs in the stomach except that catalyzed by lingual lipase. Lingual lipase originates from glands in the back of the mouth and under the tongue. This lipase is active in the acid environment of the stomach. However, because of the tendency of lipid to coalesce and form a separate phase, this lipase has limited opportunity to attack triacylglycerols. Those that are attacked release a single fatty acid, usually a short or medium chain one. The remaining diacylglycerol is subsequently hydrolyzed in the duodenum. In adults consuming a mixed diet, lingual lipase is relatively unimportant. However, in infants having an immature duodenal lipase, lingual lipase is quite important. In addition, this lipase has its greatest activity on the triacylglycerols commonly present in whole milk. Milk fat has more short and medium chain fatty acids than fats from other food sources.

Although the action of lingual lipase is slow relative to lipases found in the duodenum, its action to release diacylglycerol and short and medium chain fatty acids serves another function — these fatty acids serve as surfactants. Surfactants spontaneously adsorb to the water-lipid interface conferring a hydrophilic surface to lipid droplets and thereby provide a stable interface with the aqueous environment. The dietary surfactants are the free fatty acids, lecithin, and the phospholipids. The action of acid stable lingual lipase provides more fatty acids to supplement the dietary supply. All together these surfactants plus the churning action of the stomach produce an emulsion which is then expelled into the duodenum as chyme.

Once the chyme enters the duodenum, its entry stimulates the release into the blood stream of the gut hormone cholecystokinin. Cholecystokinin stimulates the gall bladder to contract and release bile. Bile salts serve as emulsifying agents and serve to further disperse the lipid droplets at the lipid-aqueous interface facilitating the hydrolysis of the glycerides by the pancreatic lipases. The bile salts impart a negative charge to the lipids which in turn attracts the pancreatic enzyme, colipase.

Pancreozymin stimulates the exocrine pancreas to release pancreatic juice which contains three lipases (lipase, lipid esterase, colipase) which act at the water-lipid interface of the emulsion particles. One lipase acts on the fatty acids esterified at positions 1 and 3 of the glycerol backbone leaving a fatty acid esterified at carbon 2. This 2 monoacylglyceride can isomerize, and the remaining fatty acid can move to carbon 1 or 3. The pancreatic juice contains another less specific lipase (called a lipid esterase) which cleaves the fatty acid from cholesterol esters, monoglycerides, or esters such as vitamin A ester. Its action requires the presence of the bile salts. The lipase that is specific for the ester linkage at carbons 1 and 3 does not have a requirement for the bile salts and, in fact, is inhibited by them. The inhibition of pancreatic lipase by the bile salts is relieved by the third pancreatic enzyme, colipase. Colipase is a small protein (mol. wt. 12,000 Da) which binds to both the water-lipid interface and to lipase thereby anchoring and activating the lipase. The products of the lipase catalyzed reaction, a reaction that favors the release of fatty acids having 10 or more carbons, are these fatty acids and monoacylglyceride. The products of the lipid esterase catalyzed reaction are cholesterol, vitamins, fatty acids, and glycerol. Phospholipids present in food are attacked by phospholipases specific to each of the phospholipids. The pancreatic juice contains these lipases as prephospholipases which are activated by the enzyme trypsin.

LIPIDS

The lipids comprise a group of compounds which are, in general, insoluble in water and soluble in such solvents as diethyl ether, carbon tetrachloride, hot alcohol, chloroform, and benzene. They are present in various amounts in all living mammalian cells. Nerve cells and adipose cells are rich in lipid; muscle cells and epithelial cells have considerably less.

In addition to being a very important source of energy, lipids serve a variety of other needs. They perform a basic role in the structure and function of biological membranes. In the body, they are the precursors of a variety of hormones and important cellular signals. They help to regulate the uptake and excretion of nutrients by the cell. Each cell has a characteristic lipid content. The lipids are energetically more dense than carbohydrate having an average energy value of 37.7 kJ/g. Some lipids are saponifiable; others are not. Saponifiable lipids, when treated with alkali, undergo hydrolysis at the ester linkage resulting in the formation of an alcohol and a soap. Triacylglycerol (triglyceride), for example, when treated with sodium hydroxide is hydrolyzed yielding a mixture of soaps and free glycerol. Traditionally, lipids have been classified into three groups, each with subgroups.

- A. Simple lipids — esters of fatty acids with various alcohols.
    1. Fats — esters of fatty acids with glycerol (acylglycerols).
    2. Waxes — esters of fatty acids with long chain alcohols.
    3. Cholesterol esters.
- B. Compound Lipid — esters of fatty acid which contain chemical groups in addition to fatty acids and alcohol.
    1. Phospholipids — esters of fatty acids, alcohol, a phosphoric acid residue, and usually an amino alcohol, sugar, or other substituent.
    2. Glycolipids — esters of fatty acids which contain carbohydrates and nitrogen (but not phosphoric acid) in addition to fatty acids and alcohol.
    3. Lipoproteins — loose combinations of lipids and proteins.
- C. Derived Lipids — substances derived from the above groups by hydrolysis. They are the results of saponification.

LIPOFUSCIN

Granules of pigments found in aging tissues; highly insoluble lipid-protein complexes held together by multiple cross linkages.

LIPOGENESIS

The synthesis of fatty acids, triacylglycerols, cholesterol, and phospholipids (see fatty acid synthesis, Figure 31; cholesterol synthesis, Figure 14; triacylglyceride and phospholipid synthesis, Figure 28).

LIPOIC ACID

A critical coenzyme in the oxidative decarboxylation of pyruvate and α ketoglutarate.

LIPOLYSIS

The hydrolysis of triacylglycerides and subsequent oxidation of fatty acids (see fatty acid oxidation, Figures 29 and 30).

LIPOMA

An adipose tissue tumor; a nonmalignant neoplasm composed of mature fat cells.

LIPOPROTEIN LIPASE

Enzyme which catalyzes the initial step of hydrolyzing the fatty acids from the glycerol backbone.

LIPOPROTEINS

A conjugated protein containing lipid and protein moieties having a density of 1.006 to 1.063.

LIQUID DIET

A wide variety of diets fit this category. Clear liquids include broths, clear juices, tea, jello; full liquids includes such items as ice cream, pureed soups, etc. Formulated products are available that provide all the needed nutrients for individuals who cannot chew or digest foods in the normal state. These are appropriate for long term use by such patients.

LITHIASIS

The process of stone formation in the gall bladder, bile duct, kidney, ureters, or urinary bladder.

LITHIUM

A mineral used to treat mania; interferes with the activity of the Na^+K^+ dependent ATPase on the plasma membranes of nerve cells.

LITHOTRIPSY

Procedure of shattering calculi via high frequency sound in the kidney, urinary tract, and gallbladder.

LIVER DISEASE

A generic term that covers a variety of pathologic states of the liver.

LIVER FAILURE

The liver ceases to function.

LNAA

Large neutral amino acids; branched chain and aromatic amino acids.

LOCUS

The position of a chromosome occupied by a gene or its allele.

LONGEVITY

Life span.

LOW BIRTH WEIGHT INFANT

An infant whose weight at the end of gestation is less than expected based on the mother's size and the duration of pregnancy.

LOW DENSITY LIPOPROTEIN (LDL)

A lipid protein complex consisting of a carrier protein, triglycerides, and cholesterol. Elevated LDL levels are associated with an increased risk of coronary vessel disease.

LOW FAT DIET

Therapeutic diet characterized by significantly fewer fat containing foods than the usual diet; most low fat diets contain 10–20% of total energy from fat daily.

LOW FIBER DIET

Therapeutic diet characterized by significantly fewer fiber containing foods than the usual diet; most low fiber diets contain less than 10–20 g of mixed fiber daily.

LOW RESIDUE DIET

Diet characterized by significantly fewer residue producing foods than the usual diet; most low residue diets also include foods low in fiber. In addition to restrictions found on the low fiber diet, the low residue diet typically restricts milk and milk products to one or two servings daily.

LOW SODIUM DIET

Diet characterized by significantly less sodium containing foods than the usual diet; low sodium diets range from a "no added salt diet" with approximately 4000 mg/day (174 mEq) to a severe restriction at 500 mg/day (22 mEq).

LUMEN

Interior aspect of a vessel.

LUPUS ERYTHEMATOSUS

An autoimmune disease that affects the skin, joints, blood vessels, heart, kidneys, lungs, and brain.

LUXUS CONSUMPTION

Consumption of food beyond basic needs.

LYCOPENE

A carotene-like compound that has no vitamin activity.

LYMPH

Fluid present in the vessels of the lymphatic system; newly absorbed lipid is carried via the lymphatic system from the small intestine to the jugular where the thoracic duct joins this vein.

LYSINE

An essential amino acid (see Table 1).

LYSOSOMES

Intracellular structures that contain digestive enzymes that attack material taken into the cells.

μ

Greek letter prefix which indicates 10^{-6} fraction of a liter or gram.

MACROBIOTIC (ZEN) DIET

A diet that is based on brown rice and can be deficient in a number of essential nutrients.

MACROCYTE

Immature red blood cell.

MACROCYTIC ANEMIA

An anemia characterized by large red cells (see anemia, Table 8).

MACROPHAGES

Cells of the immune system that are the first line of defense against pathogens. These cells are large mononuclear phagocytes that work by engulfing the foreign substance and neutralizing it.

MACRONUTRIENTS

Major sources of energy and building materials for the organism. The macronutrients include fats, carbohydrates, proteins, and water (see carbohydrates, fats, protein, water).

MACROSOMIA

Enlarged cells; also used to describe a very large infant born to a mother with gestational diabetes.

MAGNESIUM

An essential mineral which serves as a cofactor in phosphatase and kinase catalyzed reactions; these are the reactions that result in the hydrolysis of ATP to ADP and Pi. One of the most important of these is the activation of amino acids for protein synthesis through the action of the enzyme aminoacyl-t-RNA synthetase. Another involves the attachment of mRNA to the ribosome. A third is the phosphorylation of glucose to form glucose-6-phosphate (see minerals, Table 29).

MAGNETIC RESONANCE IMAGING

A technology allowing the imaging of a body without radiation hazard.

MAILLARD REACTION

A nonenzymatic browning reaction of reducing sugars, in which they condense with amino acids. It is a sequence of reactions, resulting in the formation of a mixture of insoluble dark-brown polymeric pigments, known as melanoidins. In the early steps of the reaction, a complex mixture of carbonyl compounds and aromatic substances is formed. These products are water-soluble and mostly colorless. They are called premelanoidins. Animal studies have indicated that large intakes of premelanoidins inhibit growth, disturb reproduction, and cause liver damage. Further, certain types of allergic reactions have been attributed to Maillard reaction products. Maillard reactions can be prevented by using the additive power of the carbonyl group in reducing sugars. Regulation of the temperature, pH, and water content can additionally inhibit Maillard reactions. Maillard reactions account for the browning of bread during baking and the browning of meat through exposure to high heat. Foods prepared in this manner provide very little premelanoidins.

MALABSORPTION

A condition where nutrients are not absorbed normally. May be due to a nutrient intolerance or some other disease which causes the intestinal cells to lose their absorptive capacity.

MALAISE

A feeling of illness or depression.

MALATE

A four carbon intermediate in the citric acid cycle.

MALATE ASPARTATE SHUTTLE

A shuttle for moving reducing equivalents into the mitochondria from the cytosol. Shown in Figure 42; has rate limiting properties in gluconeogenesis.

MALIGNANCY

An uncontrolled growth of cells; cancer.

MALNUTRITION

Inadequate or unbalanced intake of essential nutrients. The physical signs associated with malnutrition are listed in Table 28.

MALTITOL

An alcohol of maltose.

MALTOSE

A disaccharide consisting of two molecules of glucose joined by an α 1,4 linkage.

MANGANESE

An essential mineral which serves as a cofactor for the enzymes pyruvate carboxylase (converts pyruvate to oxalacetate) and superoxide dismutase. The latter enzyme also requires copper as a cofactor (see minerals, Table 29).

MANNITOL

An alcohol of mannose.

MANNOSE

A six carbon sugar that can be converted to fructose via phosphorylation and isomerization.

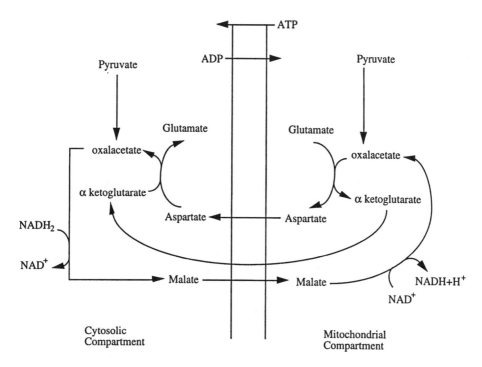

FIGURE 42 Malate aspartate shuttle.

MAO

Monoamine oxidase. A copper-containing enzyme which catalyzes the removal of oxygen from epinephrine, tyramine, and serotonin, inactivating them and reducing neuronal activity. Inhibitors of MAO are valuable drugs for treating depression.

MAPLE SYRUP URINE DISEASE

A genetic disease due to a mutation in the genes which code for the branch chain amino acid dehydrogenases. Characterized by mental retardation, ketoacidosis, and early death. The urine of such patients smells like maple syrup, hence the name.

MARASMUS

Condition of deficient energy and protein intake. Also called protein calorie malnutrition (PCM).

Although children of all ages and adults can suffer from a deficiency of both energy and protein, the marasmic child is usually less than one year old. In developing countries, a common cause for marasmus is a cessation of breast feeding. Milk production by the mother may have stopped because of the mother's poor health, or the mother may have died, or, there may be a desire on the part of the mother to bottle feed her infant rather than breast feed. This decision to bottle feed may be made for a variety of reasons. The mother may view bottle feeding as a status symbol, or she may be forced to work to earn a living and may be unable to have her baby with her, or she may not be able to lactate. While under optimal conditions of economics and sanitation, the bottle-fed child may be well fed, in emerging nations this is not always true. The mother may not be able to buy the milk formula in sufficient quantities to adequately nourish the child, she may overdilute the milk, or she

TABLE 28
Physical Signs Which Are Often Associated With Malnutrition

Area of Body Examined	Normal Appearance	Common Signs of Malnutrition	Other Causes of These Clinical Signs
Appearance in General	Normal weight for age, sex, and height. Alert and emotionally stable. No areas of edema.	Significant overweight or underweight. Apathetic or hyperirritable. Loss or slowness of ankle or knee reflexes. Pitting edema.	Non-nutritional metabolic disorders. Endocrine disease.
Eyes	Shiny and free from areas of abnormal pigmentation, opacity, vascularization, and dryness.	Paleness, dryness, redness or pigmenation of membranes (conjunctiva). Foamy patches or conjunctiva (Bitot's spots). Dullness, softness, or vascularization of the cornea. Redness or fissures on eyelids.	Exposure to environmental or chemical irritants. Tissue changes accompanying aging.
Face	Skin is clear and uniform in color, free of all except minor blemishes. Free of swollen or lumpy areas.	Skin has lighter (depigmentation) and darker (over cheeks and under eyes) area. Greasy scales around nose and lips. Swollen or lumpy areas.	Poor hygiene. Cushing's disease (moonface).
Glands	No swollen areas on face or neck.	Swelling of parotids (enlarged "jowls") or thyroid (front of neck near its base).	Mumps. Inflammation, tumor, or hyperfunction of the thyroid.
Gums	Red, free from bleeding or swelling.	Receded. "Spongy" and bleeding. Swelling of the gingiva.	Medication. Periodontal disease. Poor oral hygiene.
Hair	Shiny, firmly attached to scalp (not easily plucked without pain to patient).	Dullness, may be brittle and easily plucked without pain. Sometimes lighter in color than normal (depigmentation may be bandlike when hair is held up to a source of light).	Endocrine disorders.
Lips	Smooth, not chapped, cracked, or swollen.	Swollen, red, corners, cracked (cheilosis).	Herpes (blisters). Exposure to strong sunshine, dry or cold climates.
Muscles	Muscles are firm and of normal size.	Wasting and flabbiness of muscle. Bleeding into muscle.	Wasting diseases. Trauma.
Nails	Firm, pink.	Spoon-shaped nails. Brittle and ridged nails.	Cardiopulmonary disease.
Organs, internal	Normal heart rate and rhythm. Normal blood pressure. Internal organs cannot be palpated (except the liver in children).	Racing heartbeat (over 100 beats per minute). Abnormal rhythm of heart. High blood pressure. Palpable enlargement of liver or spleen.	Rheumatic fever. Non-nutritional diseases of the heart, liver, spleen, and kidneys.
Skeleton	Bones have normal sizes and shapes.	Softening, swelling, or distorted shapes of bones and joints.	Non-nutritional connective tissue disorders. Age change in porosity.
Skin	Smooth, free of rashes, swellings, and discoloration.	Roughness (follicular hyperkeratosis), dryness, or flakiness. Irregular pigmentation, black and blue marks, "crazy pavement" lesions. Symmetrical, reddened lesions. Looseness of skin (lack of subcutaneous fat).	Secondary syphilis. Poor or improper hygiene. Environmental irritants. Trauma. Anticoagulant therapy.

TABLE 28 (CONTINUED)
Physical Signs Which Are Often Associated With Malnutrition

Area of Body Examined	Normal Appearance	Common Signs of Malnutrition	Other Causes of These Clinical Signs
Teeth	Enamel is unbroken and unspotted. None or a few small cavities.	Caries. Mottled or darkened areas of enamel.	Developmental abnormalities. Stains from foods or cigarettes.
Tongue	Normal size of papillae (no atrophy or hypertrophy. Color is uniform and deep red. Sense of taste is normal.	Atrophy of papillae (the tongue is smooth) or hypertrophy of papillae. Irregularly shaped and distributed white patches. Swollen, scarlet, magenta (purple colored), or raw tongue.	Dietary irritants. Colors or dyes from food. Non-nutritional anemias. Antibiotics. Uremia. Malignancy.

Adapted from Ensminger et al., *Foods and Nutrition Encyclopedia*, 2nd ed., CRC Press, Boca Raton, FL, 1994, pp. 1351–1352.

may use unsafe water and unsanitary conditions to prepare the formula for the child. This, plus the insufficient nutrient content, often precipitously leads to the development of marasmus, a form of starvation characterized by **growth failure** with prominent ribs, a characteristic monkey-like face, and match stick limbs with little muscle or adipose tissue development; **tissue wastage** but not edema is present. Whereas the kwashiorkor child has a poor appetite, the marasmus child is **eager to eat**. The child is **mentally alert** but not irritable. **Anemia** and **diarrhea** are present for the same reasons as in kwashiorkor. The skin and hair appear to be of normal color.

The treatment of both kwashiorkor and marasmic children must be approached with due care and caution. Because their enzymes for digestion and their protein absorption and transport systems are less active, feeding these children with large quantities of good quality protein would be harmful. Their diets must be gradually enriched with these proteins to allow their bodies sufficient time to develop the appropriate metabolic pathways to handle a better diet. Giving these children solutions of either predigested proteins or solutions of amino acids may be of benefit initially, but these solutions, too, must be used with care. If the amino acids in excess of immediate use are deaminated and if the pathway for synthesizing urea is not fully functional, ammonia can accumulate in the child and become lethal.

Not only must one be concerned about the enzymes of the malnourished child, the protein-depleted child is also unable to synthesize adequate amounts of the protein hormones which regulate and coordinate his/her use of dietary nutrients. In addition, protein deprivation affects the structures of the cell hormone receptor sites thus further dampening the effectiveness of those hormones produced. Children with marasmus or kwashiorkor have been shown to have decreased blood sugar levels, decreased serum insulin and growth hormone levels, and, in marasmus, decreased thyroid hormone levels. Additional hormonal changes have been observed, but their relevance to treatment has not been ascertained. Most probably these changes in the levels of the protein, peptide, or amino acid derived hormones are reflective of reduced synthesis of them as a result of a shortage of incoming amino acids. Changes in the steroid hormones probably reflect the response of the child to the stress of deprivation.

MASTITIS
Inflammation of the mammary gland.

MATRIX

Center or formative section of a tissue such as bone.

MCARDLE'S DISEASE

One of the glycogen storage diseases which develops because of a mutation in the gene for hepatic phosphorylase; characterized by hepatomegaly, lipemia, and growth retardation.

MCV

Mean Corpuscular Volume. The ratio of the volume of packed cells to the volume of the blood sample; an indirect measure of the number of red blood cells in the blood sample.

MEAN

Average value for a group of values.

MEAN ARTERIAL PRESSURE

The average of the diastolic and systolic pressures.

MECHANICAL SOFT DIET

Diet characterized by foods that have been altered in texture or form to make them easier to chew and swallow.

MECONIUM

Stool produced by the fetus typically expelled during the first days of life.

MEDIAN

Value where half the values fall below and half fall above this value.

MEDICAL NUTRITION THERAPY

An integral part of the medical treatment for a specific disease state that improves the outcome and speeds recovery. Components of medical nutrition therapy include: Nutrition Screening, Nutrition Assessment, and Nutrition Treatment.

MEDICINAL PLANTS

Plants that have medicinal value. Some are recognized remedies while others are folklore. Table 29 lists some of these plants. Excess intake of some of these may be toxic.

MEDIUM CHAIN TRIGLYCERIDES

Fatty acids containing 8–12 carbon atoms.

MEGADOSE

Very large dose.

MEGALOBLAST

Large immature red blood cell.

TABLE 29
Some Common Medicinal Plants

Common and Scientific Name	Description	Production	Part(s) of Plant Used	Reported Uses
Agrimony *Agrimonia gryposepala*	Small yellow flowers on a long spike; leaves hairy and at least 5 in. (13 cm) long, narrow and pointed; leaf edges toothed; a perennial.	Needs good soil and sunshine; grows in New England and Middle Atlantic states.	Whole plant including roots.	A tonic, alterative, diuretic, and astringent; infusions from the leaves for sore throats; treatment of kidney and bladder stones; root for jaundice.
Aletris root (whitetube star-grass) *Aletris farinosa*	Grasslike leaves in a flat rosette around a spike-like stem; white to yellow tubular flowers along stem.	Moist locations in woods, meadows, or bogs; New England to Michigan and Wisconsin; south to Florida and west to Texas.	Leaves; roots.	Poultice of leaves for sore breast; liquid from boiled roots for stomach pains, tonic, sedative, and diuretic.
Alfalfa *Medicago sativa*	Very leafy plant growing 1–2 ft (30–61 cm) high; small green leaves; bluish-purple flowers; deep roots.	A legume cultivated widely in the United States.	Leaves.	Powdered and mixed with cider vinegar as a tonic; infusions for a tasty drink; leaves may also be used green.
Aloe vera *Aloe barbadensis*	A succulent plant with leathery sword-shaped leaves, 6–24 in. (15–61 cm) long.	A semidesert plant which grows in Mexico and Hawaii; temperature must remain above 50°F (10°C); can be a house plant.	Mucilaginous juice of the leaves.	Effective on small cuts and sunburn; speeds healing; manufactured product for variety of cosmetic purposes.
Angelica *Angelica atropurpurea*	Shrub growing to 8 ft (2.4 m) high; stem purplish with 3 toothed leaflets at tip of each leaf stem; white or greenish flowers in clusters at end of each stalk.	Grows in rich low soil near streams and swamps and in gardens; from New England west to Ohio, Indiana, Illinois, and Wisconsin; south to Delaware, Maryland, West Virginia, and Kentucky.	Roots; seeds.	Small amount of dried root or seeds for relief of flatulence; roots for the induction of vomiting and perspiration; roots for treatment of toothache, bronchitis, rheumatism, gout, fever, and to increase menstrual flow.
Anise (Anise seed) *Pimpinella anisum*	Annual plant, 1–2 ft (30–61 cm) high; belongs to carrot family; small white flowers on long hairy stalk; lower leaves egg-shaped; upper leaves feathery.	Grown all over the world; grows wild in countries around the Mediterranean; much is imported to United States.	Seed.	As a hot tea to relieve flatulence or for colic.
Asafetida *Ferula* sp.	A coarse plant growing to 7 ft (2.1 m) high with numerous stem leaves; pale green-yellow flowers; flowers and seeds borne in clusters on stalks; large fleshly root; tenacious odor.	Indigenous to Afghanistan, but some species grow in other Asiatic countries.	Gummy resin from the root.	As an antispasmodic; to ward off colds and flu by wearing in a bag around the neck.

TABLE 29 (CONTINUED)
Some Common Medicinal Plants

Common and Scientific Name	Description	Production	Part(s) of Plant Used	Reported Uses
Bayberry (Southern wax myrtle) *Myrica cerifera*	Perennial shrub growing to 30 ft (9.2 m) high; waxy branchlets; narrow evergreen leaves tapering at both ends; yellowish flowers; fruits are grayish berries.	Grows in coastal regions from New Jersey, Delaware and Maryland to Florida, Alabama, Mississippi, and Arkansas.	Root bark; leaves and stems.	Decoction of root bark to treat uterine hemorrhage, jaundice, dysentery, and cankers; leaves and stems boiled and used to treat fevers; decoction of boiled leaves for intestinal worms.
Bearberry *Arctostaphylos uva-ursi*	Creeping evergreen shrub with stems up to 6 in. (15 cm) high; reddish bark; bright green leaves, 1 in. (3 cm) long; white flowers with red markings, in clusters; smooth red fruits.	Grows in well-drained soils at higher altitudes; from Oregon, Washington, and California, to Colorado and New Mexico.	Leaves.	As a diuretic; also boiled infusions used as a drink to treat sprains, stomach pains, and urinary problems; poison oak inflammations treated with leaf decoction by pioneers.
Black cohosh *Cimicifuga racemosa*	Perennial shrub growing to 9 ft (2.7 m) or more in height; leaf has 2 to 5 leaflets; plant topped with spike of slender candlelike, white or yellowish flowers; rhizome gnarled and twisted.	Grows throughout eastern United States; commercial supply from Blue Ridge Mountains.	Rhizomes and roots.	Infusion and decoctions used to treat sore throat, rheumatism, kidney trouble, and general malaise; also used for "women's ailments" and malaria.
Black Walnut *Juglans nigra*	A tree growing up to 120 ft (36.6 m) high; leaflets alternate 12 to 23 per stem, finely toothed and about 3–3.5 in. (8–9 cm) long; nut occurs singly or in clusters with fleshy, aromatic husk.	Native to a large section of the rich woods of eastern and midwestern United States.	Bark; nut husk; leaves.	Inner bark used as mild laxative; husk of nut used for treating intestinal worms, ulcers, syphilis, and fungus infections; leaf infusion for bedbugs.
Blackberry (brambleberry, dewberry, raspberry) *Rubus*	Shrubby or viny thorny perennial; numerous species; large white flowers; red or black fruit.	Grows wild or in gardens throughout the United States; wild in old fields, waste areas, forest borders, and pastures.	Roots; root bark, leaves; fruit.	Infusion made from roots used to dry up runny noses; infusion from root bark to treat dysentery; fruit used to treat dysentery in children; leaves also used in similar manner.
Blessed thistle *Cnicus benedictus*	Annual plant growing to 2 ft (61 cm) high; spiny tooth, lobed leaves; many flowered yellow heads.	Grows along roadsides and in waste places in eastern and parts of southwestern United States.	Leaves and flowering tops in full bloom; seeds.	Infusions from leaves and tops for cancer treatment, to induce sweating, as a diuretic, to reduce fever, and for inflammations of the respiratory system; infusion of tops as Indian contraceptive; seeds induce vomiting.

TABLE 29 (CONTINUED)
Some Common Medicinal Plants

Common and Scientific Name	Description	Production	Part(s) of Plant Used	Reported Uses
Boneset *Eupatorium perfoliatum*	Perennial bush growing to 5 ft (1.5 m) in height; heavy stems with leaves opposite; purplish to white flowers borne in flat heads.	Commonly found in wet areas such as swamps, rich woods, marshes, and pastures; grows from Canada to Florida and west to Texas and Nebraska.	Leaves; flowering tops.	Infusions made from leaves used for laxative and treatment of coughs and chest illnesses — a cold remedy; Negro slaves and Indians used it to treat malaria.
Borage *Borago officinalis*	Entire plant not over 1 ft (30 cm) high; nodding heads of starlike flowers grow from clusters of hairy obovate leaves.	Introduced in United States from Europe; occasionally grows in waste areas in northern states; cultivated widely in gardens.	Leaves.	Most often used as an infusion to increase sweating, as a diuretic, or to soothe intestinal tract; can be applied to swellings and inflamed areas for relief.
Buchu *Rutaceae*	Low shrubs with angular branches and small leaves growing in opposition; flowers from white to pink.	Grown in rich soil in warm climate of South Africa.	Dried leaves.	Prepared as tincture or infusion; used for genito-urinary diseases, indigestion, edema, and early stages of diabetes.
Buckthorn *Rhamnus purshiana*	Deciduous tree growing to 25 ft (7.6 m) high; leaves 2–6 in. (5–15 cm) long; flowers small greenish yellow; fruit globular and black, about 1/4 in. (6 mm) across.	Grows usually with conifers along canyon walls, rich bottom lands, and mountain ridges in western United States.	Bark; fruit.	Bark used as a laxative and tonic; fruit (berries) used as a laxative.
Burdock *Arctium minus*	Biennial or perennial growing 5–8 ft (1.5–2.4 m) high; large leaves resembling rhubarb; tube-shaped white and pink to purple flowers in heads; brown bristled burrs contain seeds.	Grows in wastelands, fields, and pastures throughout the United States.	Root.	Infusion of roots for coughs, asthma, and to stimulate menstruation; tincture of root for rheumatism and stomachache.
Calamus (Sweet flag) *Acorus calamus*	Perennial growing 3–5 ft (1.0–1.5 m) high; long narrow leaves with sharp edges; aromatic leaves; flower stalk 2–3 in. (3–8 cm) long and clublike; greenish-yellow flowers.	Grows in swamps, edges of streams and ponds from New England west to Oregon and Montana, and from Texas east to Florida and north.	Rhizomes.	Root chewed to clear phlegm (mucous) and ease stomach gas; infusions to treat stomach distress; considered useful as tonic and stimulant.

TABLE 29 (CONTINUED)
Some Common Medicinal Plants

Common and Scientific Name	Description	Production	Part(s) of Plant Used	Reported Uses
Catnip *Nepeta cataria*	Perennial growing to 3 ft (1 m) in height; stem downy and whitish; leaves heart-shaped opposite coarsely toothed and 2–3 in. (3–8 cm) long; tubular whitish with purplish marked flowers in compact spikes.	Grows wild along fences, roadsides, waste places, and streams in Virginia, Tennessee, West Virginia, Georgia, New England, Illinois, Indiana, Ohio, New Mexico, Colorado, Arizona, Utah, and California; readily cultivated in gardens.	Entire plant.	Infusions for treating colds, nervous disorders, stomach ailments, infant colic, and hives; smoke relieves respiratory ailments; poultice to reduce swellings.
Celery *Apium graveolens*	A biennial producing flower stalk second year; terminal leaflet at end of stem; fruit brown and round.	Cultivated in California, Florida, Michigan, New York, and Washington.	Seeds.	As an infusion to relieve rheumatism and flatulence (gas); to act as a diuretic; to act as a tonic and stimulant; oil from seeds used similarly.
Chamomile *Anthemis nobilis*	Low growing, pleasantly strong-scented, downy, and matlike perennial; daisylike flowers with white petals and yellow center.	Cultivated in gardens; some wild growing which escaped from gardens.	Leaves and flowers.	Powdered and mixed with boiling water to stimulate stomach, to remedy nervousness in women, and stimulate menstrual flow, also a tonic; flowers for poultice to relieve pain; Chamomile tea known as soothing, sedative, completely harmless.
Chaparral *Croton corynbulosus*	Shrubby perennial plant of the Spurge family.	Grows in dry rock areas from Texas west.	Flowering tips.	Infusions act as laxative; some claims as cancer treatment.
Chickweed *Stellaria media*	Annual growing 12–15 in. (30–38 cm) high; stems matted to somewhat upright; upper leaves vary but lower leaves ovate; white, small individual flowers.	Grows in shaded areas, meadows, wasteland, cultivated land, thickets, gardens, and damp woods in Virginia to South Carolina and southeast.	Entire plant in full bloom.	Poultice made to treat sores, ulcers, infections, and hemorrhoids.
Chicory *Cichorium intybus*	Easily confused with its close relative the dandelion; in bloom bears blue or soft pink blooms not resembling dandelion.	Introduced from Europe, now common wild plant in United States; some grown in gardens.	Roots; leaves.	No great medicinal value; some mention of diuretic, laxative, and tonic use; mainly added to give coffee distinctive flavor.
Cinnamon *Cinnamomum zeylanicum*	An evergreen bush or tree growing to 30 ft (9 m) high.	A native plant of Sri Lanka, India, and Malaysia; tree kept pruned to a shrub; bark of lower branches peeled and dried.	Bark.	Treatment for flatulence, diarrhea, vomiting, and nausea.

TABLE 29 (CONTINUED)
Some Common Medicinal Plants

Common and Scientific Name	Description	Production	Part(s) of Plant Used	Reported Uses
Cleaver's herb (Catchweed bedstraw) *Galium aparine*	Annual plant; weak reclining bristled stem with hairy joints; leaves in whorls of 8; white flowers in broad, flat cluster; bristled fruit.	Grows in rich woods, thickets, seashores, waste areas, and shady areas from Canada to Florida and west to Texas.	Entire plant during flowering.	To increase urine formation; to stimulate appetite; to reduce fever; to remedy Vitamin C deficiency; also used to remove freckles.
Cloves *Syzygium aromaticum*	Dried flower bud of a tropical tree which is a 30-ft (9 m) high red flowered evergreen.	Tree native to Molucca, but widely cultivated in tropics; flower bud picked before flower opens and dried.	Flower bud.	To promote salivation and gastric secretion; to relieve pain in stomach and intestines; applied externally to relieve rheumatism, lumbago, toothache, muscle cramps, and neuralgia; clove oil used, too; infusions with clove powder relieves nausea and vomiting.
Colt's foot (Canada wild ginger) *Asarum canadense*	Low growing stemless perennial; heart-shaped leaves; flowers near root and brown and bell-shaped.	Found in moist woods from Maine to Georgia and west to Ohio.	Roots; leaves.	Infusion of root to relieve flatulence; powdered root to relieve flatulence, induce sweating, and to relieve aching head and eyes; leaves substitute for ginger.
Comfrey *Symphytum officinale*	A perennial which reaches about 2 ft (61 cm) in height; leaves are large and broad at base but lancelike at terminal; fine hair on leaves; tail-shaped head of white to purple flowers at terminal.	Prefers a moist environment; a European plant now naturalized in the United States.	Roots; leaves.	Numerous uses including treatments for pneumonia, coughs, diarrhea, calcium deficiency, colds, sores, ulcers, arthritis, gallstones, tonsils, cuts and wounds, headaches, hemorrhoids, gout, burns, kidney stones, anemia, and tuberculosis; used as a poultice, infusion, powder, or in capsule form.
Dandelion *Taraxacum officinale*	Biennial growing 2–12 in. (5–30 cm) high; leaves deeply serrated forming a basal rosette in spring; yellow flower but turns to gray upon maturing.	Weed throughout the United States; the bane of lawns.	Flowers; roots; green leaves.	Root uses include diuretic, laxative, tonic, and to stimulate appetite; infusion from flower for heart troubles; paste of green leaves and bread dough for bruises.

TABLE 29 (CONTINUED)
Some Common Medicinal Plants

Common and Scientific Name	Description	Production	Part(s) of Plant Used	Reported Uses
Echinacea (Purple echinacea) *Echinacea purpurea*	Perennial from 2–5 ft (0.6–1.5 m) high; alternate lance-shaped leaves; leaf margins toothed; top leaves lack stems; purple to white flower.	Grows wild on road banks, prairies, and dry, open woods in Ohio to Iowa, south to Oklahoma, Georgia, and Alabama.	Roots.	Treatment of ulcers and boils, syphilis, snake-bites, skin diseases, and blood poisoning; used as powder and in capsules.
Eucalyptus *Eucalyptus globulus*	Tall, fragrant tree growing up to 300 ft (92 m) high; reddish-brown stringy bark.	Native to Australia but grown in other semi-tropical and warm temperate regions.	Leaves and oil dis-tilled from leaves.	Antiseptic value; inhaled freely for sore throat; asthma relief; local application to ulcers; used on open wounds.
Eyebright (Indian tobacco) *Lobelia inflata*	Branching annual growing to 3 ft (1 m) high with leaves 1–3 in. (3–8 cm) long; small violet to pink-ish-white flowers in axils of leaves; seed capsules at base of flower containing many tiny brown seeds.	Roadside weed of east-ern United States, west to Kansas.	Entire plant in full bloom or when seeds are formed.	Treatment of whooping cough, asthma, epi-lepsy, pneumonia, hys-teria, and convulsion; alkaloid extracted for use in antismoking preparations.
Fenugreek *Trigonella foenum-graceum*	Annual plant similar to clover in size.	Native to the Mediter-ranean regions and northern India; widely cultivated; easily grown in home gardens.	Seed.	Poultice for wounds; gargle for sore throat.
Flax (Linseed) *Linum usitatissimum*	Herbaceous annual; slender upright plant with narrow leaves and blue flowers; grows to about 2 ft (61 cm) high.	Originated in Mediter-ranean region; culti-vated widely for fiber and oil.	Seed.	Ground flaxseed mixed with boiling water for poultice on burns, boils, carbuncles, and sores; internally as a laxative.
Garlic *Allium sativum*	Annual plant growing to 12 in. (30 cm) high; long, linear, narrow leaves; bulb composed of several bulblets.	Throughout the United States under cultiva-tion; some wild.	Entire plant when in bloom; bulbs.	Fresh poultice of the mashed plant for treat-ing snake bite, hornet stings, and scorpion stings; eaten to expel worms, treat colds, coughs, hoarseness, and asthma; bulb expressed against the gum for toothache.
Gentian (Sampson snake-root) *Gentiana villosa*	Perennial with stems growing 8–10 in. (20–25 cm) high; opposite ovate, lance-shaped leaves; pale blue flowers.	Grows wild in swampy areas Florida west to Louisiana, north to New Jersey, Pennsyl-vania, Ohio, and Indiana.	Rhizomes and roots.	Treatment of indiges-tion, gout, and rheuma-tism; induction of vomiting; aid to diges-tion; a tonic.

TABLE 29 (CONTINUED)
Some Common Medicinal Plants

Common and Scientific Name	Description	Production	Part(s) of Plant Used	Reported Uses
Ginger *Zingiber officinale*	Perennial plant; forms irregular-shaped rhizomes at shallow depth.	Native to southeastern Asia; now grown all over tropics.	Rhizome.	An expectorant; treatment of flatulence, colds, and sore throats.
Ginseng *Panax quinquefolia*	Hollow stems solid at nodes; leaves alternate; root often resembles shape of a man; small, inconspicuous flowers; vivid, shiny, scarlet berries.	Grows in eastern Asia, Korea, China, and Japan; some grown in United States.	Root.	As a tonic and stimulant; treatment of convulsions, dizziness, vomiting, colds, fevers, headaches, and rheumatism; commonly believed to be an aphrodisiac.
Goldenrod *Solidago odora*	Grows 18–36 in. (46–91 cm) high with narrow leaves scented like anise; inconspicuous head with 6 to 8 flowers.	Grows throughout the United States.	Leaves.	Infusions from dried leaves as aromatic stimulant, a carminative, and a diuretic.
Goldenseal *Hydrastis canadensis*	Perennial growing to about 1 ft (30 cm) high; one stem with 5 to 7 lobed leaves near top; several single leafstalks topped with petalless flowers; raspberrylike fruit but inedible.	Grows in rich, shady woods of southeastern and midwestern United States; grown under cultivation in Washington.	Roots; leaves, and stalks.	Root infusion as an appetite stimulant and tonic; root powder for open cuts and wounds; chewing root for mouth sores; leaf infusion for liver and stomach ailments.
Guarana *Paullinia cupana*	Climbing shrub of the soapberry family; yellow flowers; pear-shaped fruit; seed in 3-sided, 3-celled capsules.	Grows in South America, particularly Brazil and Uruguay.	Seeds.	Stimulant; seeds high in caffeine.
Hawthorn *Crataegus oxycantha*	Hardy shrub or tree depending upon growth conditions; small, berry fruit; cup-shaped flowers with 5 parts; thorny stems.	Originally grown throughout England as hedges; also grows wild; some introduced in the United States.	Berry.	Tonic for heart ailments such as angina pectoris, valve defects, rapid and feeble heart beat, and hypertrophied heart; reverses arteriosclerosis.
Hop *Humulus lupulus*	Twining, perennial growing 20 ft (6 m) or more; 3 smooth-lobed leaves 4–5 in. (10–13 cm) long; membranous, cone-like fruit.	Grows throughout the United States; often a cultivated crop.	Fruit (hops).	Straight hops or powder used; hot poultice of hops for boils and inflammations; treatment of fever, worms, and rheumatism; as a diuretic; as a sedative.
Horehound (White horehound) *Marrubium vulgare*	Shrub growing to 3 ft (1 m) in height; fuzzy ovate-round leaves which are whitish above and gray below; foliage aromatic when crushed.	Grows wild throughout most of United States in pastures, old fields, and waste places, except in arid southwest.	Leaves and small stems; bark.	Decoctions to treat coughs, colds, asthma, and hoarseness; other uses include treatment for diarrhea, menstrual irregularity, and kidney ailments.

TABLE 29 (CONTINUED)
Some Common Medicinal Plants

Common and Scientific Name	Description	Production	Part(s) of Plant Used	Reported Uses
Huckleberry (Sparkleberry) *Vaccinium arboreum*	Shrub or tree growing to 25 ft (7.6 m) high; leathery; shiny, thick leaves; white flowers; black berries; other species.	Grows wild in woods, clearings, sandy and dry woods in Virginia, Georgia, Florida, Mississippi, Indiana, Illinois, Missouri, Texas, and Oklahoma.	Leaves, root bark, and berries.	Decoctions of leaves and root bark to treat sore throat and diarrhea; drink from berry for treating chronic dysentery.
Hyssop *Hyssopus officinalis*	Hardy, fragrant, bushy plants belonging to the mint family; stem woody; leaves hairy, pointed, and about 1/2 in. (20 mm) long; blue flowers in tufts.	Grows in various parts of Europe including the Middle East; some grown in United States.	Leaves.	Infusions for colds, coughs, tuberculosis, and asthma; an aromatic stimulant; healing agent for cuts and bruises.
Juniper (Common juniper) *Juniperus communis*	Small evergreen shrub growing 12–30 ft (3.7–9.2 m) high; bark of trunk reddish-brown and tends to shred; needles straight and at right angles to branchlets; dark, purple, fleshy berrylike fruit.	Widely distributed from New Mexico to Dakotas and east; dry areas.	Fruit (berries).	Used as a diuretic, to induce menstruation, to relieve gas, and to treat snake bites and intestinal worms.
Lemon balm *Melissa officinalis*	Persistent perennial growing to 1 ft (30 cm) high; light green, serrated leaves; lemon smell and taste to crushed leaves.	Wild in much of the United States; grown in gardens.	Leaves.	Infusion used as a carminative, diaphoretic, or febrifuge.
Licorice (Wild licorice) *Glycyrrhiza lepidota*	Erect perennial growing to 3 ft (1 m) high; pale yellow to white flowers at end of flower stalks; brown seed pods resemble cockleburs.	Grows wild on prairies, lake shores, and railroad right-of-ways throughout much of the United States.	Root. **Caution:** Licorice raises the blood pressure of some people dangerously high, due to the retention of sodium.	Root extract to help bring out phlegm (mucus); treatment of stomach ulcers, rheumatism, and arthritis; root decoctions for inducing menstrual flow, treating fevers, and expulsion of afterbirth.
Marshmallow *Althaea officinalis*	Stems erect and 3–4 ft (0.9–1.2 m) high with only a few lateral branches; roundish, ovate-cordate leaves 2–3 in. (5–8 cm) long and irregularly toothed at margin; cup-shaped, pale-colored flowers.	Introduced into United States from Europe; now found on banks of tidal rivers and brackish streams; grew wild in salt marshes, damp meadows, by ditches, by the sea, and banks of tidal rivers from Denmark south.	Root.	Primarily a demulcent and emollient; used in cough remedies; good poultice made from crushed roots.

TABLE 29 (CONTINUED)
Some Common Medicinal Plants

Common and Scientific Name	Description	Production	Part(s) of Plant Used	Reported Uses
Motherwort *Leonurus cardiaca*	Perennial growing 5–6 ft (1.5–1.8 m) high; lobed, dented leaves, 5 in. (13 cm) long; very fuzzy white to pink flowers.	Grows wild in pastures, waste places, and road-sides from northeastern states west to Montana and Texas, south to North Carolina and Tennessee.	Entire plant above ground.	Used as a stimulant, tonic, and diuretic; Europeans used for asthma and heart palpitation; usually taken as an infusion.
Mullien (Aaron's rod) *Verbascum thapsus*	At base a rosette of woody, lance-shaped, oblong leaves with a diameter of up to 2 ft (61 cm); yellow flowers along a clublike spike arising from the rosette to a height of up to 7 ft (2.1 m).	Grows wild throughout the United States in dry fields, meadows, pastures, rocky or gravelly banks, burned areas, etc.	Leaves; roots; flowers.	Infusions of leaves to treat colds and dysentery; dried leaves and flowers serve as a demulcent and emollient; leaves smoked for asthma relief; boiled roots for croup; oil from flowers for earache; local applications of leaves for hemorrhoids, inflammations, and sunburn.
Nutmeg *Muristica fragrans*	Evergreen tree growing to about 25 ft (7.6 m) high; grayish-brown, smooth bark; fruit resembles yellow plum, the seed of which is known as nutmeg.	Native to Spice Islands of Indonesia; now cultivated in other tropical areas.	Seed.	For the treatment of nausea and vomiting; grated and mixed with lard for hemorrhoid ointment.
Papaya *Carica papaya*	Small tree seldom above 20 ft (6.1 m) high; soft, spongy wood; leaves as large as 2 ft (61 cm) in diameter and deeply cut into 7 lobes; fruit oblong and dingy green-yellow.	Originated in South American tropics; now cultivated in tropical climates.	Leaves.	Dressing for wounds, and aid for digestion; contains proteolytic enzyme, papain, used as a meat tenderizer.
Parsley *Petroselinum crispum*	Biennial which is usually grown as an annual; finely divided, often curled, fragrant leaves.	Originated in the Mediterranean area; now grown worldwide.	Leaves; seeds; roots.	As diuretic with aromatic and stimulating properties.
Passion flower (Maypop passion-flower) *Passiflora incarnata*	Perennial vine growing to 30 ft (9.2 m) in length; alternate leaves composed of 3 to 5 finely toothed lobes; showy, vivid, purple, flesh-colored flowers; smooth, yellow ovate fruit 2–3 in. (5–8 cm) long.	Grows wild in West Indies and southern United States; cultivated in many areas.	Flowering and fruiting tops.	Crushed parts for poultice to treat bruises and injuries; other uses include treatment of nervousness, insomnia, fevers, and asthma.

TABLE 29 (CONTINUED)
Some Common Medicinal Plants

Common and Scientific Name	Description	Production	Part(s) of Plant Used	Reported Uses
Peppermint *Mentha piperita*	Perennial growing to about 3.5 ft (1 m) high; dark, green, toothed leaves; purplish flowers in spike-like groups.	Originated in temperate regions of the Old World where most is still grown; grows in shady damp areas in many areas of the United States; grown in gardens.	Flowering tops; leaves.	Infusions for relief of flatulence, nausea, headache, and heartburn; fresh leaves rubbed into skin to relieve local pain; extracted oil contains medicinal properties.
Plantain *Plantago* sp.	Low perennial with broad leaves; flowers on erect spikes.	Grows wild throughout the United States in poor soils, fields, lawns, and edges of woods.	Leaves; seeds; root.	Infusion of leaves for a tonic; seeds for laxative; soaking seeds provides sticky gum for lotions; fresh, crushed leaves to reduce swelling of bruised body parts; fresh, boiled roots applied to sore nipples.
Pleurisy root (Butterfly milkweed) *Asclepias tuberosa*	Leafy perennial growing to 3 ft (1 m) high; alternate leaves which are 2 to 6 in. (5–15 cm) long and narrow; bright orange flowers in a cluster; root spindle-shaped with knotty crown.	Grows in sandy, dry soils; pastures, roadsides, and gardens; south to Florida and west to Texas and Arizona.	Root.	Small doses of dried root as a diaphoretic, diuretic, expectorant, and alternative; ground roots fresh or dried for poultice to treat sores.
Queensdelight *Stillingia sylvatica*	Perennial growing to 3 ft (1 m) high; contains milky juice; leathery, fleshy, stemless leaves; yellow flowers.	Grows wild in dry woods, sandy soils, and old fields; Virginia to Florida, Kansas, and Texas, north to Oklahoma.	Root.	Treatment of infectious diseases; as an alterative.
Red clover *Trifolium pratense*	Biennial or perennial legume less than 2 ft (61 cm) high; 3 oval-shaped leaflets form leaf; flowers globe-shaped and rose to purple colored.	Throughout United States; some wild, some cultivated.	Entire plant in full bloom.	Infusions to treat whooping cough; component of salves for sores and ulcers; flowers as sedative; to relieve gastric distress and improve the appetite.
Rosemary *Rosmarinus officinalis*	Low-growing perennial evergreen shrub; leaves about 1 in. (3 cm) in height; orange-yellow flowers; white, shiny seeds.	Native to Mediterranean region; now cultivated in most of Europe and the Americas.	Leaves.	Used as a tonic, astringent, diaphoretic, stimulant, carminative, and nervine.

TABLE 29 (CONTINUED)
Some Common Medicinal Plants

Common and Scientific Name	Description	Production	Part(s) of Plant Used	Reported Uses
Saffron (Safflower) *Carthamus tinctorius*	Annual with alternate spring leaves; grows to 3 ft (1 m) in height; orange-yellow flowers; white, shiny seeds.	Wild in Afghanistan; cultivated in the United States, primarily in California.	Flowers; seeds; entire plant in bloom.	Paste of flowers and water applied to boils; flowers soaked in water to make a drink to reduce fever, as a laxative, to induce perspiration, to stimulate menstrual flow, and to dry up skin symptoms of measles.
Sage (Garden sage) *Salvia officinalis*	Fuzzy perennial belonging to the mint family; leaves with toothed edges; terminal spikes bearing blue or white flowers in whorls.	Originated in the Mediterranean area where it grows wild and is cultivated; grown throughout the United States, some wild.	Leaves.	Treatment for wounds and cuts, sores, coughs, colds, and sore throat; infusions used as a laxative and to relieve flatulence; major use for treatment of dyspepsia.
Sarsaparilla *Smilax* sp.	Climbing evergreen shrub with prickly stems; leaves round to oblong; small, globular berry for fruit.	Grown in tropical areas of Central and South America and in Japan and China.	Root.	Primarily an alterative regarded as an aphrodisiac; for colds and fevers; to relieve flatulence; best used as an infusion.
Sassafras *Sassafras album*	Tree growing to 40 ft (12.2 m) high; leaves may be 3-lobed, 2-lobed, mitten-shaped, or unlobed; yellowish-green flowers in clusters; pea-sized, 1-seeded berries in fall.	Originated in New World; grows in New England, New York, Ohio, Illinois, and Michigan, south to Florida and Texas; grows along roadsides, in woods, along fences, and in fields.	Root bark.	Sassafras was formerly used for medical purposes, but the use of the roots was banned by the FDA because of their carcinogenic qualities.
Saw palmetto *Serenoa serrulata*	Low-growing fan palm; whitish bloom covers sawtoothed, green leaves; flowers in branching clusters; fruit varies in size and shape.	Grows in warm, swampy, low areas near the coast.	Fruit (berries).	To improve digestion; to treat respiratory infections; as a tonic and as a sedative.
Senna (Wild senna) *Cassia marilandica*	Perennial growing to 6 ft (1.8 m) in height; alternate leaves with leaflets in pairs of 5 to 10; bright yellow flowers.	Grows along roadsides and in thickets from Pennsylvania to Kansas and Iowa, south to Texas and Florida.	Leaves.	Infusions primarily employed as a laxative.
Skullcap *Scutellaria lateriflora*	Perennial growing 1–2 ft (30–61 cm) high; toothed, lance-shaped leaves; blue or whitish flowers.	Native to most sections of the United States; prefers moist woods, damp areas, meadows, and swampy areas.	Entire plant in bloom.	Powdered plant primarily a nervine.

TABLE 29 (CONTINUED)
Some Common Medicinal Plants

Common and Scientific Name	Description	Production	Part(s) of Plant Used	Reported Uses
Spearmint *Mentha spicata*	Perennial resembling other mints; grows to 3 ft (1 m) in height; pink or white flowers borne in long spikes.	Throughout the United States in damp places; cultivated in Michigan, Indiana, and California.	Above ground parts.	Primarily a carminative; administered as an infusion through extracted oils.
Tansy *Tanacetum vulgare*	Perennial growing to 3 ft (1 mg) in height; pungent fernlike foliage with tops of composite heads of buttonlike flowers.	Grown or escaped into the wild in much of the United States.	Leaves and flowering tops.	Infusions used as stomachic, emmenagogue, or to expel intestinal worms; extracted oil induced abortion often with fat results; poultice for sprains and bruises.
Valerian *Valeriana officinalis*	Coarse perennial growing to 5 ft (1.5 m) high; fragrant, pinkish-white flowers opposite pinnate leaves.	Native to Europe and Northern Asia; cultivated in the United States.	Root.	As a calmative and as a carminative.
Witch hazel *Hamamelis virginiana*	Crooked tree or shrub 8–15 ft (2.4–4.6 m) in height; roundish to oval leaves; yellow, threadlike flowers; fruits in clusters along the stem eject shiny, black seeds.	Found in damp woods of North America from Nova Scotia to Florida and west to Minnesota and Texas.	Leaves, bark, and twigs.	Twigs, leaves, and bark basis for witch hazel extract which is included in many lotions for bruises, sprains, and shaving; bark sometimes applied to tumors and skin inflammations; some preparations for treating hemorrhoids.
Yerba santa *Eriodictyon californicum*	Evergreen shrub with lance-shaped leaves.	Part of flora of the west coast of the United States.	Leaves.	As an expectorant; recommended for asthma and hay fever.

From Ensminger et al., *Foods and Nutrition Encyclopedia*, 2nd ed., CRC Press, Boca Raton, FL, 1994, pp. 1432–1441.

MEGALOBLASTIC ANEMIA

Anemia characterized by an abundance of large immature nucleated red blood cells. A typical feature of folacin deficiency.

MELANIN

Skin pigment.

MEMBRANE-AFFECTING BACTERIAL TOXINS

An example of bacteria producing these toxins is *Staphylococcus aureus*. They are nonmotile, gram-positive, nonspore-forming, facultative anaerobic bacteria, which produce several enzymes and toxins. The enzymes include coagulase (both free and bound to cell membrane staphylokinase), hydraluronidase, phosphatase, proteinase, lipase, and gelatinase. The toxins produced by *Staphylococcus aureus* are α exotoxin (lethal, dermonecrotic, hemolytic, and leucolytic), β exotoxin (hemolytic), γ exotoxin (hemolytic), δ exotoxin (dermonecrotic and hemolytic), leucocidin (leucolytic), exfoliative toxin (causing the scalded skin syndrome in skin infections), and enterotoxins.

Enterotoxins, which are simple proteins with molecular weights of 30,000 to 35,000, can be specified as enterotoxin type A, B, C, D, or E. Characteristics of enterotoxins are:

1. heat stability (enterotoxin B is the most heat stable: heating for 87 minutes at 99°C destroys the activity of type B, whereas only 1 minute at 100°C destroys 100% of the activity of type A and 80% of the activity of type D);
2. resistance to proteolytic enzymes such as trypsin, chymotrypsin, and papain; and
3. resistance to irradiation (type B only).

It has been observed that the type A strain is the most common, accounting for about 50% of the total number of enterotoxin-producing strains. The next most common type was D, whereas type B was less common. Strains producing both types A and D together were also significant in number (27%).The estimated toxic dose of enterotoxin for man is probably <1 µg. Concerning the enterotoxin levels in foods involved in poisoning outbreaks (canned prawns: 6–9 µg/100 g; trifles: 5 µg/100 g; tongue and beef: 4 µg/100 g; ham: 5–8 µg/100 g; cold chicken: 2–4 µg/100 g; vanilla cake: <1 µg/100 g; torta cream cake: 2 µg/100 g; ham and potato: 2.5 µg/100 g), consumption of less than 100 g of food will have enough toxin to elicit poisoning. Symptoms of enterotoxin poisoning, developing after 0.5 to 6 hours following consumption of contaminated food, include vomiting, diarrhea, and in severe cases, enteritis. Other symptoms are salivation, nausea, abdominal cramps, prostration, headache, muscular cramps, sweating, fever or hypothermia, hypotension, and mucus and blood in the vomitus and stools. The disease is rarely fatal.

Factors affecting growth of Staphylococcus aureus and production of enterotoxins include:

1. substrates and nutritional requirements (amino acids: arginine and cystine; vitamins: thiamin, nicotinic acid, biotin, and pantothenic acid; metals and other minerals: calcium, magnesium, and potassium; energy sources);
2. temperature (growth of Staphylococci and toxin production occurs between 10 and 45°C; the optimum temperature is 35–37°C);
3. acidity (toxin production occurs between pH 5 and pH 9);
4. effects of salts (*Staphylococcus aureus* is very salt resistant: growth can occur in the presence of NaCl levels up to 14%);
5. effect of moisture content (aerobic growth occurs with a water activity between 0.86 and 0.99) and drying (*Staphylococcus aureus* is resistant to drying or a dry environment);
6. effects of other microorganisms growing with *Staphylococcus aureus* on specific substrates (*Staphylococcus aureus* cannot compete effectively with other microorganisms growing on food);
7. other inhibitors (antibiotics such as streptomycin inhibit toxin production without interfering in the growth).

Sources of enterotoxins of *Staphylococcus aureus* include nose and throat discharges; hands and skin; and infected cuts, wounds, burns, boils, pimples, acne, and feces. The principal food types in which bacterial contamination of *Staphylococcus aureus* occurs are cooked ham and other meat products; cream-filled pastry; potato, ham, poultry, and fish salads; milk, cheese, shrimp; and other low acid food stored and served between 5 and 55°C. Prevention of Staphylococcal food poisoning is focusing on three factors:

1. the human contaminator (adequate personal hygiene, cleanliness, and good disinfection practice);
2. the food product (heating); and
3. the storage and handling of food products prior to consumption (refrigerated storage and, if possible, avoidance of preparation of food products in multiple steps, in large quantities, and far in advance).

MEMBRANES

The physical boundaries of cells and cell compartments. The membranes exist as a lipid bilayer because the phospholipids have amphipathic characteristics. They have both polar (the phosphorylated substituent at carbon 3) and nonpolar (the fatty acids) regions. The polar region is hydrophilic and is positioned such that it is in contact with the aqueous media around and within the cells. The nonpolar or fatty acid region is oriented toward the center of the bilayer so that it is protected from contact with the contents of the cell and the fluids that surround it.

Membrane composition

There are three major classes of lipids in membranes — glycolipids, cholesterol, and phospholipids. The glycolipids have a role in the cell surface-associated antigens as well as cell surface receptors, whereas cholesterol serves to regulate fluidity. The phospholipids have fatty acids attached at carbons 1 and 2. It is usual to find a saturated fatty acid attached at carbon 1 and an unsaturated fatty acid at carbon 2. In addition, phosphatidylethanolamine and phosphatidylserine usually have fatty acids that are more unsaturated than phosphatidylinositol and phosphatidylcholine. Less than 10% of the membrane phospholipid is phosphatidylinositol. Plasma membranes have no cardiolipin, and the mitochondrial membranes have very little phosphatidylserine. Several of these phospholipids have important roles in the signal transduction processes that mediate the action of a variety of hormones. Phosphatidylinositol and its role in the phosphatidylinositol cycle is one of the most important. Phosphatidylcholine and phosphaditylethanolamine also play a role in these systems. The PIP cycle functions in moving the calcium ion from its intracellular store to the inner aspect of the cell membrane where it stimulates protein kinase C. Phosphatidylinositol also serves to anchor glycoproteins to the membrane. Glycoproteins are tethered to the external aspect of the plasma membrane and play a role in the cell recognition process. Antigens, pathogens, and foreign proteins are recognized by these structures.

MENADIONE

Synthetic Vitamin K; K_3.

MENAQUINONE

Vitamin K_2; form found in animal cells (see Table 49).

MENARCHE

Beginning of estrus cycles.

MENKES DISEASE

A genetic disorder of copper absorption. The defect is in the mechanism for copper absorption by the enterocyte. Symptoms are those of copper deficiency (see Table 30).

MENOPAUSE

Cessation of estrus cycles.

MESSENGER RNA (mRNA)

A single strand of purine and pyrimidine bases synthesized in the nucleus so that its base sequence complements DNA. The mRNA leaves the nucleus, attaches to the ribosome, and provides the code for the synthesis of a single protein. Each protein has its own mRNA template.

METABOLIC ACIDOSIS

Acid-base imbalance associated with shock, diabetes, starvation, alcoholism, renal failure, or severe diarrhea and characterized by shortness of breath, lethargy, confusion, drowsiness, flushed and warm skin, hypotension, stupor, and coma.

METABOLIC ALKALOSIS

Acid-base imbalance associated with vomiting and gastric drainage, prolonged diuretic therapy, Cushing's syndrome, or excessive ingestion of bicarbonate and characterized by slow and shallow respirations, dizziness, paresthesia, confusion, agitation, seizures, and coma.

METABOLIC CONTROL

The regulation of the rates at which metabolic pathways function and interact.

METABOLIC REACTION

A food-intolerance reaction resulting from the effect of a food product on a metabolic abnormality of the host. The most important in this respect are enzyme deficiencies. An example is lactase deficiency, frequently occurring in Asian and African countries, leading to intolerance of lactose (a carbohydrate in milk or milk products). After lactose is ingested, it is not metabolized in the usual way and therefore not taken up by the gut mucosa. Because lactose remains in the intestinal tract it has a hyperosmotic effect and causes diarrhea. Some of the lactose is metabolized by intestinal flora which produce gas and thus flatulence is another characteristic of lactose intolerance.

METABOLIC WATER

Water formed as a result of metabolic reactions.

METABOLISM

The sum of all the anabolic and catabolic reactions that take place in the body.

METABOLITE

An intermediate formed in the course of a metabolic pathway.

METALLOENZYME

An enzyme containing a mineral as an integral part of its structure.

METALLOTHIONEIN

A carrier for certain minerals.

METHIONINE

An essential amino acid (see Table 5). Methionine serves as an essential methyl donor for the synthesis of many compounds. Through its interconversion to cysteine, sulfur is conserved as shown in Figure 43.

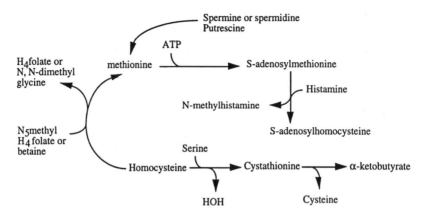

FIGURE 43 Conservation of SH groups via methionine cysteine interconversion.

METHYLMALONIC ACIDEMIA

Accumulation of methyl malonic acid in the blood; can be due to a genetic error but also is a characteristic of vitamin B_{12} deficiency.

MICELLES

Aggregates of bile salts, phospholipids, glycerides, and cholesterol. They range in size from 40–600 Å. Micelles are structured such that the hydrophobic portions (triglycererols, cholesterol esters, etc.) are toward the center of the structure while the hydrophilic portions (phospholipids, short chain fatty acids, bile salts) surround this center. The micelles contain many different lipids. Mixed micelles have a disc-like shape wherein the lipids form a bilayer and the bile acids occupy edge positions rendering the edge of the disc hydrophilic. During the process of lipase and esterase digestion of the lipids in the chyme, the water-insoluble lipids are rendered soluble and transferred from the lipid emulsion of the chyme to the micelle. In turn, these micelles transfer the products of digestion (free fatty acids, glycerol, cholesterol, etc.) from the intestinal lumen to the surface of the epithelial cells where absorption takes place. The micellar fluid layer next to this cell surface is homogenous, yet, the products of lipid digestion are presented to the cell surface and, by passive diffusion, these products are transported into the absorptive cell. Thus, the degree to which dietary lipid is absorbed once digested depends largely on the amount of lipid to be absorbed relative to the amount of bile acid available to make the micelle. This, in turn, is dependent on the rate of bile acid synthesis by the liver and bile release by the gall bladder. Once the fat has been absorbed, the bile acids pass on through the intestine where they are either reabsorbed for reuse or conjugated and excreted in the feces.

MICROANGIOPATHY

Thickening of the capillary basement membrane.

MICROCYTIC HYPOCHROMIC ANEMIA

Anemia characterized by a low number of small red cells which contain less than normal amounts of hemoglobin (see Table 8).

MICROFLORA

Advantageous bacteria that thrive in the gastrointestinal tract.

MICRONUTRIENTS

A group of nutrients (vitamins and minerals) required in small amounts.

MICROVASCULAR

Capillaries; vessels of a diameter sufficient for the passage of red blood cells one at a time.

MID-ARM CIRCUMFERENCE

An anthropometric measure used to calculate total arm area as part of an estimate of body fat and muscle mass.

MILK ALKALI SYNDROME

Condition resulting from excessive ingestion of milk and absorbable antacids which causes increased serum calcium and renal dysfunction.

MILLIEQUIVALENT

A measurement of the concentration of electrolytes in solution that is determined by multiplying the milligrams per liter by the valence of the chemical and dividing by the molecular weight of the substance:

$$mEq/L = \frac{(mg/L) \cdot Valence}{molecular\ weight}$$

A measurement of the osmotic activity of a solution that is determined by dividing the milliequivalent value by its valence.

MINERALS

Mineral salts comprise a large number of elements necessary for growth and maintenance of the cellular and metabolic systems. An important factor in the toxicity of minerals is their solubility in an aqueous environment, e.g., the contents of the digestive tract. Sodium and potassium salts are readily soluble in water and thus available for uptake from the intestine. Several other elements, such as iron, calcium, and phosphorus, are present in complex salts which are relatively insoluble. These elements are not easily absorbed from the gut. After intake, the major part of the insoluble salts appears in the feces. Minerals are important constituents of bones and teeth. Minerals may be integral parts of biologically important compounds such as hemoglobin and the cytochromes. Minerals also serve as required cofactors for enzymatic reactions. Minerals may be divided into two groups based on the levels at which they occur in the body: (1) elements that are present in considerable amounts (e.g., iron, calcium, sodium, potassium, chloride, magnesium, and phosphorus; combined mass: ± 3 kg); and 2) elements which are required in very small amounts only, the so-called trace elements (e.g., zinc, iodine, selenium, copper, manganese, fluorine, chromium, and molybdenum; combined mass: ± 30 g). Table 30 lists these minerals and their functions.

MITOCHONDRION

Organelle in the cell responsible for respiration coupled with ATP synthesis; fatty acid oxidation; initiation of urea synthesis (see Table 14 and Figure 13).

MITRAL INSUFFICIENCY

Failure of the mitral valve of the heart to close completely causing blood to flow backward from left ventricle to left atrium during ventricular contraction.

TABLE 30
Minerals as Essential Dietary Components

Function	Deficiencies and Toxicity Symptoms	Sources	Comments
	Macrominerals		
Calcium (Ca) The primary function of calcium is to build the bones and teeth and to maintain the bones. Other functions are: 1. Blood clotting. 2. Muscle contraction and relaxation, especially the heartbeat. 3. Nerve transmission. 4. Cell wall permeability. 5. Enzyme activation. 6. Secretion of a number of hormones and hormone-releasing factors.	Deficiency symptoms: 1. Stunting of growth. 2. Poor quality bones and teeth. 3. Malformation of bones — rickets. The clinical manifestations of calcium related diseases are: 1. Rickets in children. 2. Osteomalacia, the adult counterpart of rickets. 3. Osteoporosis, a condition of too little bone, resulting when bone resorption exceeds bone formation. 4. Hypercalcemia, characterized by high serum calcium. 5. Tetany, characterized by muscle spasms and muscle pain. 6. Kidney stones. Toxicity — Normally, the small intestine prevents excess calcium from being absorbed. However, a breakdown of this control may raise the level of calcium in the blood and lead to calcification of the kidneys and other internal organs. High calcium intake may cause excess secretion of calcitonin and very dense bones. High calcium intakes have also been reported to cause kidney stones.	Cheeses, wheat-soy flour, blackstrap molasses, milk, and milk products.	Calcium is the most abundant mineral in the body. It comprises about 40% of the total mineral present; 99% of it is in the bones and teeth. Generally, nutritionists recommend a calcium–phosphorus ratio of 1.5:1 in infancy, decreasing to 1:1 at 1 year of age and remaining at 1:1 throughout the rest of life; although they consider ratios between 2:1 and 1:2 as satisfactory.

Phosphorus (P)

Essential for bone formation and maintenance. Important in the development of teeth. Essential for normal milk secretion. Important in building muscle tissue. As a component of nucleic acids (RNA and DNA), which are important in genetic transmission and control of cellular metabolism. Maintenance in many metabolic functions especially:
1. Energy utilization.
2. Phospholipid formation;
3. Amino acid metabolism; protein formation.
4. Enzyme systems.

Deficiency symptoms — General weakness, loss of appetite, muscle weakness, bone pain, and loss of calcium. Severe and prolonged deficiencies of phosphorus may be manifested by rickets, osteomalacia, and other phosphorus related diseases.
Toxicity — There is no known phosphorus toxicity per se. However, excess phosphate consumption may cause hypocalcemia (a deficiency of calcium in the blood).

Cocoa powder, cottonseed flour, fish flour, peanut flour, pumpkin and squash seeds, rice bran, rice polish, soybean flour, sunflower seeds, wheat, and bran.

Phosphorus comprises about 1/4 the total mineral matter in the body. Eighty percent of the phosphorus is in the bones and teeth in inorganic combination with calcium. Normally, 70% of the ingested phosphorus is absorbed. Generally, nutritionists recommend a calcium–phosphorus ratio of 1.5:1 in infancy, decreasing to 1:1 at 1 year of age, and remaining at 1:1 throughout the rest of life, although they consider ratios between 2:1 and 1:2 as satisfactory.

Sodium (Na)

Helps to maintain the balance of water, acids, and bases in the fluid outside the cells. As a constituent of pancreatic juice, bile, sweat, and tears. Associated with muscle contraction and nerve functions. Plays a specific role in the absorption of carbohydrates.

Deficiency symptoms — Reduced growth, loss of appetite, loss of body weight due to loss of water, reduced milk production of lactating mothers, muscle cramps, nausea, diarrhea, and headache. Excess perspiration and salt depletion may be accompanied by heat exhaustion.
Toxicity — Salt may be toxic when (1) a high intake is accompanied by a restriction of water, (2) when the body is adapted to a chronic low salt diet, or (3) when it is fed to infants or others whose kidneys cannot excrete the excess in the urine.

Table salt, processed meat products, and pickled/cured products.

Deficiencies of sodium may occur when there has been heavy, prolonged sweating, diarrhea, vomiting, or adrenal cortical insufficiency. In such cases, extra salt should be taken.

Chlorine (Cl)

Plays a major role in the regulation of osmotic pressure, water balance, and acid-base balance. Required for the production of hydrochloric acid in the stomach; this acid is necessary for the proper absorption of Vitamin B-12 and iron, for the activation of the enzyme that breaks down starch, and for suppressing the growth of microorganisms that enter the stomach with food and drink.

Deficiency symptoms — Severe deficiencies may result in alkalosis (an excess of alkali in the blood), characterized by slow and shallow breathing, listlessness, muscle cramps, loss of appetite, and, occasionally, by convulsions. Deficiencies of chloride may develop from prolonged and severe vomiting, diarrhea, pumping of the stomach, injudicious use of diuretic drugs. Toxicity — An excess of chlorine ions is unlikely when the kidneys are functioning properly.

Table salt (sodium chloride) and foods that contain salt.

Persons whose sodium intake is severely restricted (owing to diseases of the heart, kidney, or liver) may need an alternative source of chloride; a number of chloride-containing salt substitutes are available for this purpose.

TABLE 30 (CONTINUED)
Minerals as Essential Dietary Components

Function	Deficiencies and Toxicity Symptoms	Sources	Comments
Magnesium (Mg) Constituent of bones and teeth. Essential element of cellular metabolism, often as an activator of enzymes involved in phosphorylated compounds and of high energy phosphate transfer of ADP and ATP. Involved in activating certain peptidases in protein digestion. Relaxes nerve impulse, functioning antagonistically to calcium which is stimulatory.	Deficiency symptoms — A deficiency of magnesium is characterized by (1) muscle spasms (tremor, twitching) and rapid heartbeat; (2) confusion, hallucinations, and disorientation; and (3) lack of appetite, listlessness, nausea, and vomiting. Toxicity — Magnesium toxicity is characterized by slowed breathing, coma, and sometimes death.	Rich sources — Coffee (instant), cocoa powder, cottonseed flour, peanut flour, sesame seeds, soybean flour, spices, wheat bran, and wheat germ.	Overuse of such substances as "milk of magnesia" (magnesium hydroxide) or "Epsom salts" (magnesium sulfate) may lead to deficiencies of other minerals or even to toxicity.
Potassium (K) Involved in the maintenance of proper acid-base balance and the transfer of nutrients in and out of individual cells. Relaxes the heart muscle — action opposite to that of calcium which is stimulatory. Required for the secretion of insulin by the pancreas in enzyme reactions involving the phosphorylation.	Deficiency symptoms — Potassium deficiency may cause rapid and irregular heartbeats and abnormal electrocardiograms; muscle weakness, irritability, and occasionally paralysis; and nausea, vomiting, diarrhea, and swollen abdomen. Extreme and prolonged deficiency of potassium may cause hypokalemia, culminating in the heart muscles stopping. Toxicity — Acute toxicity from potassium (known as hyperpotassemia or hyperkalemia) can result when kidneys are not functioning properly. The condition may prove fatal due to cardiac arrest.	Dehydrated fruits, molasses, potato flour, rice bran, seaweed, soybean flour, spices, sunflower seeds, and wheat bran.	Potassium is the third most abundant element in the body, after calcium and phosphorus, and it is present in twice the concentration of sodium
Cobalt (Co) The only known function of cobalt is that of an integral part of Vitamin B-12, an essential factor in the formation of red blood cells.	A cobalt deficiency as such has never been produced in humans. The signs and symptoms that are sometimes attributed to cobalt deficiency are actually due to lack of Vitamin B-12, characterized by pernicious anemia, poor growth, and occasionally neurological disorders.	Cobalt is present in many foods.	Cobalt is an essential constituent of Vitamin B-12 and must be ingested in the form of vitamin molecule inasmuch as humans synthesize little of the vitamin. (A small amount of Vitamin B-12 is synthesized in the human colon by *E. coli*, but absorption is very limited.)

Copper (Cu)

Facilitating the absorption of iron from the intestinal tract and releasing it from storage in the liver and the reticuloendothelial system. Essential for the formation of hemoglobin, although it is not a part of hemoglobin as such. Constituent of several enzyme systems. Development and maintenance of the vascular and skeletal structures (blood vessels, tendons, and bones).

Structure and function of the central nervous system. Required for normal pigmentation of hair. Component of important copper-containing proteins. Reproduction (fertility).

Deficiency symptoms — Deficiency is most apt to occur in malnourished children and in premature infants fed exclusively on modified cow's milk and in infants breast fed for an extended period of time.

Deficiency leads to a variety of abnormalities, including anemia, skeletal defects, demyelination and degeneration of the nervous system, defects in pigmentation and structure of the hair, reproductive failure, and pronounced cardiovascular lesions.

Toxicity — Copper is relatively nontoxic to monogastric species, including man. The recommended copper intake for adults is in the range of 2–3 mg/day. Daily intakes of more than 20–30 mg over extended periods would be expected to be unsafe.

Black pepper, blackstrap molasses, Brazil nuts, cocoa, liver, and oysters (raw).

Most cases of copper poisoning result from drinking water or beverages that have been stored in copper tanks and/or pass through copper pipes.

Dietary excesses of calcium, iron, cadmium, zinc, lead, silver, and molybdenum plus sulfur reduce the utilization of copper.

Fluorine (F)

Constitutes 0.02–0.05% of the bones and teeth. Necessary for sound bones and teeth. Assists in the prevention of dental caries.

Deficiency symptoms — Excess dental caries. Also, there is indication that a deficiency of fluorine results in osteoporosis in the aged.

Toxicity — Deformed teeth and bones, and softening, mottling, and irregular wear of the teeth.

Fluorine is found in many foods, but seafoods and dry tea are the richest food sources.

Fluoridation of water supplies to bring the concentration of fluoride to 1 ppm.

Large amounts of dietary calcium, aluminum, and fat will lower the absorption of fluorine. Fluoridation of water supplies (1 ppm) is the simplest and most effective method of providing added protection against dental caries.

Iodine (I)

The sole function of iodine is making the iodine-containing thyroid hormones.

Deficiency symptoms — Iodine deficiency is characterized by goiter (an enlargement of the thyroid gland at the base of the neck), coarse hair, obesity, and high blood cholesterol.

Iodine-deficient mothers may give birth to infants with a type of dwarfism known as cretinism, a disorder characterized by malfunctioning of the thyroid gland, goiter, mental retardation, and stunted growth. A similar disorder of the thyroid gland, known as myxedema, may develop in adults.

Toxicity — Long-term intake of large excesses of iodine may disturb the utilization of iodine by the thyroid gland and result in goiter.

Among natural foods the best sources of iodine are kelp, seafoods, and vegetables grown in iodine-rich soils and iodized salt. Stabilized iodized salt contains 0.01% potassium iodide (0.0076% I), or 76 mcg of iodine per gram.

Certain foods (especially plants of the cabbage family) contain goitrogens, which interfere with the use of thyroxine and may produce goiter. Fortunately, goitrogenic action is prevented by cooking.

TABLE 30 (CONTINUED)
Minerals as Essential Dietary Components

Function	Deficiencies and Toxicity Symptoms	Sources	Comments
Iron (Fe) Iron (heme) combines with protein (globin) to make hemoglobin, the iron-containing compound in red blood cells which transports oxygen. Iron is also a component of enzymes which are involved in energy metabolism.	Deficiency symptoms — Iron-deficiency (nutritional) anemia, the symptoms of which are: paleness of skin and mucous membranes, fatigue, dizziness, sensitivity to cold, shortness of breath, rapid heartbeats, and tingling of the fingers and toes. An excess of iron in the diet can tie up phosphorus in an insoluble iron-phosphate complex, thereby creating a deficiency of phosphorus.	Red meat, egg yolk, and dark green, leafy vegetables.	About 70% of the iron is present in the hemoglobin, the pigment of the red blood cells. The other 30% is present as a reserve store in the liver, spleen, and bone marrow.
Manganese (Mn) Formation of bone and the growth of other connective tissues. Blood clotting. Insulin action. Cholesterol synthesis. Activator of various enzymes in the metabolism of carbohydrates, fats, proteins, and nucleic acids.	Deficiency symptoms — No clear deficiency disease in man has been reported. Toxicity — Toxicity in man as a consequence of dietary intake has not been observed. However, it has occurred in workers (miners and others) exposed to high concentrations of manganese dust in the air. The symptoms resemble those found in Parkinson's and Wilson's disease.	Rice (brown), rice bran and polish, walnuts, wheat bran, and wheat germ.	In average diets, only about 45% of the ingested magnesium is absorbed. The manganese content of plants is dependent on soil content.
Molybdenum (Mo) As a component of three different enzyme systems which are involved in the metabolism of carbohydrates, fats, proteins, sulfur-containing amino acids, nucleic acids (DNA and RNA), and iron. As a component of the enamel of teeth.	Deficiency symptoms — Naturally occurring deficiency in man is not known. Molybdenum-deficient animals are especially susceptible to the toxic effects of bisulfite, characterized by breathing difficulties and neurological disorders. Severe molybdenum toxicity in animals (molybdenosis), particularly cattle, occurs throughout the world wherever pastures are grown on high-molybdenum soils. The symptoms include diarrhea, loss of weight, decreased production, fading of hair color, and other symptoms of copper deficiency.	The concentration of molybdenum in food varies considerably, depending on the soil in which it is grown. Most of the dietary molybdenum intake is derived from organ meats, whole grains, leafy vegetables, legumes, and yeast.	The utilization of molybdenum is reduced by excess copper, sulfate, and tungsten. In cattle, a relationship exists between molybdenum, copper, and sulfur. Excess molybdenum will cause copper deficiency. However, when the sulfate content of the diet is increased, the symptoms of toxicity are avoided inasmuch as the excretion of molybdenum is increased.

Selenium (Se)			
Component of the enzyme glutathione peroxidase, the metabolic role of which is to protect against oxidation of polyunsaturated fatty acids and resultant tissue damage.	Deficiency symptoms — There are no clear-cut deficiencies of selenium, because this mineral is so closely related to vitamin E that it is difficult to distinguish deficiency due to selenium alone. Toxicity — Poisonous effects of selenium are manifested by (1) abnormalities of the hair, nails, and skin; (2) garlic odor on the breath; (3) intensification of selenium toxicity by arsenic or mercury; and (4) higher than normal rates of dental caries.	The selenium content of plant and animal products is affected by the selenium content of the soil and animal feed, respectively. Brazil nuts, butter, flour, fish, lobster, and smelt.	The high selenium areas are in Great Plains and the Rocky Mountain states — especially in parts of the Dakotas and Wyoming.
Zinc (Zn) Needed for normal skin, bones, and hair. As a component of several different enzyme systems which are involved in digestion and respiration. Required for the transfer of carbon dioxide in red blood cells; for proper calcification of bones; for the synthesis and metabolism of proteins and nucleic acids; for the development and functioning of reproductive organs; for wound and burn healing; for the functioning of insulin; and for normal taste acuity.	Deficiency symptoms--Loss of appetite, stunted growth in children, skin changes, small sex glands in boys, loss of taste sensitivity, lightened pigment in hair, white spots on the fingernails, and delayed healing of wounds. In the Middle East, pronounced zinc deficiency in man has resulted in hypogonadism and dwarfism. In pregnant animals, experimental zinc deficiency has resulted in malformation and behavioral disturbances in offspring. Toxicity — Ingestion of excess soluble salts may cause nausea, vomiting, and purging.	Beef, liver, oysters, spices, and wheat bran.	The biological availability of zinc in different foods varies widely; meats and seafoods are much better sources of available zinc than vegetables. Zinc availability is adversely affected by phytates (found in whole grains and beans), high calcium, oxalates (in rhubarb and spinach), high fiber, copper (from drinking water conveyed in copper piping), and EDTA (an additive used in certain canned foods).

Adapted from Ensminger et al., *Foods and Nutrition Encyclopedia*, 2nd ed., CRC Press, Boca Raton, FL, 1994, pp. 1511–1521.

MITRAL STENOSIS

Failure of the mitral valve of the heart to open completely from severe narrowing of the mitral valve orifice.

MITRAL VALVE PROLAPSE

A form of mitral insufficiency that occurs when one or more of the mitral leaflets of this valve protrudes into the left atrium during systole leading to blood regurgitation from the left ventricle into the left atrium.

MOBILE GLUCOSE TRANSPORTERS

Glucose specific transport proteins, sequestered in the cell which, when needed, migrate to the cell surface, bind to glucose, and transport it through the plasma membrane to its site of use. There are several different proteins involved. They are identified as GLUT 1, 2, 3, 4, and 5 (see Tables 24 and 25).

MOLYBDENUM

An essential mineral; serves as a cofactor for xanthine oxidase, aldehyde oxidase, and sulfate oxidase. High intakes of molybdenum increase copper excretion (see minerals, Table 30).

MONOAMINE OXIDASE INHIBITORS

Group of medications used to treat depression. If consumed with tyramine-containing foods can cause severe hypertension.

MONOGLYCERIDE (MONOACYLGLYCEROL)

A glycerol having only one fatty acid esterified to it.

MONOMERIC FORMULA

Specialized formulation of hydrolyzed macronutrients.

MONOSACCHARIDE

A simple sugar containing only one saccharide unit.

MONOSODIUM GLUTAMATE (VE-TSIN, MSG)

An additive involved in idiosyncratic food intolerance reactions. Salts of glutamic acid are used as flavorings, for instance in chinese food, soup, meat products, and heavily spiced foods. Well-known is the "Chinese restaurant syndrome." Symptoms can include tightness of the chest, headache, nausea, vomiting, abdominal cramps, and even shock. In asthmatic patients, ve-tsin may cause bronchoconstriction. The first symptoms may appear after 15 min, while an interval of 24 hours has also been described. The mechanism underlying this syndrome is not known.

MONOUNSATURATED FATTY ACID

A fatty acid having only one double bond; a common one is oleic acid (16 carbons; one double bond). Olive oil contains oleic acid.

mRNA

Messenger RNA. Short lived species of RNA which carries the code for the synthesis of specific compounds (peptides or proteins) from the nucleus to the ribosome.

MORBIDITY
Illness leading to death.

MORTALITY
Cause of death.

MUCOPOLYSACCHARIDE
A group of complex carbohydrates containing hexosamine; a thick gelatinous material.

MUCOSA
Mucus secreting membrane.

MUCUS
A polypeptide containing a carbohydrate, usually a hexosamine.

MUCUS MEMBRANE
A membrane lining the cavities and canals of the body kept moist by the secretion of mucus.

MULTIPAROUS
A woman who has had more than one pregnancy.

MULTIPLE SCLEROSIS
A chronic disease characterized by demyelination of nerve fibers with accompanying motor and sensory deficits.

MUSCULAR DYSTROPHY
An inherited disorder characterized by a gradual muscle wasting and loss.

MUSH
A hot cereal made by boiling cornmeal in water.

MUTAGENS
Chemicals which cause changes in the base sequence of DNA.

MUTATION
When the sequence of bases in the DNA is disturbed by either a deletion or substitution of one or more of the bases, the code is said to be mutated and the protein coded by this sequence will not be synthesized in its normal amino acid sequence. The amino acid sequence determines the shape and function of the protein. Many mutations occur that have an effect on this sequence but have **no effect** on function because the substitution or deletion does not occur in the active or working part of the protein molecule.

MUTTON
Meat from mature sheep.

MUTUAL SUPPLEMENTATION
Food blends that provide the optimal array of essential amino acids.

MYASTHENIA GRAVIS

Autoimmune disease characterized by chronic, progressive muscle fatigue and weakness, especially in the face and throat.

MYCOTOXINS

Secondary metabolites of fungi which can induce acute as well as chronic toxic effects (i.e., carcinogenicity, mutagenicity, teratogenicity, and estrogenic effects) in animals and man. According to habitat, mycotoxin-producing fungi can be classified as: (1) fungi infecting living plants (e.g., *Aspergillus flavus, Claviceps purpurea,* and *Fusarium graminearum*); (2) fungi infecting stored food products (e.g., *Aspergillus flavus, Aspergillus ochraceus,* and *Aspergillus parasiticus, Fusarium graminearum, Penicillium expansum, Penicillium viridicatum*); and (3) fungi infecting decaying organic matter (e.g., *Fusarium graminearum*). Some important mycotoxins are aflatoxins, sterigmatocystin, ochratoxins, patulin, trichothecenes, zearalenone, and ergot alkaloids. Toxic syndromes resulting from the intake of mycotoxins by animals and man are known as mycotoxicoses. Well-known examples of mycotoxicoses include "Holy Fire" in Europe caused by the mould *Claviceps purpurea,* "Alimentary Toxic Aleukia" in the Soviet Union caused by *Fusarium* spp., and "Yellow Rice Disease" in Japan caused by *Penicillium* spp. Factors affecting mould growth, mycotoxin production, and infection of foods and feeds are:

1. moisture (growth — in general, water activity ≥0.80);
2. temperature (growth — psychrophile moulds [optimum temperature: <10°C]; mesophile moulds [optimum temperature: 10–40°C]; and thermophile moulds [optimum temperature: >40°C]);
3. mechanical, insect, and mould damage;
4. time (in general, there is a lag between mould growth and mycotoxin production);
5. types of substrates and nutritional factors;
6. atmospheric oxygen and carbon dioxide levels (moulds are highly aerobic and require a minimum amount of atmospheric oxygen for growth and efficient mycotoxin production);
7. chemical treatment;
8. presence of other moulds; and
9. geographical location.

Thus, mycotoxin contamination of food and feed depends on the environmental conditions that lead to mould growth and toxin production. The detectable presence of live moulds in food does not automatically indicate that mycotoxins have been produced. On the other hand, the absence of viable moulds in foods does not necessarily mean that there are no mycotoxins. The latter could have been formed at an earlier stage, prior to food processing. Because of their chemical stability, several mycotoxins persist during food processing, while the moulds are destroyed. Since the discovery of the aflatoxins, probably no commodity can be regarded as absolutely free from mycotoxins. Also, mycotoxin production can occur in the field, during harvest, processing, storage, and shipment of a given commodity.

MYELIN

The fatty coating of nerves.

MYOCARDIAL INFARCTION

Heart attack. Occurs when one or more of the coronary vessels is occluded and heart muscle fails to receive sufficient oxygen and dies. The term infarction refers to the fact that the depolarization of the muscle just prior to contraction (a part of the pumping action of the heart) cannot spread across this dead part of the muscle. The presence of this infarction can be detected by an electrocardiograph which documents the depolarization and repolarization of the heart muscle.

MYOCARDIUM

Heart muscle.

MYOGLOBIN

Iron-containing globulin in muscle.

MYOSIN

Muscle cell protein which (with actin) plays a role in muscle contraction and relaxation.

MYRISTICIN

A methylenedioxyphenyl substance. It is found in nutmeg and mace, and in lesser quantities in black pepper, parsley, celery, dill, and carrots. Nutmeg produces effects similar to alcoholic intoxication. Reportedly these spices have been frequently used as narcotics by prison inmates. Around 5–15 g of nutmeg powder can produce euphoria, hallucinations, and narcosis. The side effects however, are very unpleasant and severe — headache, nausea, abdominal pain, delirium, hypotension, depression, acidosis, stupor, shock and, in large doses, liver damage and death.

MYXEDEMA

Advanced deficiency of thyroxine.

N

Na⁺K⁺ PUMP

See active transport. An energy dependent pump that operates to keep Na⁺ on the outside of cells and K⁺ on the inside of cells.

NAD, NADH, NADP, NADPH

Niacin-containing coenzymes which function as carriers for hydrogen ions in dehydrogenase catalyzed reactions.

NAPTHAQUINONE

A derivative of quinone that has some Vitamin K activity.

NASOGASTRIC TUBE

Tube inserted through the nose and ending in the stomach that carries liquid nourishment.

NATIONAL CENTER FOR HEALTH STATISTICS (NCHS) (U.S.)

An agency which collects data on the causes of death and disease in the United States as well as in other nations.

NATIONAL HEALTH EXAMINATION SURVEY (NHANES) (U.S.)

Data collected at intervals to document the usual types and amounts of food consumed as related to a variety of measurements of body size and body function. Assessments of health status are part of this survey.

NATIONAL RESEARCH COUNCIL (NRC)

A division of the U.S. National Academy of Sciences established in 1916 to promote the effective utilization of scientific and technical resources.

NATIONAL SCIENCE FOUNDATION (NSF) (U.S.)

A U.S. government funding organization for the basic sciences

NATIONWIDE FOOD CONSUMPTION SURVEY (NFCS) (U.S.)

Data collected to document the kinds and amounts of food consumed in the United States.

NATURALLY OCCURRING TOXICANTS

Products of the metabolic processes of animals, plants, and microorganisms from which the food products are derived.

NAUSEA

Upset stomach associated with the urge to vomit.

NECROSIS

Cellular changes that occur and are indicative of cellular death.

NEONATAL

The first 4 weeks after birth.

NEONATAL JAUNDICE

An accumulation of bilirubin under the skin of the newborn infant giving the infant a yellowish hue.

NEONATAL HEMORRHAGING

Excessive blood loss by the neonate.

NEONATE

A newborn animal. In the human, a neonate is an infant of <4 weeks of age.

NEPHRON

The basic structural unit of the kidney which functions to filter the blood of waste products for excretion in the urine. This unit reabsorbs water and conserves sodium under the influence of antidiuretic hormone (ADH). The nephron consists of a tuft of capillaries known as the glomerulus and the renal tubule. The average adult human kidney contains about one million glomeruli.

NEPHROSCLEROSIS

Hardening of the vessels (arteries) of the kidney.

NEPHROTIC SYNDROME

Kidney damage characterized by increased permeability in renal tubules and loss of protein in the glomerular filtrate.

NEURITIS

Inflammation of nerve endings.

NEUROTRANSMITTER

A chemical signal for nerve action. Serotonin, epinephrine, and acetylcholine, for example, are neurotransmitters.

NEUTROPENIA

Elevated levels of neutrophils in blood.

NIACIN (B3)

A vitamin which serves as an essential component of the coenzymes NAD and NADP and can be synthesized from tryptophan. Nicotinamide is the active form of vitamin in the body. Can also exist as nicotinic acid (see vitamins, Table 49).

NIACINAMIDE

See Niacin (see vitamins, Table 49).

NICKEL

A mineral which may or may not be essential to the human. It is needed in trace amounts by growing chicks.

NICOTINIC ACID

See Niacin (see vitamins, Table 49).

NIEMAN PECK DISEASE

A genetic disease in which a mutation in the gene for sphingolipid degradating enzyme (sphingomylinase) has occurred. The disease is characterized by CNS degeneration and very early (under 3 years) death.

NIGHT BLINDNESS

First symptom of Vitamin A deficiency. The individual is unable to adapt to changes in light intensity. Is reversible if the vitamin is provided (see vitamins, Table 49).

NIH — NATIONAL INSTITUTES OF HEALTH (U.S.)

Located primarily in Bethesda, Maryland. One of the largest U.S. government funded health and disease research centers.

NITRATE (NO₃⁻)

The principal natural source of nitrate in the biosphere is microbial nitrification. This process is responsible for the nitrate conversion of ammonia in fertilizers, used either as such or in the form of urea, derived from the decomposition of human and animal waste matter. The nitrification reaction is a two-step process: (1) $2NH_4^+ + 3O_2$ becomes $2NO_2^- + 2H_2O + 4H^+$ (by chemoautotrophic nitrifiers, e.g., species of Nitrosomonas, Nitrospira, and Nitrosolabus); and (2) $NO_2^- + 1/2\ O_2$ becomes NO_3^- (by nitrite oxidizers, e.g., species of Nitrobacter, Nitrospira, and Nitrococcus). Counteracting the accumulation of nitrate in the biosphere are the denitrifying bacteria and fungi, which are capable of reducing nitrate to nitrite, or in some cases to ammonia. Because contamination with nitrogen compounds results in an increase of the nitrate concentration of ground water, levels of nitrate in drinking water and foods (of plant origin) can be increased as well. Nitrate has been reported to occur in several foods, such as vegetables (e.g., asparagus, beets, beans, broccoli, cabbage, carrots, celery, corn, cucumbers, eggplant, lettuce, melons, onion, peas, sweet peppers, pickles, potatoes, pumpkin, spinach, sauerkraut, and tomatoes), breads, all fruits, juices, cured meats, milk and milk products, and water. Since the nitrate content of the reported foods varies greatly, the level of consumption is also important. Foodstuffs contributing most to the total nitrate intake include potatoes (14.2 mg/person/day), lettuce (18.9 mg/person/day), and celery (16.0 mg/person/day). Oral toxicity of nitrate can be due to the nitrate ion per se or to the microbial conversion of nitrate to nitrite *in situ* in the food and in the mouth or gastrointestinal tract. In general, nitrate has a low oral toxicity because it is rapidly excreted in the urine. Repeated large doses of nitrate can cause dyspepsia, mental depression, headache, and weakness. The intake of nitrate via food consumption is estimated at 1.4–2.5 mg/kg/day and from water at 0.3 mg/kg/day. The acceptable daily intake of nitrate is 3.64 mg/kg/day.

NITRITE (NO$_2^-$)

Produced by bacterial reduction of nitrate which may be present as a contaminant or food additive. The toxicological significance of nitrate lies in its easy conversion to nitrite by nitrifying bacteria that may be present in foodstuffs, the saliva, and in the gastrointestinal tract. Populations that are particularly at risk are: (1) those that lack the NADH-dependent methemoglobin reductase activity (e.g., infants under 1 year of age, subjects with hereditary familial methemoglobinemia), (2) those lacking erythrocyte glucose-6-phosphate dehydrogenase activity (e.g., certain Mediterranean and Middle-Eastern populations), (3) pregnant women, and (4) those with decreased stomach acidity as a result of such diseases as pernicious anemia, chronic gastritis, stomach ulcer, and cancer. An important toxic effect of nitrite is methemoglobinemia (i.e., an increased level of methemoglobin in the blood). Iron in hemoglobin is in the ferrous state (Fe^{2+}). When it is oxidized (e.g., by nitrite) to the ferric state (Fe^{3+}), hemoglobin is transformed to methemoglobin, which is incapable of transporting oxygen. There is normally a small amount of methemoglobin (1.7%) in the blood, and this level is maintained by methemoglobin reductase in the presence of NADH. At levels below 5%, no symptoms have been observed. Levels of 5–20% are associated with mild cyanosis; 20–40% with marked cyanosis, fatigue, and dyspnea; 40–60% with severe cyanosis, tachypnea, serious cardiopulmonary signs, tachycardia, and depression; and >60% with ataxia, coma, and death. Another important effect of nitrite is the formation of nitrosamine.

NITROGEN

An essential element that is a component of amino acids.

NITROGEN BALANCE

When the intake of protein is equal to the excretion of nitrogen in the urine and feces, the individual is in nitrogen balance. When excretion exceeds intake, negative nitrogen balance occurs. Positive balance is when intake exceeds excretion. This happens in growth while the former happens in tissue wasting or when intake is of poor quality or quantity of protein. The concept of nitrogen balance is illustrated in Figure 44.

NITROGLYCERINE

A vasodilator used to ease the pain of angina pectoris (pain in the chest due to insufficient oxygen supply to the heart).

NITROSAMINES

Formed outside or inside the body from precursors like amines, amides, and nitrites. The fundamental requirements are a secondary amino nitrogen and nitrous acid. Three types of nitrosamines can be distinguished: (1) dialkyl nitrosamines (e.g., dimethylnitrosamine, diethylnitrosamine), (2) cyclic nitrosamines (e.g., N-nitrosopiperidine, N-nitrosopyrrolidine), and (3) acylalkyl nitrosamines or nitrosamides (different types of nitrosoureas, thioureas, carbamates, carboxamides, and guanidines). The conditions in the alimentary tract from the mouth to the anus are conducive to nitrosamine formation. The most important factor inhibiting nitrosamine formation is ascorbic acid, which rapidly reacts with nitrite to form nitric oxide and dehydroascorbic acid. Other inhibitors are gallic acid, sodium sulfite, cysteine, tannins, and urea (only effective at pH 1–2). Occurrence of the different nitrosamines has been reported in several foodstuffs: (1) dimethylnitrosamine (e.g., fried bacon, luncheon meat, salami, sausages, fish [raw sable, salmon, and shad; smoked sable and salmon; smoked and nitrate or nitrite-treated sable, salmon, shad and salted marine fish], fish sauce, cheese, baby

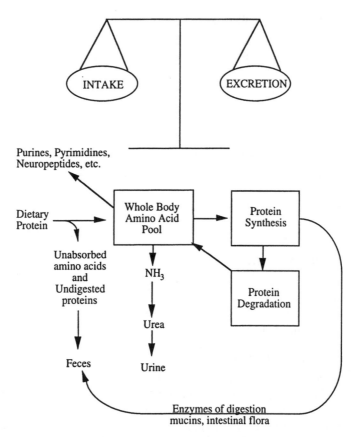

FIGURE 44 Nitrogen balance exists when the diet contains sufficient high-quality protein to provide amino acids for the synthesis of proteins lost through degradation. (From Berdanier, C.D., *Advanced Nutrition: Macronutrients*, CRC Press, Boca Raton, FL, 1994, 115.)

foods, dried shrimps, shrimp sauce, squid, uncooked canned meats, uncooked ham and other pork products, uncooked beef products, light and dark beers, and Scotch whisky); (2) diethyl-nitrosamine (e.g., fried bacon, luncheon meat, salami, and wheat flour); (3) nitrosopiperidine (e.g., fried bacon); and (4) nitrosopyrrolidine (e.g., fried bacon, fish sauce, dried shrimps, and squid). In animals, a large number of N-nitroso compounds have been shown to be carcinogenic. Factors enhancing the carcinogenicity of N-nitroso compounds are hormones, other carcinogens or toxicants, viral or bacterial infections, metals, and nutritional factors. The inhibitory factors can be identified as: (1) those that decrease the metabolism of the carcinogen (e.g., aminoacetonitrile [affects dimethylnitrosamine], dibenamine [affects dimethylnitrosamine], and phenobarbitone [affects diethylnitrosamine]); and (2) those that retard or interfere in the formation of the carcinogen (e.g., ascorbic acid, tannins, sulfite, and cysteine). Since no animal species that has been tested so far is resistant to dimethylnitro-samine or diethylnitrosamine, it is expected that humans are not resistant to the nitrosamines either. When the amounts of total nitrosamines in food, water, and other sources are added to those formed throughout the alimentary tract, the total nitrosamine load could be considerable.

NITROUS OXIDE (N₂O)

An inhalation anesthetic.

NO-OBSERVED-EFFECT LEVEL (NOEL)

The highest concentration of a substance which may be administered to a test animal in any way without causing that animal to be distinguishable from a control to which the substance is not administered.

NOCTURIA

Excessive urination during the night.

NONCALORIC SWEETENERS

See non-nutritive sweeteners, cyclamate, saccharine, and aspartame.

NONESSENTIAL AMINO ACIDS (NEAA)

Those amino acids that the body can synthesize in sufficient quantity to meet its need.

NONEXPERIMENTAL STUDIES

Studies in which the exposure is "chosen' by the subjects themselves. The investigator confines him/herself to observe the subjects and to collect data on their exposure and disease, without interfering with their way of life. Also known as observational studies. In general, four types of nonexperimental studies can be identified: (1) cross-sectional studies (possibilities — estimation of prevalence of exposure or disease; limitations — distinction between cause and effect is difficult); (2) follow-up or cohort studies (possibilities — (a) a large number of exposures and diseases can be studied, (b) exposure is determined before onset of the disease, and (c) estimation of the incidence of a disease; limitations — (a) during the follow-up period the investigators must keep track of all study subjects, (b) expensive (time and money), and (c) only suitable for frequently occurring diseases); (3) case-control studies (possibilities — (a) a large number of exposures can be studied — (b) the number of study subjects may be relatively small, and (c) suitable for rare diseases; limitations — exposure is determined after onset of the disease and reporting of exposure by the respondents might be affected by the disease), and (4) ecological studies (possibilities — can be used when information is only available on an aggregated level; limitations: ecological fallacy). The rank order from weak suggestions to strong evidence of a causal relation in the studies would be — ecological studies, cross-sectional studies, case-control studies, and finally follow-up or cohort studies.

NONHEME IRON

Iron in the body not associated with the heme of hemoglobin. Some of the cytochromes have iron as part of their active site.

NONIMMUNOLOGICAL DEFENSE MECHANISM

One of the defense mechanisms is the digestive tract, which forms a physical barrier against unwanted effects of food. The mucus membrane of the gut forms a protective barrier against penetration of pathogenic microorganisms and allergens. Also, the secretion of certain enzymes and gastric acid (which may lead to degradation of unwanted substances) and the enteric motility (which prevents excessive proliferation of bacteria in the small intestine as well as absorption of macromolecules through the digestive mucosa) contribute to the non-immunological defense.

NONINSULIN-DEPENDENT DIABETES MELLITUS (NIDDM)

A disease of aberrant glucose metabolism that can usually be managed without hormone replacement. A genetic disease. The range of disorders in man and laboratory animals that fit the description for NIDDM is far greater than that for IDDM. The disorders are summarized in Table 31. For most of the NIDDM disorders, obesity is a concurrent feature. This obesity either precedes or accompanies the development of abnormal glucose tolerance. The animals that are genetically obese usually overeat, and studies of the neuroendocrine influence on food intake have suggested that, in part, the genetic error in these animals may reside in the satiety signalling system in the brain. One feature of obesity that is common to NIDDM, is the resistance of the peripheral fat cell to the effects of insulin. The plasma membrane receptor on the fat cell may be aberrant in structure or number. If abnormal in structure, insulin may not bind efficiently to it. This may occur either because the receptor protein is abnormal or because the fat cell is enlarged by its stored fat and the receptor structure is distorted. When the fat cell shrinks, i.e., when the obese person loses a large percentage of excess stored fat, insulin binding is normalized. Insulin binding, in this instance, is directly related to fat cell size, which in turn is directly related to the size of its fat store. The insulin resistance, thus observed, refers to the particular abnormality of the fat cell insulin receptor conferred upon it by its excess fat store. Other abnormalities include mutations in the pancreatic insulin release mechanisms and mutations in one or more of the mobile glucose transporters.

TABLE 31
Abnormalities in Cells, Tissues, or Systems that are Associated with NIDDM

Abnormality[a]	Result
Amino acid substitution in A or B chains of insulin	Major, minor, or no effect on insulin activity
Amino acid substitution in C chain of proinsulin	No C chain cleavage to produce insulin
β cell glucokinase	Inability to recognize the glucose signal for insulin release
Obesity	Distortion of fat cell membrane insulin receptor; tissue insensitivity to insulin
Insulin receptor protein	Defective structure fails to fully bind insulin to the target cell membrane and/or fails to send signal to mobilize glucose transporters; tissue insensitivity to insulin
Mobile glucose transporters	Failure to move glucose into target cell
Intracellular enzymes	Failure to process glucose appropriately

[a] Within each of these disorders, several different mutations causing the same clinical state have been found.

From Berdanier, C.D., *Advanced Nutrition: Macronutrients*, CRC Press, Boca Raton, FL, 1994, 196.

Although mutations associated with diabetes mellitus are many and are of clinical and scientific interest, the management of the disease varies little. People with noninsulin-dependent diabetes mellitus are counseled to keep their body weight within the range of desirable weights for their height and sex, to maintain as much physical activity as possible, and, if needed, monitor their insulin needs according to their blood glucose levels.

NONINVASIVE TECHNIQUE

A medical treatment or procedure that does not involve surgery. X-rays, for example, are in this category of techniques.

NONSTEROIDAL ANTI-INFLAMMATORY DRUGS

Aspirin, indomethacin, and phenylbutazone; These drugs block the action of cyclooxygenase by acetylating the enzyme. While occasional use of these drugs for the occasional injury or headache is harmless, long term, chronic use can result in untoward effects. Long term, chronic use of aspirin, for example, can affect vascular competence and blood clotting. People consuming large amounts of aspirin over long periods of time may find an increase in bruises (subcutaneous hemorrhages). Small contact injuries that normally would not result in a bruise will do so in these people. Gastric bleeding is another possible complication with long term, chronic aspirin ingestion. Aplastic anemia can result from long term phenylbutazone therapy.

NONTROPICAL SPRUE

Malabsorption/diarrhea due to localized reaction to certain foods. See gluten-sensitive enteropathy.

NOREPINEPHRINE

A neurotransmitter released in response to stress; part of the "fight or flight" response. Acts as a vasoconstrictor. Produced by the adrenal medulla and the sympathetic nervous system. It is released by the nerve endings and crosses the nerve junctions to stimulate subsequent neural fibers.

NORMAL CLINICAL VALUES FOR BLOOD

See Table 32.

NOSOCOMIAL INFECTION

Infection that originated in a hospital.

NOSTRUM

Folk remedy which may be ineffective in treatment of a clinical condition.

NOVEL FOOD

A food that the consumer has never eaten or a food newly developed by food manufacturers.

NPU

Net protein use. A measure of the biological value of a dietary protein based on the amount of protein retained in the body as a percentage of that consumed.

NDp CAL %

Net protein calories percent. The percent of the total energy value of the diet provided by the protein.

NUCLEIC ACIDS

Chains of nucleotides whose function is to store and transmit the genetic information from one generation to the next. A nucleotide contains a ribose, 1–3 phosphate groups, and either a purine (adenine or guanine) or a pyrimidine (cytosine, uracil, or thymine).

TABLE 32
Normal Clinical Values for Blood

	Common Units or SI Units
Ammonia	22–39 μmol/l
Calcium	8.5–10.5 mg/dl or 2.25–2.65 mmol/l
Carbon dioxide	24–30 meq/l or 24–29 mmol/l
Chloride	100–106 meq/l or mmol/l
Copper	100–200 μg/dl or 16–31 μmol/l
Iron	50–150 μg/dl or 11.6–31.3 μmol/l
Lead	50 μg/dl or less
Magnesium	1.5–2.0 meq/l or 0.75–1.25 mmol/l
P CO_2	35–40 mm Hg
pH	7.35–7.45
Phosphorus	3.0–4.5 mg/dl or 1–1.5 mmol/l
PO_2	75–100 mm Hg
Potassium	3.5–5.0 meq/l or 2.5–5.0 mmol/l
Sodium	135–145 meq/l or 135–145 mmol/l
Acetoacetate	<2 mmol
Ascorbic acid	0.4–15 mg/dl or 23–85 μmol/l
Bilirubin	0.4–0.6 mg/dl or 1.71–6.84 μmol/l
Carotinoids	0.8–4.0 mg/ml
Creatinine	0.6–1.5 mg/dl or 60–130 μmol/l
Lactic acid	0.6–1.8 meq/l or 0.44–1.28 mmol/l
Cholesterol	120–220 mg/dl or 3.9–7.3 mmol/l
Triglycerides	40–150 mg/dl or 6–18 mmol/l
Pyruvic acid	0–0.11 meq/l or 79.8–228.0 μmol/l
Urea nitrogen	8–25 mg/dl or 2.86–7.14 mmol/l
Uric acid	3.0–7.0 mg/dl or 0.18–0.29 mmol/l
Vitamin A	0.15–0.6 μg/dl
Albumin	3.5–5.0 g/dl
Insulin	6–20 μU/dl
Glucose	70–100 mg/dl or 4–6 mmol/l

NUCLEUS

An organelle in the cell containing DNA, the genetic material plus the enzymes, coenzymes, and cofactors needed to synthesize mRNA which transfers genetic messages from the DNA to the ribosome where proteins are synthesized.

NUTRIENT DENSITY

The nutrient composition of food expressed in terms of nutrient quantity per 1000 kcal or 4200 kJ.

NUTRIENT REQUIREMENTS

The amounts of nutrients absolutely required by an individual to avoid the symptoms of deficiency disease and to optimize health and well being.

NUTRIENTS

The chemical substances present in food that are utilized by the body as components for synthesizing needed materials and for fuel.

NUTRITION SCREENING

Process of identifying characteristics associated with dietary and nutritional problems.

NUTRITION THERAPY

A component of medical treatment that includes enteral and parenteral nutrition as well as disease-specific therapeutic diets.

NUTRITION TREATMENT

Intervention, management, and counseling of individuals on appropriate food choices to meet their nutrient needs.

NUTRITIONAL ADEQUACY

A measure of the health and well being of the individual in relation to the intake of essential nutrients.

NUTRITIONAL ASSESSMENT

Measurement of indicators of dietary status and the nutrition-related health status of individuals or populations (see Tables 28 and 32).

NUTRITIONAL STATUS

The health of the individual with respect to nutrient intake

NUTRITIVE VALUE OF FOODS

The content of essential nutrients as assessed in an analytical laboratory. The nutrient content of many foods humans consume can be found in Tables of Composition compiled by The United States Department of Agriculture (Handbooks 8–15, U.S. Government Printing Office, Washington, D.C. 20402). Other tables are also available.

O

OBESITY

Excess accumulation of body fat (more than 20% of the body as fat). Although excess body fat stores, or obesity, is considered a risk factor in a number of diseases, we have no permanent cure for the disorder. Listed in Table 33 are some of the reasons why excess body fatness develops.

Research on the genetic basis for excess body fatness is very active. Several investigators have shown that the familial trait for body fatness has a much stronger influence on body composition than environmental influences such as culture, socioeconomic status, or food intake patterns. Studies of monozygotic and dizygotic twins reared by their biological parents or by adoptive parents have been conducted. In one study, adopted children and their biological and adoptive parents were compared with respect to body weight and body fatness while in other studies twins reared together or apart were compared. All these studies showed that the genetic influence far outweighed the environmental influence. Further, a number of genetically obese rats, mice, dogs, and desert animals have been described. In the rodent species, the mode of inheritance and, in some instances, the chromosomal location of genes for obesity have been identified. Obesity can be inherited via an autosomal-recessive, dominant, or sex-linked trait. There are several mutations that are phenotypically expressed as obesity. In each of these mutations, an error occurs that affects energy balance. Errors in the perception of hunger and/or satiety by the brain can explain the excess food intake (hyperphagia) that characterizes several of these mutants. Both inappropriate hunger signals and satiety signals have been implicated. Higher than normal food intake may also characterize the genetically obese human. Yet, there are many over fat people who are not hyperphagic. There are those who cannot dissipate their surplus intake energy as heat, i.e., thermogenesis (see section on brown fat thermogenesis). These individuals do not tolerate cold well either. The common

---

TABLE 33
Suggested Reasons Why Obesity May Develop

Genetic Errors

(a) Satiety signal not sent or perceived
(b) Inability to utilize stored energy
(c) Inability to increase thermogenesis to get rid of excess intake energy

Hormonal Imbalance

(a) Excess glucocorticoids
(b) Hypothyroidism
(c) Hyperinsulinism
(d) Inappropriate neuropeptide levels

Other Causes

(a) Injury to hypothalamus
(b) Sociocultural feeding behaviors

---

thread to these two conditions is the apparent inability of tissues to regulate the degree of uncoupling of its mitochondria so as to release more heat and synthesize less ATP. This ATP is used for the synthesis of macromolecules. It has also been attributed to a failure of the brown fat cell to respond to the stimulatory effects of epinephrine and is associated with an anomalous central regulation of the sympathetic input to this tissue.

Lastly, there are social and cultural influences that can ensure or potentiate genetic tendencies to develop obesity. Anthropologists and medical historians have identified examples of cultural groups that consider excess body fat as a mark of beauty as well as an indication of economic status within their society.

Morbidity of severely obese people

Health care professionals have observed countless instances of the codevelopment of excess body fat with diabetes mellitus, hypertension, and cardiovascular disease. Epidemiologists have reported that obesity and overweight are risk factors in the development of these diseases. However, there are some inconsistencies with respect to the relationship of obesity to cardiovascular disease and total mortality. Studies by the CDC and others suggest that weight loss by the obese does not positively affect lifespan. Long term studies of mortality by formerly obese people conducted by Williamson et al. of the CDC suggest the reverse. Their preliminary report indicates an increase in mortality in people who have consciously reduced their body fat and remained lean. This report has raised serious questions about the efficacy of weight loss with respect to lifespan extension.

Treatment of obesity

In almost no other area of medicine have there been so many failures as have occurred in the treatment of obesity. Fully 90% of all those who lose weight regain it.

The effects of weight cycling on energy efficiency may be due to the composition of the weight loss during calorie restriction. One of the consequences of rapid weight loss, especially when induced by very low calorie, low carbohydrate diets, is the loss of body protein or lean body mass (LBM). This is especially true when the individuals are physically inactive. Maintenance of LBM is an energy expensive process. Lean body mass is the most metabolically active tissue in the body with respect to energy demands, accounting for the majority of calories to support the basal energy requirement (i.e., 60–70% of daily basal energy requirements for adults). Therefore, the less body protein, the lower the energy requirement. If weight loss consists of significant amounts of body protein, then the formerly overfat person will have a lower basal energetic requirement and an increased energy efficiency in terms of the weight regain as fat.

Exercise on a regular basis stimulates muscle protein development as well as increases energy expenditure. Exercise can be a useful adjunct to energy intake restriction because it redirects energy loss from the lean body mass. In the sedentary individual, weight loss occurs at the expense of both fat and protein components of the body. In the exercising, food-restricted individual, the weight loss is primarily fat loss. Further, mild to moderate exercise seems to suppress food intake. Thus, food restriction together with exercise are additive in a beneficial way with respect to the loss and regain of body fat.

OBLIGATORY LOSS

Usually refers to the excretion of the products of one way reactions, as for example, the loss of nitrogen in creatinine, the product of the one way conversion of creatine to creatinine.

OCHRATOXINS

Mycotoxins produced by *Aspergillus ochraceus*, *Aspergillus* spp., and *Penicillium viridicatum*. They can be categorized as ochratoxin A, B, and C and 4-hydroxyochratoxin A.

Ochratoxin A, the most important ochratoxin, is a fairly stable substance which is not easily metabolized. It is a potent hepatotoxin (in rats, ducklings, and Babcock cockerels) and a nephrotoxin (in rats and pigs). The primary target organ is the developing central nervous system. Furthermore, it was reported to be teratogenic in mice and rats, whereas it was noncarcinogenic to rats by both oral and subcutaneous administration. Ochratoxin A production in cereals is favored under humid conditions at moderate temperatures. Occurrence of ochratoxin A has been reported in grains and, following transfer, in the organs and blood of a number of animals, especially pigs.

ODDS RATIO (OR)

A good approximation of the relative risk. It compares the ratio of exposed/unexposed individuals among the diseased with the ratio of exposed/unexposed individuals among the controls. The odds ratio is a measure that is used in case-control studies, where cases and controls are selected at the same time.

ODYNOPHAGIA

Pain associated with swallowing.

OILS

Fats that are liquid at room temperature (20–22°C). Usually of vegetable origin with the exception of the marine oils. These are the fats extracted from sea creatures and which are rich in the long chain polyunsaturated fatty acids.

OLESTRA

A synthetic fat that is a sucrose polyester. It has the texture of fat but does not have the energy value of fat.

OLIGURIA

Decreased urine production.

OMEGA-3 FATTY ACIDS

See fatty acids. Fatty acids having one or more double bonds in the omega-3 (N-3) position. The numbers begin at the methyl end of the molecule.

OMEGA-6 FATTY ACIDS

See fatty acids. Fatty acids having one or more double bonds in the omega-6 (N-6) position.

ONCOTIC PRESSURE

The pressure exerted by the plasma proteins on the walls of the vascular system. These proteins are too large to pass through the capillaries hence this pressure is noted only in the large vessels.

OPHTHALMIA

Inflammation of the conjunctiva (membrane that lines the eyelid) of the eye.

OPSIN

A protein which combines with retinal (Vitamin A aldehyde) to form rhodopsin (visual purple). Rhodopsin bleaches upon exposure to bright light and breaks apart. It is reformed and this process is called the visual cycle. The cycle does not function in the Vitamin A-deficient individual.

ORAL
Pertaining to the mouth.

ORGANELLE
A discrete structure within the cell.

ORGANIC
Substances containing carbon that originates from living creatures.

ORGANIC FOOD
A term usually taken to mean a food grown without the aid of fertilizers, herbicides, and pesticides. This is a misnomer since all foods are comprised of organic molecules and hence are organic.

ORGANOGENESIS
The development of specific organs in the course of embryonic and fetal development.

ORGANOLEPTIC
Features of a food perceived by the senses of taste, smell, sound, vision, and tactile, or feel.

ORNITHINE CYCLE
See urea cycle.

ORTHOSTATIC HYPOTENSION
Hypotension that results from standing and often associated with dehydration.

OSMOLALITY
Quantity of solutes per liter of solution that contributes to the pressure of that solution on a membrane.

OSMOSIS
The passage of solvents across a membrane so as to equalize the concentrations of solutes on each side of the membrane

OSMOTIC EFFECT
The effects of solutes on water passage.

OSMOTIC PRESSURE
The pressure that must be applied to prevent the passage of a solvent. Only those solutes that cannot pass through a membrane can contribute to osmotic pressure.

OSSIFICATION
The process of bone formation.

OSTEOARTHRITIS

Degenerative bone and joint disease due to wear and tear; age-associated.

OSTEOBLASTS

Bone forming cells.

OSTEOCALCIN

A protein whose synthesis is dependent on Vitamin K and which acts to promote mineral deposition in bone. This protein contains numerous glutamic acid residues which are carboxylated post-translationally through the action of the Vitamin K-dependent epoxide cycle.

OSTEOCLASTS

Cells responsible for bone remodeling. These cells mobilize bone mineral.

OSTEOMALACIA

A condition characterized by a weakening and softening of the bone and in which the bending of long bones can develop. Associated with Vitamin D deficiency.

OSTEOPENIA

Decreased bone mass.

OSTEOPOROSIS

Disease in which the bone loses its mineral content and becomes porous; associated with aging, particularly in females lacking estrogen.

OVALBUMIN

Egg albumin. The major protein in egg white.

OVERHYDRATION

Extracellular fluid volume excess.

OVERWEIGHT

A body weight in excess of that thought to be normal for height.

OVOLACTOVEGETARIAN

An individual who includes fruits, milk, vegetables, milk products, eggs, and cheese in the diet but not meat.

OVOMUCOID

A minor protein in egg white which contains carbohydrate as part of its structure.

OXALATES

See type B antinutritives.

OXALIC ACID

A two carbon dicarboxylate found in foods especially rhubarb, spinach, parsley, cocoa, and tea. Can bind divalent minerals and make them biologically unavailable.

OXALOACETATE

A labile metabolic intermediate. See citric acid cycle.

OXIDASE

An enzyme group responsible for oxygen removal; catalyzes oxidation/reduction reactions using oxygen as the electron acceptor.

OXIDATION

The removal of electrons using oxygen as the electron acceptor.

The process may not always involve an enzyme. It may occur spontaneously and when this occurs, it is called auto-oxidation. In food, auto-oxidation occurs and is responsible for the deterioration of food quality. The discoloration of red meat upon exposure to air at room temperature is an indication of the auto-oxidation process. The off odor that accompanies this discoloration is the result of the auto-oxidation of the fatty acids in the meat fat. In living systems, the process of auto-oxidation is suppressed to a large extent, because the products of this oxidation, fatty acid peroxides, can be very damaging. Peroxides denature proteins rendering them inactive and attack the DNA in the nucleus and mitochondria resulting in base pair deletions or breaks in the DNA which, in turn, result in mutations or errors in this DNA. In the nucleus, these breaks or deletions can be repaired. In the aging animal, the repair mechanism loses its efficiency. One of the characteristics of aged cells is the loss of its DNA repair ability. Mitochondria have no DNA repair mechanism so base pair deletions occurring as a result of free radical attack cannot be reversed. Fortunately, there are many mitochondria (up to 50,000) in each cell so that if a few are damaged in this way, the effect is not as devastating as happens with unrepaired DNA damage in the nucleus.

To prevent wide-spread damage to cellular proteins and DNA by these radicals, there is a potent antioxidation system in all cells. This antioxidation system includes the selenium-containing enzyme, glutathione peroxidase, catalase, and superoxide dismutase. These enzymes are found in the peroxisomes. Superoxide dismutase is also found in the mitochondria. All of these components serve to suppress free radical formation.

The free radical chain reaction is shown in Figure 45. Free radicals can form when the oxygen atom is excited by a variety of drugs and contaminants and by ultraviolet light. The excited oxygen atom is called singlet oxygen (O_2^-). Pollutants such as the oxides of nitrogen or carbon tetrachloride can provoke this reaction. *In vivo*, the detoxification reactions catalyzed by the cytochrome P450 enzymes generate free radicals. In the respiratory chain of the mitochondria, the possibility of oxygen radical production exists, and it is for this reason the mitochondria possess a particularly potent peroxide suppressor, superoxide dismutase or SOD. SOD in the mitochondria requires the manganese ion as a cofactor. The cytosol also has SOD, but this enzyme requires the copper and zinc ions. Both forms of the enzyme catalyze the reaction $O_2^- + O_2^- + 2H^+ \rightarrow H_2O_2 + O_2$. Two superoxides and two hydrogen ions are joined to form one molecule of hydrogen peroxide and a molecule of oxygen. In turn, the peroxide can be converted to water through the action of the enzyme catalase. Peroxides can also be "neutralized" through the action of glutathione s-transferase. This reaction requires two moles of reduced glutathione and produces two molecules of oxidized glutathione and two molecules of water. Fatty acid radicals can also be neutralized by glutathione peroxidase producing a molecule of an alcohol with the same chain length as the fatty acid. Glutathione-S-transferase can duplicate the action of glutathione peroxidase. These enzymes and the reactions they catalyze are listed in Table 34.

In addition to the reactions that counteract the *in vivo* formation of oxygen radicals or fatty acid peroxides, certain of the vitamins have this role as well. Ascorbic acid has an antioxidant function as it can donate reducing equivalents to a peroxide converting it to an

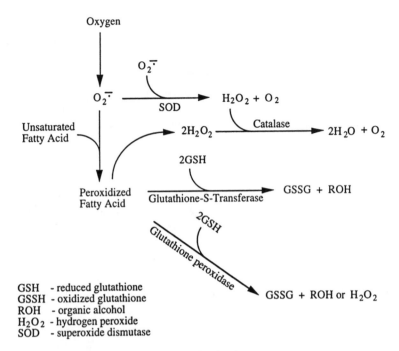

GSH   - reduced glutathione
GSSH - oxidized glutathione
ROH   - organic alcohol
H_2O_2 - hydrogen peroxide
SOD   - superoxide dismutase

FIGURE 45 Free radical formation and suppression *in vivo.*

alcohol. β carotene can quench singlet oxygen and thus convert it into O_2. Vitamin E is perhaps the best known antioxidant vitamin, and its action is similar to that of ascorbic acid. It donates reducing equivalents to a peroxide converting it to an alcohol.

Although the foregoing has emphasized the negative aspects of the partial reduction products of oxygen, there is some evidence that peroxide formation has some benefit. For example, leukocytes produce peroxides as a means of killing invading bacteria. Other examples no doubt will emerge as scientists struggle to understand the role of peroxidation (and the peroxisomes) in mammalian metabolism.

TABLE 34
Antioxidant Enzymes Found in Mammalian Cells

Enzyme	Required Mineral Cofactor	Reaction Catalyzed
Superoxide dismutase	CuZn	$2O_2^- + 2H^+ \rightarrow + H_2O_2$
Glutathione peroxidase	Se	$H_2O_2 + 2GSH \rightarrow GSSG + 2H_2O$
		$ROOH + 2GSH \rightarrow GSSG + ROH + H_2O$
Catalase	Fe	$2H_2O_2 \rightarrow 2H_2O + O_2$
Glutathione-S-transferases	—	$ROOH + 2GSH \rightarrow GSSG + ROH + H_2O$

OXIDATION/REDUCTION

Reactions in which electrons are lost by one reactant and gained by another.

OXIDATIVE DEAMINATION

The removal of an amino group together with the loss of electrons which are accepted by oxygen.

OXIDATIVE DECARBOXYLATION

The removal of a carboxyl group together with the loss of electrons accepted by oxygen.

OXIDATIVE PHOSPHORYLATION (OXPHOS)

Two processes whereby water and ATP are synthesized simultaneously. One, respiration, joins hydrogen and oxygen ions to make water, and the other, ATP synthesis, uses some of the energy so released to synthesize ATP. These coupled processes occur in the mitochondria of the cell.

OXIDATIVE RANCIDITY

Caused by products from reactions of fatty acids with atmospheric oxygen. Oxidation of fats and oils usually results in the formation of a variety of toxic substances. Three types of oxidation can be identified: (1) auto oxidation; (2) photo-oxidation; and (3) enzymatic oxidation.

OXYTOCIN

Hormone that stimulates uterine contractions as part of the parturition process.

P

PACEMAKER

Electrical device used to maintain a normal sinus rhythm of myocardial contraction by electrically stimulating the heart muscle.

PANCREATIN

Extract of pancreas; contains pancreatic enzymes.

PANCREATITIS

Inflammation of the pancreas; associated with alcoholism or biliary tract obstruction. If untreated the exocrine pancreas becomes necrotic and characteristic disturbances in digestion occur together with progressive decline of health. This can be life threatening.

PANCREOZMIN

A hormone (also called cholecystokinin) secreted by endocrine cells lining the duodenum. Its release is stimulated by the presence of lipid in the chyme. It signals the exocrine pancreas to release pancreatic enzymes (pancreatic juice) and stimulates the release of bile from the gall bladder.

PANTOTHENIC ACID

An essential B vitamin that is an integral part of coenzyme A which is essential for the synthesis of fatty acids. In food it is found free and also as part of phosphopantetheine (see vitamins, Table 48).

$$-O-\overset{\overset{O}{\|}}{C}-CH_2-CH_2-NH-\overset{\overset{O}{\|}}{C}-\underset{\underset{OH}{|}}{CH}-\underset{\underset{CH_3}{|}}{\overset{\overset{CH_3}{|}}{C}}-CH-OH$$

PAPAIN

A proteolytic enzyme found in papaya.

PARA AMINO BENZOIC ACID

A growth factor for bacteria; an integral part of folacin (see Vitamins, Table 49).

PARALYTIC SHELLFISH TOXINS (PSTs)

Neurotoxins which are among the most potent of the known low molecular weight toxins. Paralytic shellfish poisoning is attributed to the consumption of shellfish that have become contaminated with a toxin or group of toxins on the ingestion of toxic plankton, in particular of toxic dinoflagellates. The shellfish involved are pelecypods, a family of mollusks, including mussels and clams. The paralytic toxins from dinoflagellates can be categorized in two groups; (1) water soluble toxins, responsible for almost all types of paralytic shellfish poisoning in humans, and (2) lipid soluble toxins, found in oysters and clams. So far, seven different kinds of paralytic shellfish toxins have been identified and characterized: (1) saxitoxin, (2) neosaxitoxin (1-hydroxysaxitoxin), (3) gonyautoxin-I (11α-neosaxitoxin sulfate), (4) gonyautoxin-II (11α-saxitoxin sulfate), (5) gonyautoxin-III (11β-saxitoxin sulfate), (6) gonyautoxin-IV (11β-neosaxitoxin sulfate), and (7) gonyautoxin-V (structure unknown). Two major effects of the paralytic shellfish toxins are noted: (1) effects on peripheral and central nervous system, and (2) systemic effects. The initial symptoms (within 30 min) of paralytic shellfish poisoning in humans include tingling, burning sensation, and numbness (lips, gums, tongue, face, and fingertips). Then, similar sensations spread to the neck, arms, and legs, and general muscular incoordination ensues. Other symptoms may also be present, such as weakness, dizziness, malaise, prostration, headache, salivation, rapid pulse, intense thirst, dysphagia, perspiration, anuria, impairment of vision, or even temporary blindness. Depending on the amount of toxin ingested, death following respiratory paralysis may occur within 2–12 hr. The risk of contamination and poisoning is highest during a so-called red tide. In many parts of the world, the sea sometimes suddenly becomes colored, as a result of dinoflagellate bloom. The phenomenon is referred to as red tide, although the bloom may also be yellow or brown. In spite of the frequent occurrence of red tide and the high toxicity of the paralytic shellfish toxins, intoxication rarely happens. This is largely due to the strict regulations set by many countries and the awareness of people in coastal areas of the risks associated with eating shellfish during red tides. Although ordinary cooking destroys up to 70% of the toxin(s) and pan-frying even more, there may be sufficient toxin left in the mollusks to cause serious poisoning.

PARATHORMONE

A hormone synthesized and released by the parathyroid glands located in the thyroid gland. This hormone is involved in the regulation of blood calcium levels.

PARATHYROIDECTOMY

Removal of parathyroid glands.

PARENTERAL NUTRITION

Nutritional support furnished through the vascular system.

PARESTHESIA

A sensation of burning, numbness, or tingling usually associated with damage to sensory nerve.

PARIETAL CELLS

Stomach cells that secrete hydrochloric acid.

PARTS PER MILLION (PPM)

Expression of concentration of a solute in a solution.

PASSIVE DIFFUSION

A process for the passage of solutes across a membrane which does not involve a carrier or energy.

PASTEURIZATION

Process of applying heat to a liquid to destroy harmful organisms.

PATHOGENS

Microorganisms that cause disease.

PATULIN

A mycotoxin produced by *Penicillium urticae*, *Penicillium patulum*, *Penicillium expansum*, 12 other species of *Penicillium* and *Aspergillus*, and *Byssochlamus nivea*. It is a wide-spectrum toxicant which is poisonous to mammals, plants, and many lower forms of life. Patulin is stable under conditions required for fruit juice production and preservation. In experimental animals, it has been shown to cause hemorrhages, formation of edema, and dilatation of the intestinal tract. In subchronic studies, hyperemia of the epithelium of the duodenum and kidney function impairment were observed as main effects. Factors involved in fungal growth and patulin production include moderate temperature, high moisture content, and a pH between 3 and 5. Occurrence of patulin is mainly reported in fruits, such as apples, peaches, pears, apricots, and cherries. Patulin is an indicator of poor manufacturing practice (use of mouldy raw material) and can pose a serious threat to human and animal health.

PBB

Polybrominated biphenyl. An environmental contaminant.

PBI TEST

A test which measures thyroid activity by measuring the amount of protein bound iodine in the blood.

PCB

Polychlorinated biphenyl. An environmental contaminant.

PECTIN

A type of water-soluble fiber found in many fruits. When hydrolyzed it forms a gel.

PEDIATRICS

A specialty having to do with children.

PELLAGRA

Niacin deficiency disorder.

PENTOSE

A five carbon sugar found in plums and cherries.

PENTOSE PHOSPHATE PATHWAY

See hexose monophosphate shunt (Figure 41).

PENTOSURIA

A genetic disease due to a mutation in the gene for the NADP-linked enzyme xylose/xylulose dehydrogenase and characterized by the presence of xylose or xylulose in the urine instead of xylitol. This has no clinical significance.

PEP

Phosphoenopyruvic acid. A key intermediate in glucose synthesis and in glycolysis.

PEPCK

Phosphoenolpyruvate carboxykinase. Rate-limiting enzyme in gluconeogenesis.

PEPSIN

A protein digestive enzyme released by gastric cells as pepsinogen and activated by hydro-chloric acid.

PEPSINOGIN

The inactive form of pepsin.

PEPTIC ULCER

Chronic lesions found in the gastrointestinal tract in locations exposed to hydrochloric acid or pepsin. The most common locations are the duodenum and stomach. Lesions are due to a penicillin sensitive organism, *H. pylorii.*

PEPTIDE BOND

The bond formed between the amino group of one amino acid and the carboxyl group of another. A molecule of water is formed as a byproduct of this reaction.

PEPTIDES

Single chains of amino acids joined together by peptide bonds (see protein structure).

PEPTONES

A secondary protein derivative formed during protein digestion in the stomach.

PER OS

By mouth.

PERCUTANEOUS TRANSLUMINAL CORONARY ANGIOPLASTY (PTCA)

See cardiovascular tests and therapies.

PERICARDITIS

Inflammation of the sac enclosing the heart and its vessels known as the pericardium.

PERINATAL

Period of time occurring before and immediately after birth.

PERIODONTAL DISEASE

Inflammation of the gums.

PERIPHERAL VASCULAR DISEASE

Atherosclerotic changes in the vessels of the limbs.

PERISTALSIS

The rhythmic contractions of the smooth muscles which surround the gastrointestinal tract.

PERITONEAL DIALYSIS

Therapy useful in treating renal failure in which toxic substances are removed from the body by using the peritoneum as a semipermeable membrane.

PERNICIOUS

Adjective that describes a fatal (usually) disease.

PERNICIOUS ANEMIA

Disease of Vitamin B_{12} deficiency. Characterized by low numbers of red blood cells that are poorly formed and by demyelination of the sheaths of nerve cells.

PEROXIDATION

Oxidation to the point of forming peroxides (see free radicals and autooxidation).

PESTICIDES

See contamination with organic chemicals. Chemicals used to reduce the population of plant and animal insects, fungi, molds, and parasites.

PETECHIAE

Minute hemorrhagic spots in the skin.

PGI, PGE

Prostaglandins in the I or E series.

pH

The numerical representation of the hydrogen ion concentration in a solution. A low pH represents an acid solution while a high pH represents a basic or alkaline solution. Physiological pH is 7.4.

PHARMACOLOGICAL REACTION

A food-intolerance reaction resulting from the pharmacological effect of a food component. A well-known example is caffein, a methylxanthine derivative present in tea and coffee. Its biological action includes stimulation of the heart muscle, the central nervous system, and the production of gastrin. Symptoms associated with a high coffee intake are restlessness, tremors, weight loss, palpitations, and alterations in mood. Other biologically active substances are histamine, tyramine, phenylethylamine, and histamine releasers.

PHENFORMIN

An oral hypoglycemic agent that works by decreasing the rate of intestinal glucose uptake.

PHENOL OR PHENYL OXIDASES

Copper-containing enzymes responsible for the browning of fruit at the cut surface. These enzymes can be inhibited by ascorbic acid or by heating.

PHENOTYPE

A category or group to which an individual is assigned based on one or more inherited characteristics; the overt expression of the genotype.

PHENYLALANINE

An essential amino acid containing a phenyl group and alanine; a precursor to tyrosine (see amino acids, Table 5).

PHENYLETHYLAMINE

A biologically active substance, which can be involved in the pharmacological reactions of food intolerance. It occurs in chocolate, old cheese, and red wine and can provoke migraine attacks. It is the amine form of phenylalanine which forms when phenylalanine hydroxylase does not metabolize all of the phenylalanine present.

PHENYLKETONURIA (PKU)

A genetic disease due to a mutation in the gene for the enzyme phenylalanine hydroxylase. Several variants have been described. The phenotypic expression of the genotype includes mental retardation. Expression can be prevented by early diagnosis and use of a low phenylalanine diet.

PHOSPHATASE

An enzyme which catalyzes the removal of a phosphoryl group from a substrate.

PHOSPHATE

A molecule (PO_4) containing phosphorus and oxygen.

PHOSPHATIDYL CHOLINE

A phospholipid commonly known as lecithin.

PHOSPHATIDYL ETHANOLAMINE

A phospholipid in membranes; important component (cephalin) of the brain lipids.

PHOSPHATIDYL INOSITOL

A phospholipid in the plasma membrane which is an important component of the second messenger system called the PIP cycle. This is shown in Figure 46.

Peptide and polypeptide hormones bind to their cognate receptors lodged in the plasma membrane. These receptors generally penetrate the membrane and have a tyrosine rich tail protruding into the cytosol. Part of the hormone-receptor binding and subsequent cellular events involve G proteins. The G protein is a protein which has a high affinity for GTP

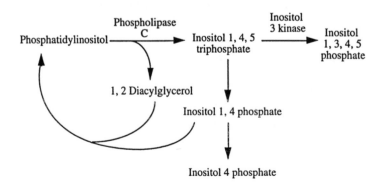

FIGURE 46 Phosphatidylinositol (PIP) cycle.

(guanine triphosphate). It serves as the signal transducer for the hormone. The G proteins have several subunits which interact and then react with enzymes such as adenyl cyclase or phospholipase C. This process is illustrated in Figure 47. These enzymes may be either activated or inhibited depending on the hormone in question. Both adenyl cyclase and phospholipase C are components of the intracellular signalling system, the former is a component cyclic AMP or protein kinase system and the latter, a component of the phosphatidylinositol (PIP) system. The former leads to a cellular effect such as the release of cortisol when ACTH binds to the receptor on the membrane of the adrenocortical cell while the latter leads to the release of calcium from intracellular stores. The calcium ion in turn plays a role in exocytosis or may be active in the exchange of metabolites across intracellular membranes.

PHOSPHOCREATINE

See creatine phosphate.

PHOSPHOGLUCONATE PATHWAY

See hexose monophosphate shunt.

PHOSPHOGLYCERIDE

A lipid containing a glycerol backbone, one or two fatty acids, and a phosphate group.

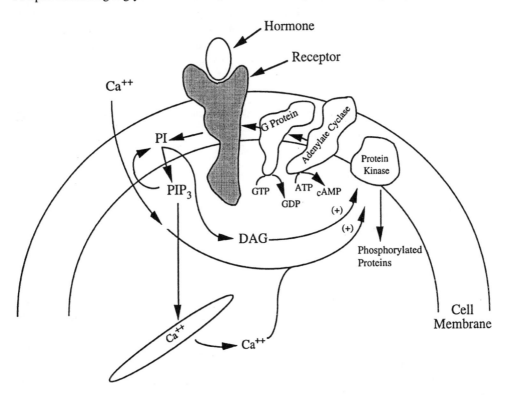

FIGURE 47 Hormone-receptor reaction that involves the G proteins, adenylate cyclase, proteins, the PIP cycle, and cAMP. When the hormone binds to the receptor, the G protein moves over to the receptor protein and binds to GTP. Adenylate cyclase moves over and binds to the G protein and ATP is converted to cAMP. (From Berdanier, C.D., *Advanced Nutrition: Macronutrients*, CRC Press, Boca Raton, FL, 1994, 125.)

PHOSPHOLIPID

A family of compounds containing a glycerol or sphingosine backbone plus one or two fatty acids and a phosphate group linked to one of the following — choline, inositol, ethanolamine, or serine.

PHOSPHORUS

An essential mineral component of bone tissue, where it occurs in the mass ratio of 1 phosphorus to 2 calcium. Phosphorus is present in nearly all foods. The mean daily intake is estimated at about 1500 mg, while the Recommended Dietary Allowance is 1200 mg. In a number of species, excess phosphorus, i.e., a calcium–phosphorus ratio of 0.5, leads to a decrease in the blood calcium level and secondary hyperparathyroidism with loss of bone. The phosphorus levels in normal diets are not likely to be harmful (see minerals, Table 30).

PHOSPHORYLATION

The addition of a phosphate group.

PHOTO-OXIDATION

Oxidative degradation of a substance by photoreaction. (Poly)unsaturated fatty acids can undergo two types of photo-oxidation: (1) a free-radical chain reaction, which starts from the excited state of another molecule, and (2) a singlet oxygen ($^1O_2$) reaction in which the absorption of photons by molecules of another food component is followed by energy transfer to ground-state oxygen, leading to the formation of singlet oxygen. Photo-oxidation of foods can be prevented by using packaging materials that absorb the photochemically active light and by removing endogenous photosensitizers and oxygen from the food.

PHOTOSYNTHESIS

The process whereby plants convert CO_2 and water into carbohydrates with the energy provided by ultraviolet light.

PHYLLOQUINONE

Vitamin K from plant sources.

PHYSIOLOGICAL FUEL VALUE

The energy provided by food with a correction for the energy lost through digestion and absorption.

PHYTIC ACID

A component of plants which can bind divalent ions. Phytate is a form of inositol that is phosphorylated in all six positions of the carbons; when calcium and magnesium are bound it becomes an insoluble salt called phytin (see type B antinutrients).

PHYTOBEZOAR

A mass of food in the stomach, usually vegetable type food, that does not pass into the intestine.

PHYTOSTEROL

A sterol related to cholesterol found in plants.

PICA

The consumption of items of no nutritional value. The habit is called pica after the Latin word for magpie. The magpie is a bird which will consume all manner of food and nonfood items. Pica has been observed for centuries and was described by Aetius of Amida in 1542. Many different items are consumed; however, the most common are clay (geophagia), laundry starch (amylophagia), or ice (pagophagia). A number of studies on the prevalence of pica have shown that up to 70% of some population groups may have this habit. Pregnant women as well as children are the most frequently affected, and black women were 3 to 4 times more affected than white women of the same socioeconomic group. The most common cravings were for laundry starch (as much as 8 oz. a day) and clay. When both men and women were studied, few men exhibited the practice and it has been suggested that men use liquor or tobacco to meet their nonfood oral needs.

The question of why pica exists has not been satisfactorily answered. From the various epidemiological studies, age, sex, social status, and race appear to be important factors in the development of the habit. Several studies have noted that pica was associated with anemia. Reynolds et al. reported that frequent nosebleeds and other spontaneous losses of blood accompanied or preceded an increased craving for certain food and nonfood items. Clay, rice, French fries, ice, green vegetables, bread, hot tea, and grapefruit were mentioned as being consumed in large quantities by these patients. The patients were treated for their anemias by iron supplements and were tested for their iron-binding capacity. Some of the patients had low uptakes of iron while others were normal. Those with poor iron-binding capacities were usually the clay eaters; those with normal iron-binding capacities were ice or ice cream eaters. Clay, even the small amount residing in the gastrointestinal tract of patients having no access to clay while hospitalized, could have adsorbed the oral iron supplements. Thus, it seems unlikely that an innate lowered iron-binding capacity was responsible for either the anemia or the pica. However, pica does appear to **follow** the development of anemia rather than precede it.

In addition to anemia, other conditions have been observed in pica patients. Muscular weakness and low serum potassium levels have been reported in geophagic patients. Both these conditions could be attributed to the binding of potassium in the intestine by the clay. This may also be true in patients consuming large quantities of laundry starch.

PIGMENTATION

Coloration of skin related to the amount of melanin present.

PINOCYTOSIS

Engulfing process in which cells absorb or ingest nutrients and fluid before hydrolysis.

PITUITARY GLAND

The master endocrine gland located at the base of the brain; secretes a number of trophic hormones which activate other endocrine organs. ACTH (adrenalcorticotrophic hormone) is an example. The pituitary gland also releases growth hormone as well as a number of other hormones that have direct action on metabolic processes.

PLACEBO

An inert preparation given for its psychological effect.

PLACENTA

The organ which surrounds the unborn child and serves as a barrier between the two. It is permeable to a large number of solutes. The umbilical cord connects the placenta to the child.

PLANTAIN

Banana.

PLASMA

The fluids surrounding the red blood cells.

PLASMALOGENS

An acetyl phosphatide.

PLATELETS

Small, rod-shaped blood cells which, when meshed together, help form a clot.

PLP

Pyridoxal phosphate. A coenzyme required in amino acid metabolism and which contains the vitamin pyridoxine in the aldehyde form.

PLUMBISM

Consumption of paint chips. If the paint contains lead oxide as the pigment, lead intoxication can develop. This is characterized by anemia, low serum iron and copper values, growth depression, ataxia, kidney damage, coma, convulsions, and death. The ataxia, stupor, coma, and convulsions reflect the effect of lead on the central nervous system. This can be understood as the effect of lead on hemoglobin synthesis. Both copper and iron utilization is impaired and the anemia typical of lead intoxication is microcytic and hypochromic in character. In addition, lead may replace either copper, iron, or calcium in a number of tissues and, because it is metabolically inert, inhibit the functionality of that tissue. In the case of hemoglobin synthesis, it becomes obvious that the oxygen carrying capacity of the red blood cells is decreased. Those tissues with a high oxygen requirement, i.e., the neural tissue, will be the most affected. Thus, one can understand the neuromuscular response to chronic lead ingestion. If neuronal tissue suffers from prolonged oxygen deprivation, it will die and this damage is irreversible. Subjects with lead poisoning can be treated with compounds such as EDTA which will bind the circulating lead and allow the body to excrete the EDTA-lead complex. It is not possible, however, to rid the body of all of its accumulated lead nor to protect the patients from future ill effects of their lead-induced pathology. Lead will remain in its storage sites like bone and, when mobilized, will have untoward effects.

In the United States today, the majority of lead intoxication cases are young children ages 1 to 6, with pica. Adults who work in lead-related industries or consume lead-contaminated illicit beverages are also affected. Increasing the levels of lead exposure generally increases the blood and tissue lead levels, yet, individual variation due to age, sex, and nutritional status occurs. The factors which determine the fractions of the body where lead is deposited have not been determined. It is known that well-nourished individuals are more resistant to the deleterious effects of lead than are poorly nourished individuals.

PNEUMOTHORAX

Collection of air or gas in the pleural space between the visceral and parietal pleurae of the lungs.

POACH

A method of cooking using water heated to a temperature just below boiling.

POISONOUS PLANTS

Plants which contain toxic materials sufficient to cause serious symptoms. Examples are listed in Table 35.

POLAR

A characteristic of a molecule possessing a positive or negative charge.

POLYCHLORIDE BIPHENYL

A plasticizer and insulator material used in the electronics industry found to be a very long-lived toxic environmental contaminant.

POLYCHLORINATED DIBENZODIOXINS

See contamination with organic chemicals.

POLYCHLORINATED DIBENZOFURANS

See contamination with organic chemicals.

POLYNEURITIS

Inflammation of many nerve endings.

POLYPEPTIDE

A string of amino acids in excess of 8. See protein structure.

POLYSACCHARIDE

A string of monosaccharides joined together. If the linkage is an α 1,4 or α 1,6, mammalian enzymes can break the bond. If the linkage is a β linkage, mammalian enzyme cannot sever it.

POLYUNSATURATED FATTY ACID

A fatty acid having more than one double bond.

POLYURIA

Excessive urination.

POMPE'S DISEASE

A genetic disease due to a mutation in the gene for the enzyme α 1,4 glucosidase. Characterized by excess glycogen stores in the muscle.

PONDERAL INDEX

An expression of leanness: height (inches) / $\sqrt[3]{\text{weight (lbs)}}$.

TABLE 35
Some Important Poisonous Plants of North America

Common and Scientific Name	Description; Toxic Parts	Geographical Distribution	Poisoning; Symptoms	Remarks
Baneberry *Actaea* sp.	Description — Perennial herb growing to 3 ft (1 m) tall from a thick root; compound leaves; small, white flowers; white or red berries with several seeds borne in short, terminal clusters. Toxic parts — All parts, but primarily roots and berries.	Native in rich woods occurring from Canada south to Georgia, Alabama, Louisiana, Oklahoma, and the northern Rockies; red-fruited western baneberry from Alaska to central California, Arizona, Montana, and South Dakota.	Poisoning — Attributed to a glycoside or essential oil which causes severe inflammation of the digestive tract. Symptoms — Acute stomach cramps, headache, increased pulse, vomiting, delirium, dizziness, and circulatory failure.	Only 6 berries can cause symptoms persisting for hours. Treatment may be a gastric lavage or vomiting. Bright red berries attract children.
Buckeye; Horsechestnut *Aesculus* sp.	Description — Shrub or tree; deciduous, opposite, palmately, divided leaves with 5 to 9 leaflets on a long stalk; red, yellow, or white flowers; 2- to 3-valved, capsule fruit; with thick, leathery husk enclosing 1 to 6 brown shiny seeds. Toxic parts — Leaves, twigs, flowers, and seeds.	Various species throughout the United States and Canada; some cultivated as ornamentals, others growing wild.	Poisoning—Toxic parts contain the glycoside, esculin. Symptoms — Nervous twitching of muscles, weakness, lack of coordination, dilated pupils, nausea, vomiting, diarrhea, depression, paralysis, and stupor.	By making a "tea" from the leaves and twigs or by eating the seeds, children have been poisoned. Honey collected from the buckeye flower may also cause poisoning. Roots, branches, and fruits have been used to stupefy fish in ponds. Treatment usually is a gastric lavage or vomiting.
Buttercup *Ranunculus* sp.	Description — Annual or perennial herb growing to 16–32 in. (41–81 cm) high; leaves alternate entire to compound, and largely basal; yellow flowers borne singly or in clusters on ends of seed stalks; small fruits, 1-seeded pods. Toxic parts — Entire plant.	Widely distributed in woods, meadows, pastures, and along streams throughout temperate and cold locations.	Poisoning — The alkaloid, protoanemonin which can injure the digestive system and ulcerate the skin. Symptoms — Burning sensation of the mouth, nervousness, nausea, vomiting, low blood pressure, weak pulse, depression, and convulsions.	Sap and leaves may cause dermatitis. Cows poisoned by buttercups produce bitter milk or milk with a reddish color.

	Description / Toxic parts	Habitat	Poisoning / Symptoms	Notes
Castor bean *Ricinus communis*	Description — Shrublike herb 4-12 ft. (1.2–3.7 m) tall; simple, alternate, long-stalked leaves with 5 to 11 long lobes which are toothed on margins; fruits oval, green, or red, and covered with spines; 3 elliptical, glossy, black white, or mottled seeds per capsule. Toxic parts — Entire plant, especially the seeds.	Cultivated as an ornamental or oilseed crop primarily in the southern part of the United States and Hawaii.	Poisoning — Seeds, pressed cake, and leaves poisonous when chewed; contain the phytotoxin, ricin. Symptoms — Burning of the mouth and throat, nausea, vomiting, severe stomach pains, bloody diarrhea, excessive thirst, prostration, dullness of vision, and convulsions; kidney failure and death 1–12 days later.	Fatal dose for a child is 1 to 3 seeds, and for an adult 2 to 8 seeds. The oil extracted from the seeds is an important commercial product. It is not poisonous and it is used as a medicine (castor oil), for soap, and as a lubricant.
Chinaberry *Helia azedarach*	Description — Deciduous tree 20–40 ft (6–12 m) tall; twice, pinnately divided leaves and toothed or lobed leaflets, purple flowers borne in clusters; yellow, wrinkled, rounded berries which persist throughout the winter. Toxic parts — Berries, bark, flowers, and leaves.	A native of Asia introduced as an ornamental in the United States; common in the southern United States and lower altitudes in Hawaii; has become naturalized in old fields, pastures, around buildings, and along fence rows.	Poisoning — Most result from eating pulp of berries; toxic principle is a resinoid with narcotic effects. Symptoms — Nausea, vomiting, diarrhea, irregular breathing, and respiratory distress.	Six to eight berries can cause the death of a child. The berries have been used to make insecticide and flea powder.
Death camas *Zigadenus paniculatus*	Description — Perennial herb resembling wild onions but the onion odor lacking; long, slender leaves with parallel veins; pale yellow to pink flowers in clusters on slender seedstalks; fruit a 3-celled capsule. Toxic parts — Entire plant, especially the bulb.	Various species occur throughout the United States and Canada; all are more or less poisonous.	Poisoning — Due to the alkaloids, zygadenine, veratrine, and others. Symptoms — Excessive salivation, muscular weakness, slow heart rate, low blood pressure, subnormal temperature, nausea, vomiting, diarrhea, prostration, coma, and sometimes death.	The members of Lewis and Clark Expedition made four from the bulbs and suffered the symptoms of poisoning. Later some pioneers were killed when they mistook death camas for wild onions or garlic.

TABLE 35 (CONTINUED)
Some Important Poisonous Plants of North America

Common and Scientific Name	Description; Toxic Parts	Geographical Distribution	Poisoning; Symptoms	Remarks
Dogbane (Indian hemp) *Apocynum cannabinum*	Description — Perennial herbs with milky juice and somewhat woody stems; simple, smooth, and oppositely paired leaves; bell-shaped, small, white to pink flowers borne in clusters at ends of axillary stems; paired, long, slender seed pods. Toxic parts — Entire plant.	Various species growing throughout North America in fields and forests, and along streams and roadsides.	Poisoning — Only suspect since it contains the toxic glycoside, cymarin, and is poisonous to animals. Symptoms — In animals, increased temperature and pulse, cold extremities, dilation of the pupils, discoloration of the mouth and nose, sore mouth, sweating, loss of appetite, and death.	Compounds extracted from roots of dogbane have been used to make a heart stimulant.
Foxglove *Digitalis purpurea*	Description — Biennial herb with alternate, simple, toothed leaves; terminal, showy raceme of flowers, purple, pink, rose, yellow, or white; dry capsule fruit. Toxic parts — Entire plant, especially leaves, flowers, and seeds.	Native of Europe commonly planted in gardens of the United States; naturalized and abundant in some parts of the western United States.	Poisoning — Due to digitalis component. Symptoms — Nausea, vomiting, dizziness, irregular heartbeat, tremors, convulsions, and possible death.	Foxglove has long been known as a source of digitalis and steroid glycosides. It is an important medicinal plant when used correctly.
Henbane *Hyoscyamus niger*	Description — Erect annual or biennial herb with coarse, hairy stems 1–5 ft (30–152 cm) high; simple, oblong, alternate leaves with a few, coarse teeth, not stalked; greenish-yellow or yellowish with purple vein flowers; fruit a rounded capsule. Toxic parts — Entire plant.	Along roads, in waste places across southern Canada and northern United States, particularly common in the Rocky Mountains.	Poisoning — Caused by the alkaloids, hyoscyamine hyoscine, and atropine. Symptoms — Increased salivation, headache, nausea, rapid pulse, convulsions, coma, and death.	A gastric lavage of 4% tannic acid solution may be used to treat the poisoning.

	Description / Toxic parts	Distribution	Poisoning / Symptoms	Comments
Iris (Rock Mountain Iris) *Iris missouriensis*	Description — Lilylike perennial plants often in dense patches; long, narrow leaves; flowers blue-purple; fruit a 3-celled capsule. Toxic parts — Leaves, but especially the root stalk.	Wet land of meadows, marshes, and along streams from North Dakota to British Columbia, Canada; south to New Mexico, Arizona, and California; scattered over entire Rocky Mountain area; cultivated species also common.	Poisoning — An irritating resinous substance, irisin. Symptoms — Burning, congestion, and severe pain in the digestive tract; nausea and diarrhea.	Rootstalks have such an acrid taste that they are unlikely to be eaten.
Jasmine *Geisemium sempervirens*	Description — A woody, trailing, or climbing evergreen vine; opposite, simple, lance-shaped, glossy leaves; fragrant, yellow flowers; flattened 2-celled, beaked capsule fruits. Toxic parts — Entire plant, but especially the root and flowers.	Native to the southeastern United States; commonly grown in the Southwest as an ornamental.	Poisoning — Alkaloids, geisemine, gelseminine, and gelsemoidine found throughout the plant. Symptoms — Profuse sweating, muscular weakness, convulsions, respiratory depression, paralysis, and death possible.	Jasmine has been used as a medicinal herb, but overdoses are dangerous. Children have been poisoned by chewing on the leaves.
Jimmyweed (Rayless goldenrod) *Haplopappus heterophyllus*	Description — Small, bushy, half-shrub with erect stems arising from the woody crown to a height of 2–4 ft (61–122 cm); narrow, alternate, sticky leaves; clusters of small, yellow flower heads at tips of stems. Toxic parts — Entire plant.	Common in fields or ranges around watering sites and along streams from Kansas, Oklahoma, and Texas to Colorado, New Mexico, and Arizona.	Poisoning — Contains higher alcohol, tremetol, which accumulates in the milk of cows and causes human poisoning known as "milk sickness."	Other species of Haplopappus probably are equally dangerous. White snakeroot also contains tremetol and causes "milk sickness."
Jimsonwood (Thornapple) *Datura stramonium*	Description — Coarse, weedy plant with stout stems and foul-smelling foliage; large, oval leaves with wavy margins; fragrant, large, tubular, white to purple flowers; round, nodding or erect prickly capsule. Toxic parts — Entire plant, particularly the seeds and leaves.	Naturalized throughout North America; common weed of fields, gardens, roadsides, and pastures.	Poisoning — Due to the alkaloids, hyoscyamine, atropine, and hyoscine (scopolamine). Symptoms — Dry mouth, thirst, red skin, disturbed vision, pupil dilation, nausea, vomiting, headache, hallucination, rapid pulse, delirium, incoherent speech, convulsion, high blood pressure, coma, and possibly death.	Sleeping near the fragrant flowers can cause headache, nausea, dizziness, and weakness. Children pretending the flowers were trumpets have been poisoned.

TABLE 35 (CONTINUED)
Some Important Poisonous Plants of North America

Common and Scientific Name	Description; Toxic Parts	Geographical Distribution	Poisoning; Symptoms	Remarks
Lantana (Red Sage) *Lantana camara*	Description — Perennial shrub with square twigs and a few spines; simple, opposite or whorled oval-shaped leaves with tooth margins; white, yellow, orange, red, or blue flowers occurring in flat-topped clusters; berry-like fruit with a hard, blue-black seed. Toxic parts — All parts, especially the green berries.	Native of the dry woods in the southeastern United States; cultivated as an ornamental shrub in pots in the northern United States and Canada; or a lawn shrub in the southeastern coastal plains, Texas, California, and Hawaii.	Poisoning — Fruit contains high levels of an alkaloid, lantanin or lantadene A. Symptoms — Stomach and intestinal irritation, vomiting, bloody diarrhea, muscular weakness, jaundice, and circulatory collapse; death possible but not common.	In Florida, these plants are considered a major cause of human poisoning. The foliage of lantana may also cause dermatitis.
Larkspur *Delphinium* sp.	Description — Annual or perennial herb 2–4 ft (61–122 cm) high; finely, palmately, divided leaves on long stalks; white, pink, rose, blue, or purple flowers each with a spur; fruit a many-seeded, 3-celled capsule. Toxic parts — Entire plant.	Native of rich or dry forest and meadows throughout the United States but common in the West; frequently cultivated in flower gardens.	Poisoning — Contains the alkaloids, delphinine, delphinidine, ajacine, and others. Symptoms — Burning sensation in the mouth and skin, low blood pressure, nervousness, weakness, prickling of the skin, nausea, vomiting, depression, convulsions, and death within 6 hours if eaten in large quantities.	Poisoning potential of larkspur decreases as it ages, but alkaloids still concentrated in the seeds. Seeds are used in some commercial lice remedies.
Laurel (Mountain laurel) *Kalmia latifolia*	Description — Large evergreen shrubs growing to 35 ft (11 m) tall; alternate leaves dark green on top and bright green underneath; white to rose flowers in terminal clusters; fruit in a dry capsule. Toxic parts — Leaves, twigs, flowers, and pollen grains.	Found in moist woods and along streams in eastern Canada southward in the Appalachian Mountains and Piedmont, and sometimes in the eastern coastal plain.	Poisoning — Contains the toxic resinoid, andromedotoxin. Symptoms — Increased salivation, watering of eyes and nose, loss of energy, slow pulse, vomiting, low blood pressure, lack of coordination, convulsions, and progressive paralysis until eventual death.	The Mountain laurel is the state flower of Connecticut and Pennsylvania. By making "tea" from the leaves or by sucking on the flowers, children have been poisoned.

Plant	Description	Distribution	Poisoning / Symptoms	Notes
Locoweed (Crazyweed) *Oxtropis* sp	Description — Perennial herb with erect or spreading stems; pealike flowers and stems — only smaller.	Common throughout the southwestern United States.	Poisoning — Contains alkaloidlike substances — a serious threat to livestock. Symptoms — In animals, loss of weight, irregular gait, loss of sense of direction, nervousness, weakness, and loss of muscular control.	Locoweeds are seldom eaten by humans, hence, they are not a serious problem. There are more than 100 species of locoweeds.
Lupine (Bluebonnet) *Lupinus* sp.	Description — Annual or perennial herbs; digitately divided, alternate leaves; peak-shaped blue, white, red, or yellow flowers borne in clusters at ends of stems; seeds in flattened pods. Toxic parts — Entire plant, particularly the seeds.	Wide distribution but most common in western North America; many cultivated as ornamentals.	Poisoning — Contains lupinine and related toxic alkaloids. Symptoms — Weak pulse, slowed respiration, convulsions, and paralysis.	Rarely have cultivated varieties poisoned children. Not all lupines are poisonous.
Marijuana (hashish, Mary Jane, pot, grass)	Description — A tall coarse, annual herb; palmately divided and long stalked leaves; small, green flowers clustered in the leaf axils. Toxic parts — Entire plant, especially the leaves, flowers, sap and resinous secretions.	Widely naturalized weed in temperate North America; cultivated in warmer areas.	Poisoning — Various narcotic resins but mainly tetrahydrocannabinol (THC) and related compounds. Symptoms — Exhilaration, hallucinations, delusions, mental confusion, dilated pupils, blurred vision, poor coordination, weakness, and stupor; coma and death in large doses.	Poisoning results form drinking the extract, chewing the plant parts, or smoking a so-called "reefer" (joint). The hallucinogenic and narcotic effects of marijuana have been known for more than 2,000 years. Laws in the United States and Canada restrict the possession of living or dried parts of marijuana.
Mescal bean (Frijolito) *Sophora secundiflora*	Description — Evergreen shrub or small tree growing to 40 ft (12 m) tall; stalked, alternate leaves 4–6 in. (10–15 cm) long, which are pinnately divided and shiny, yellow-green above and silky below when young; violet-blue, pealike flowers; bright red seeds. Toxic parts — Entire plant, particularly the seed.	Native to southwestern Texas and southern New Mexico; cultivated as ornamentals in the southwestern United States.	Poisoning — Contains cytisine and other poisonous alkaloids. Symptoms — Nausea, vomiting, diarrhea, excitement, delirium, hallucinations, coma, and death; deep sleep lasting 2–3 days in nonlethal doses.	One seed, if sufficiently chewed, is enough to cause the death of a young child. The Indians of Mexico and the Southwest have used the seeds in medicine as a narcotic and as a hallucinatory drug. Many necklaces have been made from the seeds.

TABLE 35 (CONTINUED)
Some Important Poisonous Plants of North America

Common and Scientific Name	Description; Toxic Parts	Geographical Distribution	Poisoning; Symptoms	Remarks
Mistletoes *Phoradendron serotinum*	Description — Parasitic evergreen plants that grow on trees and shrubs; oblong, simple, opposite leaves, which are leathery; small, white berries. Toxic parts — All parts, especially the berries.	Common on the branches of various trees from New Jersey and southern Indiana southward to Florida and Texas; other species throughout North America.	Poisoning — Contains the toxic amines, beta-phenylethylamine and trysamine. Symptoms — Gastrointestinal pain, diarrhea, slow pulse, and collapse; possibly nausea, vomiting, nervousness, difficult breathing, delirium, pupil dilation, and abortion; in sufficient amounts, death within a few hours.	Mistletoe is a favorite Christmas decoration. It is the state flower of Oklahoma. Poisonings have occurred when people eat the berries or make "tea" from the berries. Indians chewed the leaves to relieve toothache.
Monkshood (Wolfsbane) *Aconitum columbianum*	Description — Perennial herb about 2–5 ft (61–152 cm) high; alternate, petioled leaves which are palmately divided into segments with pointed tips; generally dark blue flowers with a prominent hood; seed in a short-beaked capsule. Toxic parts — Entire plant, especially roots and seeds.	Rich, moist soil in meadows and along streams from western Canada south to California and New Mexico.	Poisoning — Due to several alkaloids, including aconine and aconitine. Symptoms — Burning sensation of the mouth and skin; nausea, vomiting, diarrhea, muscular weakness, and spasms, weak, irregular pulse, paralysis of respiration, dimmed vision, convulsions, and death within a few hours.	Small amounts can be lethal. Death in humans reported from eating the plant or extracts made from it. It has been mistaken for horseradish.

	Description / Toxic parts	Distribution	Poisoning / Symptoms	Remarks
Mushrooms (toadstools) *Amanita muscaria, Amanita verna, Chlorophyllum molybdites*	Description — Common types with central stalk, and cap; flat plates (gills) underneath cap; some with deeply ridged, cylindrical top rather than cap. Toxic parts — Entire fungus.	Various types throughout North America.	Poisoning — Depending on type of mushroom; complex polypeptides such as amanitin and possibly phalloidin; a toxic protein in some; the poisons ibotenic acid, muscimol, and related compounds in others. Symptoms — Vary with type of mushroom but include deathlike sleep, manic behavior, delirium, seeing colored visions, feeling of elation, explosive diarrhea, vomiting, severe headache, loss of muscular coordination, abdominal cramps, and coma and death from some types; permanent liver, kidney, and heart damage from other types.	Wild mushrooms are extremely difficult to identify and are best avoided. There is no simple rule of thumb for distinguishing between poisonous and nonpoisonous mushrooms — only myths and nonsense. Only one or two bites are necessary for death from some species. During the month of December 1981, three people were killed and two hospitalized in California after eating poisonous mushrooms.
Nightshade *Solanum nigrum, Solanum elaeagnifolium*	Description — Annual herbs or shrublike plants with simple alternate leaves; small, white, blue, or violet flowers; black berries or yellow to yellow-orange berries depending on species. Toxic parts — Primarily the unripe berries.	Throughout the United States and southern Canada in waste places, old fields, ditches, roadsides, fence rows, or edges of woods.	Poisonings — Contains the alkaloid, solanine; possibly saponin, atropine, and perhaps high levels of nitrate. Symptoms — Headache, stomach pain, vomiting, diarrhea, dilated pupils, subnormal temperature, shock, circulatory and respiratory depression, and possible death.	Some individuals use the completely ripe berries in pies and jellies. Young shoots and leaves of the plant have been cooked and eaten like spinach.

TABLE 35 (CONTINUED)
Some Important Poisonous Plants of North America

Common and Scientific Name	Description; Toxic Parts	Geographical Distribution	Poisoning; Symptoms	Remarks
Oleander *Nerium oleander*	Description — An evergreen shrub or small tree growing to 25 ft. (8 m) tall; short-stalked, narrow, leathery leaves, opposite or in whorls of 3; white to pink to red flowers at tips of twigs. Toxic parts — Entire plant, especially the leaves.	A native of southern Europe but commonly cultivated in the southern United States and California.	Poisoning — Contains the poisonous glycosides, oleandrin and nerioside, which act similar to digitalis. Symptoms — Nausea, severe vomiting, stomach pain, bloody diarrhea, cold feet and hands, irregular heartbeat, dilation of pupils, drowsiness, unconsciousness, paralysis of respiration, convulsions, coma, and death within a day.	One leaf of an oleander is said to contain enough poison to kill an adult. In Florida, severe poisoning resulted when oleander branches were used as skewers. Honey made form oleander flower nectar is poisonous.
Peyote (Mescal buttons) *Lophophora williamsii*	Description — Hemispherical, spineless member of the cactus family growing from carrot-shaped roots; low, rounded sections with a tuft of yellow-white hairs on top; flower from the center of the plant, white to rose-pink; pink berry when ripe; black seeds. Toxic parts — Entire plant, especially the buttons.	Native to southern Texas and northern Mexico; cultivated in other areas.	Poisoning — Contains mescaline, lophophorine and other alkaloids. Symptoms — Illusions and hallucinations with vivid color, anxiety, muscular tremors and twitching, vomiting, diarrhea, blurred vision, wakefulness, forgetfulness, muscular relaxation, and dizziness.	The effects of chewing fresh or dried "buttons" of peyote are similar to those produced by LSD, only milder. In some states, peyote is recognized as a drug. Peyote has long been used by the Indians and Mexicans in religious ceremonies.

Plant	Description / Toxic parts	Distribution	Poisoning / Symptoms	Remarks
Poison hemlock (poison parsley) *Conium maculatum*	Description — Biennial herb with a hairless purple-spotted or lined, hollow stem growing up to 8 ft (2.4 m) tall; turniplike, long, solid taproot; large, alternate, pinnately divided leaves; small, white flowers in umbrella-shaped clusters, dry; ribbed, 2-part capsule fruit. Toxic parts — Entire plant, primarily seeds and root.	A native of Eurasia, now a weed in meadows and along roads and ditches throughout the United States and southern Canada where moisture is sufficient.	Poisoning — The poisonous alkaloid, coniine and other related alkaloids. Symptoms — Burning sensation in the mouth and throat, nervousness, uncoordination, dilated pupils, muscular weakness, weakened and slowed heartbeat, convulsions, coma, and death.	Poisoning occurs when the leaves are mistaken for parsley, the roots for turnips, or the seeds for anise. Toxic quantities seldom consumed because the plant has such an unpleasant odor and taste. Assumed by some to be the poison drunk by Socrates.
Poison ivy (poison oak) *Toxicodendron radicans*	Description — A trailing or climbing vine, shrub, or small tree; alternate leaves with 3 leaflets; flowers and fruits hanging in clusters; white to yellowish fruit (drupes). Toxic parts — Roots, stems, leaves, pollen, flowers, and fruits.	An extremely variable native weed throughout southern Canada and the United States with the exception of the west coast; found on flood plains, along lake shores, edges of woods, stream banks, fences, and around buildings.	Poisoning — Skin irritation due to an oil-resin containing urushiol. Symptoms — Contact with skin causes itching, burning, redness, and small blisters; severe gastric disturbance and even death by eating leaves or fruit.	Almost half of all persons are allergic to poison ivy. Skin irritation may also result form indirect contact such as animals (including dogs and cats), clothing, tools, or sports equipment.
Pokeweed (Pokeberry) *Phytolacca americana*	Description — Shrublike herb with a large fleshy taproot; large, entire, oblong leaves which are pointed; white to purplish flowers in clusters at ends of branches; mature fruit a dark purple berry with red juice. Toxic parts — Rootstalk, leaves, and stems.	Native to the eastern United States and southeastern Canada.	Poisoning — Highest concentration of poison mainly in roots; contains the bitter glycoside, saponin and a glycoprotein. Symptoms — Burning and bitter taste in mouth, stomach cramps, nausea, vomiting, diarrhea, drowsiness, slowed breathing, weakness, tremors, convulsions, spasms, coma, and death if eaten in large amounts.	Young tender leaves and stems of pokeweed are often cooked as greens. Cooked berries are used for pies without harm. It is one of the most dangerous poisonous plants because people prepare it improperly.

TABLE 35 (CONTINUED)
Some Important Poisonous Plants of North America

Common and Scientific Name	Description; Toxic Parts	Geographical Distribution	Poisoning; Symptoms	Remarks
Poppy (common poppy) *Papaver somniferum*	Description — An erect, annual herb with milky juice; simple, coarsely toothed, or lobed leaves; showy red, white, pink, or purple flowers; fruit an oval, crowned capsule; tiny seeds in capsule. Toxic parts — Unripe fruits of their juice.	Introduced from Eurasia and widely grown in the United States until cultivation without a license became unlawful.	Poisoning — Crude resin from unripe seed capsule source of narcotic opium alkaloids. Symptoms — From unripe fruit, stupor, coma, shallow and slow breathing, and depression of the central nervous system; possibly nausea and severe retching (straining to vomit).	The use of poppy extracts is a double edged sword — addictive narcotics and valuable medicines. Poppy seeds which are used as toppings on breads are harmless.
Rhododendron; azaleas *Rhododendron* sp.	Description — Usually evergreen shrubs; mostly entire, simple, leathery leaves in whorls or alternate; showy white to pink flowers in terminal clusters; fruit a wood capsule. Toxic parts — Entire plant.	Throughout the temperate parts of the United States as a native and as an introduced ornamental.	Poisoning — Contains the toxic resinoid, andromedotoxin. Symptoms — Watering eyes and mouth, nasal discharge, nausea, severe abdominal pain, vomiting, convulsions, lowered blood pressure, lack of coordination and loss of energy; progressive paralysis of arms and legs until death, in severe cases.	Cases of poisoning are rare in this country but rhododendrons should be suspected of possible danger.
Rosary pea (precatory pea) *Abrus precatorius*	Description — A twining, more or less, woody perennial vine; alternate and divided leaves with small leaflets; red to purple or white flowers; fruit a short pod containing ovoid seeds which are glossy, bright scarlet over 3/4 of their surface, and jet black over the remaining 1/4. Toxic parts — Seeds.	Native to the tropics, but naturalized in Florida and the Keys.	Poisoning — Contains the phytotoxin, abrin and tetanic glycoside, abric acid. Symptoms — Severe stomach pain, in 1–3 days, nausea, vomiting, severe diarrhea, weakness, cold sweat, drowsiness, weak, fast pulse, coma, circulatory collapse, and death.	The beans are made into rosaries, necklaces, bracelets, leis, and various toys which receive wide distribution. Seeds must be chewed and swallowed to cause poisoning. Whole seeds pass through the digestive tract without causing symptoms. One thoroughly chewed seed is said to be potent enough to kill an adult or child.

Snow-on-the-mountain *Euphorbia marginata*	Description — A tall annual herb, growing up to 4 ft (122 cm) high; smooth, lance-shaped leaves with conspicuously white margins; whorls of white petal-like leaves border flowers; fruit a 3-celled, 3-lobed capsule. Toxic parts — Leaves, stems, and milky sap.	Native to the western, dry plains and valleys from Montana to Mexico; sometimes escapes in the eastern United States.	Poisoning — Toxins causing dermatitis and severe irritation of the digestive tract. Symptoms — Blistering of the skin, nausea, abdominal pain, fainting, diarrhea, and possibly death in severe cases.	Milky juice of this plant is very caustic. Outwardly, snow-on-the-mountain resembles a poinsettia.
Skunkcabbage *Veratrum californicum*	Description — Tall, broadleaved herbs of the lily family, growing to 6 ft (183 cm) high; large, alternate pleated, clasping, and parallel-veined leaves; numerous whitish to greenish flowers in large terminal clusters; 3-lobed, capsule fruit. Toxic parts — Entire plant.	Various species throughout North America in wet meadows, forests, and along streams.	Poisoning — Contains such alkaloids as veradridene and veratrine. Symptoms — Nausea, vomiting, diarrhea, stomach pains, lowered blood pressure, slow pulse, reduced body temperature, shallow breathing, salivation, weakness, nervousness, convulsions, paralysis, and possibly death.	These plants have been used for centuries as a source of drugs and as a source of insecticide. Since the leaves resemble cabbage, they are often collected as an edible wild plant, but with unpleasant results.
Tansy *Tanacetum vulgare*	Description — Tall, aromatic herb with simple stems to 3 ft (91 cm) high; alternate, pinnately divided, narrow leaves; flower heads in flat-topped clusters with numerous small, yellow flowers. Toxic parts — Leaves, stems, and flowers.	Introduced from Eurasia; widely naturalized in North America; sometimes found escaped along roadsides, in pastures, or other wet places; grown for medicinal purposes.	Poisoning — Contains an oil, tanacetin, or oil of tansy. Symptoms — Nausea, vomiting, diarrhea, convulsions, violent spasms, dilated pupils, rapid and feeble pulse, and possibly death.	Tansy and oil of tansy are employed as a herbal remedy for nervousness, intestinal worms, to promote menstruation, and to induce abortion. Some poisonings have resulted from the use of tansy as a home remedy.

TABLE 35 (CONTINUED)
Some Important Poisonous Plants of North America

Common and Scientific Name	Description; Toxic Parts	Geographical Distribution	Poisoning; Symptoms	Remarks
Waterhemlock *Cicuta* sp.	Description — A perennial with parsleylike leaves; hollow, jointed stems and hollow, pithy roots; flowers in umbrella clusters; stems streaked with purple ridges; 2–6 ft (61–183 cm) high. Toxic parts — Entire plant, primarily the roots and young growth.	Wet meadows, pastures, and flood plains of western and eastern United States, generally absent in the plains states.	Poisoning — Contains the toxic resinlike higher alcohol, cicutoxin. Symptoms — Frothing at the mouth, spasms, dilated pupils, diarrhea, convulsions, vomiting, delirium, respiratory failure, paralysis, and death.	One mouthful of the waterhemlock root is reported to contain sufficient poison to kill a man. Children making whistles and peashooters from the hollow stems have been poisoned. The waterhemlock is often mistaken for the edible wild artichoke or parsnip. However, it is considered to be one of the most poisonous plants of the North Temperate Zone.
White snakeroot *Eupatorium rogosum*	Description — Erect perennial with stems 1–5 ft. (30–152 cm) tall; opposite oval leaves with pointed tips and sharply toothed edges, and dull on the upper surface but shiny on the lower surface; showy, snow white flowers in terminal clusters. Toxic parts — Entire plant.	From eastern Canada to Saskatchewan and south to Texas, Louisiana, Georgia, and Virginia.	Poisoning — Contains the higher alcohol, tremetol and some glycosides. Symptoms — Weakness, nausea, loss of appetite, vomiting, tremors, labored breathing, constipation, dizziness, delirium, convulsions, coma, and death.	Recovery from a nonlethal dose is a slow process, due to liver and kidney damage. Poison may be in the milk of cows that have eaten white snakeroot — "milk sickness."

From Ensminger et al., *Foods and Nutrition Encyclopedia*, 2nd ed., CRC Press, Boca Raton, FL, 1994, pp. 1776–1785.

PORK

Meat from a pig.

PORPHYRIN

An iron-containing ring structure that is part of hemoglobin.

PORTAL HYPERTENSION

Increased pressure in the portal vein resulting from an obstruction of blood flow through the liver.

PORTAL VEIN

The vein which carries the absorbed nutrients from the intestinal tract to the liver.

POSTPRANDIAL

After a meal.

POTASSIUM (K⁺)

An essential mineral. Main intracellular cation; plays an important role in the Na^+K^+ pump, and in the maintenance of cell volume, acid-base balance, muscle contraction, nerve conductance, and protein synthesis (see minerals, Table 30).

POTASSIUM 40 (K^{40})

Naturally occurring nonradioactive isotope of potassium.

PPC_{10}

The concentration at which in 10% of the population the critical organ is affected.

PREALBUMIN

A blood protein smaller than albumin which migrates ahead of it when a sample of blood proteins are separated by electrophoresis.

PRECISION

No random errors in the measurements. Also referred to as reproducibility. The reproducibility of a measurement is high, if there is good concordance between repeated measurements.

PRECURSOR

A predecessor molecule.

PREECLAMPSIA

Toxemia of pregnancy characterized by hypertension, albuminuria, edema of the lower extremities, and headaches that must be corrected to avoid true eclampsia.

PREGNANCY INDUCED ANEMIA

Dilution of the red cell number due to the increase in blood volume associated with pregnancy.

PREGNANCY INDUCED HYPERGLYCEMIA

Abnormal glucose tolerance which occurs (gestational diabetes) during gestation but not before or after.

PREGNANCY INDUCED HYPERTENSION

An increase in blood pressure due to pregnancy. If markedly elevated, is a sign of pending toxemia.

PREMATURE BABIES

Infants born before their prenatal development is complete; infants born prior to 37 weeks of gestation.

PREMELANOIDS

Precursor of the skin pigment melanin.

PRESERVATIVES

See additives, Table 4.

PRESSURE SORES

Ulceration of tissue, usually located over a bony prominence thinly covered with flesh such as the spine, heels, elbows, shoulder blades, or hip, resulting from impaired blood circulation or pressure from prolonged confinement in bed.

PREVALENCE

The number of existing cases of X in a given population at a given time.

PRIMIGRAVIDA

A woman during her first pregnancy.

PRIMIPARA

A woman who is experiencing her first pregnancy

PROBLEM ORIENTED MEDICAL RECORD (POMR)

Method of charting in a patients medical record that identifies the problems, usually in order of importance, and plans for intervention.

PROKARYOTES

Single cell organisms.

PROLACTIN

Hormone which stimulates milk production by the mammary cell.

PROLINE

A nonessential amino acid (see Table 5, Amino Acids).

PROSTAGLANDINS

See eicosanoids.

PROSTHETIC GROUP

A nonprotein component of an enzyme (or other body protein) that is necessary to the activity of that enzyme or protein.

PROTEASE

An enzyme which catalyzes the degradation of protein.

PROTEASE INHIBITORS

Compounds that inhibit the protein degradative action of the protease enzymes.

PROTECTIVE FOODS

Foods that are rich in essential nutrients. So called because they protect the body against deficiency diseases.

PROTEINS

A large group of complex molecules which are polymers of a variety of amino acids. They are classified as simple proteins (Table 36) or conjugated proteins (Table 37). Conjugated proteins have a variety of biological functions and are characterized by the type of prosthetic group attached to the protein.

Only 8 of the 100 or so carbohydrates that are known to occur in nature are found in glycoproteins (Table 38). These carbohydrates occur in chains containing no more than 15 saccharide units. Of the 20 amino acids in these proteins only four (Table 38) actually bind to the carbohydrate moiety. The carbohydrates are linked to these amino acids by a nitrogen-oxygen glucosidic bond or through an oxygen bond. Some proteins contain small amounts of carbohydrate in loose association rather than as integral and characteristic parts of their structure. An example of this association is the glycosylated hemoglobin found in the blood of poorly controlled diabetics. In diabetes, blood glucose levels may fluctuate and exceed the normal range of 80–120 mg/dl. Some of this excess of glucose may be picked up by the hemoglobin and form glycosylated hemoglobin. Levels of glycosylated hemoglobin are used as indicators of the degree of control of the diabetic state.

The function of the carbohydrate moiety of glycoproteins is not well-defined. Some of the glycoproteins, those located on the exterior aspect of the plasma membrane are part of the cell recognition system. Others are essential to the immune mechanism as a component of γ globulin. Glycoproteins are essential components of membrane transport systems and are components of many receptors.

Lipoproteins

Lipoproteins are multicomponent complexes of lipids and protein that form distinct molecular aggregates with approximate stoichiometry between each of the components. They contain polar and neutral lipids, cholesterol, or cholesterol esters in addition to protein. The protein and lipid is held together by noncovalent forces. The protein component (apolipoprotein) is located on the outer surface of the micellular lipid structure, where it serves a hydrophilic function. Lipids, primarily hydrophobic molecules, are not easily transported through an aqueous environment such as blood. However, when they combine with proteins, the resulting compound becomes hydrophilic and can be transported in the blood to tissue which can use or store these lipids.

Membrane lipoproteins, like the glycoproteins, are essential components of membrane transport systems and as such, are important in the overall regulation of cellular activity.

TABLE 36
Simple Proteins

Name	Characteristics	Example
Albumins	Soluble in water, coagulated by heat, precipitated by saturated salt solutions	Lactalbumin Serum albumin
Globulins	Soluble in salt solutions; insoluble in water; coagulated by heat	Serum globulin Ovoglobulin
Glutelins	Soluble in dilute acids and bases; insoluble in neutral solvents, coagulated by heat	Glutenin from wheat
Prolamins	Soluble in 70-80% alcohol; insoluble in absolute alcohol, water, and other neutral solvents	Zein (corn) Gliadin (wheat)
Scleroproteins	Insoluble in all neutral solvents and in dilute acids and bases	Keratin Collagen
Histones	Soluble in water and very dilute acids; insoluble in very dilute NH_4OH; not coagulated by heat; basic amino acids predominate	Nucleoproteins
Protamines	Basic polypeptides, soluble in water or in NH_4OH; not coagulated by heat; basic amino acids predominate	Eggs

From Berdanier, C.D., *Advanced Nutrition: Macronutrients*, CRC Press, Boca Raton, FL, 1994, 110.

TABLE 37
Some Conjugated Proteins

Name	Prosthetic Group	Example
Glycoproteins and Mucoproteins	Nucleic acid carbohydrates which hydrolyze to amino acid sugars; mucoproteins contain 4% hexosamines; mucin and glycoproteins contain less	Serum alpha, beta, and gamma globulins
Lipoproteins	Neutral fats, phospholipids, cholesterol	Cell membranes; Blood lipid carrying proteins
Nucleoproteins	Nucleic acid	Chromosomes
Phosphoproteins	Phosphate joined in ester linkage	Milk casein
Hemoproteins	Iron	Catalase; Hemoglobin, the Cytochromes
Flavoproteins	Flavin adenine nucleotide (FAD)	FAD linked-succinate dehydrogenase
Metalloproteins	Metals (not part of a nonprotein prosthetic group)	Ferritin

From Berdanier, C.D., *Advanced Nutrition: Macronutrients*, CRC Press, Boca Raton, FL, 1994, 110.

Nucleoproteins
Nucleoproteins are combinations of nucleic acids and simple proteins. The protein usually consists of a large number of the basic amino acids. Nucleoproteins are ubiquitous molecules that tend to have very complex structures and numerous functional activities. All living cells contain nucleoproteins.

Other conjugated proteins
The phosphoproteins and the metalloproteins are associations of proteins with phosphate groups or such ions as zinc, copper, and iron. The association may be fairly loose as with the phosphate carrying protein or tight as with the phosphate in casein and the iron in ferritin.

TABLE 38

Components of Glycoproteins

Sugars Found in Glycoproteins		Amino Acids which Bind to the Carbohydrates in Glycoproteins
Glucose	Acetylgalactosamine	Asparagine
Galactose	Arabinose	Serine
Mannose	Xylose	Threonine
Fucase (6-deoxy galactose)		Hydroxylysine
Acetylglucosamine		

From Berdanier, C.D., *Advanced Nutrition: Macronutrients*, CRC Press, Boca Raton, FL, 1994, 111.

Hemoproteins sometimes are grouped with the metalloproteins because of the iron which they contain. Flavoproteins are primarily enzymes and have as their prosthetic group a phosphate-containing adenine nucleotide which functions as an acceptor or donor of reducing equivalents.

Classification by Nutritive Value

In nutrition, we are interested in food proteins as sources of needed amino acids. Those proteins which contain the essential amino acids in the proportions needed by the body are referred to as complete proteins. They are primarily of animal origin. Eggs, milk, meat, and fish are sources of complete protein. Proteins lacking in one or more essential amino acids or which have a poor balance of amino acids relative to the body's need are incomplete or imbalanced proteins. These proteins are usually of plant origin, although some animal proteins are incomplete. The connective tissue protein called collagen, from which gelatin is isolated, lacks tryptophan; zein, the protein in corn, is low in lysine as well as tryptophan. When food selection is limited by the availability of protein-rich foods, incomplete proteins can be combined so that all of the essential amino acids are provided. For example, corn or wheat and soy or peanut proteins can be combined in the same meal so that all of the essential amino acids are provided. When these proteins are combined they will provide sufficient amounts of the needed amino acids. The combination of incomplete proteins needed to provide all the needed amino acids must be consumed within a relatively short time interval (less than four hours) to obtain the appropriate and needed amounts of amino acids. Maximum benefit is obtained when the combination is consumed at the same time. Supplementation of incomplete proteins with missing amino acids has been suggested for populations consuming diets having a single dietary item as its main protein source. This supplementation is not very practical over a long period of time due to the cost of the pure amino acid supplement. Such populations are also likely to develop other nutritional disorders when their food supply is so limited. With judicious use of a variety of foods available to these populations, amino acid deficiencies or imbalances can be overcome.

In addition to the amino acid content, protein quality, or rather the quality of the food containing the protein, is classed according to its total protein content. Potatoes, for example, contain a very good distribution of essential and nonessential amino acids, yet, because the potato contains so little protein (1.7%), it is not considered a good protein source. One would have to consume a lot of potatoes (3.18 kg or ~ 7 lb) to meet one's daily amino acid and total nitrogen requirements. Total protein content can be determined rather easily but analysis of a food to establish the individual amino acid content can be tedious and difficult.

Protein Denaturation

One of the most striking characteristics of proteins is the response to heat, alcohol, and other treatments which affect their quaternary, tertiary, and secondary structures. This characteristic response is called denaturation. Denaturation results in the unfolding of a protein molecule, thus breaking its hydrogen bonds and the associations between functional groups; as a result, the three-dimensional structure is lost. Denaturation affects many of the properties of the protein molecule. Its physical shape is changed, its solubility in water is decreased, and its reactivity with other proteins may be lost. When denatured, the protein loses its biological activity. Most proteins are denatured at temperatures greater than 50–60°C; some are denatured at temperatures less than 15°C. A very good example of protein denaturation is the coagulation of egg white when heated. Heat denaturation, unless extreme, does not affect the amino acid composition of protein and, indeed, may make these amino acids more available to the body because heating provokes the unfolding or uncoiling of the protein and exposes more of the amino acid chain to the action of the proteolytic digestive enzymes. For this reason, many cooked proteins are of higher biological value than those same proteins if consumed without heat treatment. If only mild denaturation occurs, it can be reversed. This process is called renaturation. If a protein is renatured, it will resume its original shape and biological activity.

PROTEIN ABSORPTION

See absorption of amino acids.

PROTEIN ANALYSIS (FOOD)

Total protein content is estimated from the total nitrogen content of the test sample as determined by the classical Kjeldahl method. This method also determines nonprotein nitrogen as well; however, the amount of error in the method due to the inclusion of these compounds is very small. Most proteins contain 16% nitrogen. To convert the nitrogen content to protein, one uses the following formula:

$$P_G = N_G \times \frac{100}{16} = N_G \times 6.25$$

where P_G = grams of protein in 100 grams of food and N_G = grams of nitrogen in 100 grams of food.

This conversion factor is an average factor. If one wishes more exact figures, established conversion factors for each food category are available. For example, cereals generally have less protein nitrogen and more nonprotein nitrogen, thus, the conversion factor of 5.7 is used for cereal foods. On the other hand, milk has more protein nitrogen and the factor of 6.4 may be used. Generally speaking, because humans usually consume a mixed diet, the lower and higher factors tend to average out and the value of 6.25 is correct to use when the protein intake of a day's food intake is chemically determined.

The amino acid determination of a protein has two phases — qualitative identification and quantitative estimation of the residues. The peptide bond that connects the residues is cleaved by acid, base, or enzyme-catalyzed hydrolysis to give a mixture of separated amino acids. The free amino acids are separated from one another and identified using chromatographic and/or electrophoretic techniques. Once separated and identified, each amino acid present can be determined quantitatively. Several amino acid specific reactions are available. These assays do not establish the sequence of the amino acids, nor the protein's primary structure but merely tell how much of each amino acid is present. The sequence of amino acids can be determined by cleaving, one by one, the amino acids from the protein and following this cleavage with an analysis of the individual amino acids. High performance liquid chromatography (HPLC) can be used for this analysis.

PROTEIN CONTENT IN FOODS

Foods vary in their protein content. Shown in Table 39 are a few foods and their protein content. A more complete list of foods and their nutrient content can be found in the USDA Handbooks #8–15.

TABLE 39
Protein Content of Representative Foods in the Human Diet

Food	Protein, grams
Milk, 244 g (8 oz)	8.0
Cheddar cheese, 84 g (3 oz)	21.3
Egg, 50 g (1 large)	6.1
Apple, 212 g (1–3 1/4″ diameter)	0.4
Banana, 74 g (1–8 3/4″ long)	1.2
Potato, cooked, 136 g (1 potato)	2.5
Bread, white, slice, 25 g	2.1
Fish, cod, poached, 100 g (3 1/2 oz)	20.9
Oysters, 100 g (3 1/2 oz)	13.5
Beef, pot roast, 85 g (3 oz)	22.0
Liver, pan fried, 85 g (3 oz)	23.0
Pork chop, bone in, 87 g (3.1 oz)	23.9
Ham, boiled, 2 pieces, 114 g	20.0
Peanut butter, 16 g (1 tablespoon)	4.6
Pecans, 28 g (1 oz)	2.2
Snap beans, 125 g (1 cup)	2.4
Carrots, sliced, 78 g (1/2 cup)	0.8

From Handbooks #8–15, USDA, Composition of Foods, U.S. Government Printing Office, Washington, D.C., 1986. These handbooks are periodically updated as new information becomes available.

PROTEIN DIGESTION

The degradation of food protein into its component amino acids and dipeptides.

The purpose of protein digestion is to liberate the amino acids which comprise the proteins. Protein digestion does not begin until the protein reaches the stomach and the food is acidified with the gastric hydrochloric acid. Hydrochloric acid also serves to denature the food proteins thus making them more vulnerable to attack by pepsin, an endopeptidase. Actually, pepsin is not a single enzyme. It consists of pepsin A which attacks peptide bonds involving phenylalanine or tyrosine and several other enzymes which have specific attack points. The pepsins are released into the gastric cavity as pepsinogen. Food entering the stomach stimulates HCl release, the pH of the gastric contents fall below 2, and the pepsinogen loses a 44 amino acid sequence. The activation of the pepsins from pepsinogen occurs by one of two processes. The first, called **autoactivation**, occurs when the pH drops below 5. At low pH the bond between the 44th and 45th amino acid residue falls apart and the 44 amino acid residue (from the amino terminus) is liberated. The liberated residue acts as an inhibitor of pepsin by binding to the catalytic site until pH 2 is achieved. The inhibition is relieved when this fragment is degraded, as happens at pH 2 or below or when it is attacked by pepsin. Since the fragment binds at the catalytic site of pepsin, this can happen. The other process is called **autocatalysis** and occurs when already active pepsin attacks the precursor pepsinogen. This is a self repeating process and serves to ensure ongoing catalyses of the resident protein. The cleavage of the 44 amino acid residue, in addition to providing activated pepsin, has another purpose. That is, it serves as a signal peptide for cholecystokinin release in the duodenum. This then sets the stage for the subsequent pancreatic phase of protein digestion. As described in the units on lipids and carbohydrates, cholecystokinin stimulates both the exocrine pancreas and the intestinal mucosal epithelial cell to release its digestive enzymes. The intestinal cell releases an enzyme, enteropeptidase or enterokinase, which serves to activate the protease, trypsin, released as trypsinogen by the exocrine pancreas. This trypsin not only acts on food proteins, it also acts on other pre-proteases, released by the exocrine pancreas, activating them. Thus, trypsin acts as an endoprotease on chymotrypsinogen, releasing chymotrypsin, on proelastase, releasing elastase, and on procarboxypeptidase, releasing carboxypeptidase. Trypsin, chymotrypsin, and elastase are all endoproteases each having specificity for particular peptide bonds. Each of these three proteases have serine as part of their catalytic site so any compound that ties up the serine will inhibit the activity of these proteases. Such inhibitors as diisopropylphosphofluoridate react with this serine and in so doing bring a halt to protein digestion.

The daily protein intake of about 100 g plus that protein that appears in the gut as enzymes, sloughed epithelial gut cells, and mucins is almost completely digested and absorbed. This is a very efficient process that ensures a continuous supply of amino acids to the whole body amino acid pool. Less than 1% of the total protein that passes through the gastrointestinal tract appears in the feces. If the food contributes between 70 and 100 g of protein and the endogenous protein contributes another 100 g (range: 35–200 g) then one might expect to see about 1–2 g of nitrogen in the feces. This is equivalent to 6–12 g protein. Of the dietary protein, the fecal protein might include the hard to chew/digest tough fibrous connective tissue of meat or nitrogen-containing indigestible kernel coats of grains or particles of nuts that are not attacked by the digestive enzymes. Peanuts, for example, eaten whole have a structure that is difficult to broach by the digestive enzymes. Unless chewed very finely, much of the nutritive value of this food may be lost. Peanut butter on the other hand, is very well digested because the preparation of the peanut butter ensures that its particle size is **very** small and is thus quite digestible. The enzymes which are responsible for protein digestion are listed in Table 40.

TABLE 40
Digestive Enzymes and Their Target Linkages

Enzyme	Location	Target
Pepsin	Stomach	Peptide bonds involving the aromatic amino acids
Trypsin	Small intestine	Peptide bonds involving arginine and lysine
Chymotrypsin	Small intestine	Peptide bonds involving tyrosine, tryptophan, phenylalanine, methionine, and leucine
Elastase	Small intestine	Peptide bonds involving alanine, serine, and glycine
Carboxypeptidase A	Small intestine	Peptide bonds involving valine, leucine, isoleucine, and alanine
Carboxypeptidase B	Small intestine	Peptide bonds involving lysine and arginine
Endopeptidase, Aminopeptidase, Dipeptidase	Cells of brush border	di- and tripeptides that enter the brush border of the absorptive cells

The protein hydrolases, called peptidases, fall into two categories. Those that attack internal peptide bonds and liberate large peptide fragments for subsequent attack by other enzymes are called the endopeptidases. Those that attack the terminal peptide bonds and liberate single amino acids from the protein structure are called exopeptidases. The exopeptidases are further subdivided according to whether they attack at the carboxy end of the amino acid chain (carboxypeptidases) or the amino end of the chain (aminopeptidases). The initial attack on an intact protein is catalyzed by endopeptidases while the final digestive action is catalyzed by the exopeptidases. The final products of digestion are free amino acids and some di- and tripeptides that are absorbed by the intestinal epithelial cells.

PROTEIN EVALUATION (BIOLOGICAL VALUE OF PROTEIN)

Methods for determining how well the food protein meets the biological need for protein by the consumer.

Biological value is high when the protein is rich in all the amino acids in the right amounts needed by the consumer. Several techniques have been developed for this assessment. The nitrogen balance technique for evaluating protein quality assumes that a given protein when fed at maintenance levels will completely replace the protein being catabolized during the normal course of metabolic events in the body. It also assumes that all nitrogen gain and loss can be measured. Thus, for good quality proteins, nitrogen balance (intake vs. excretion) should be zero for an adult individual and for poor quality proteins, nitrogen balance will be negative. For growing individuals, good quality proteins result in high nitrogen retentions while poor quality proteins result in low nitrogen retention. The amount of protein retained can be determined by analyzing the total nitrogen content of the food, the feces, and the urine.

The biological value (BV) was conceived as a ratio of the nitrogen absorbed to that retained multiplied by 100. In the original method, animals were fed a nitrogen-free diet for 7–10 days, then fed a diet containing the test protein at a level commensurate with their protein maintenance requirements for the same time interval. During each of these periods, the urine and feces were collected and analyzed for total nitrogen. Knowing the nitrogen intake and the nitrogen excretion during both the nitrogen-free and test periods, the biological value was calculated as follows:

$$BV = 100 \times \frac{N \text{ absorbed}}{N \text{ retained}} = 100 \times \frac{N_I - (N_{FT} - N_{FF}) - (N_{UT} - N_{UF})}{N_I - (N_{FT} - N_{FF})}$$

Where BV   = Biological value
   N_I = Nitrogen intake
   N_{FT} = Fecal nitrogen during test period
   N_{FF} = Fecal nitrogen during nitrogen-free period
   N_{UT} = Urinary nitrogen during test period
   N_{UF} = Urinary nitrogen during nitrogen-free period

This method is noninvasive and very useful for work with humans. However, nitrogen can be lost via routes other than urine and feces. In hot climates or in physically active subjects, significant nitrogen losses can occur through the sweat. On an adequate protein intake, it has been estimated that up to 1 g N/dl can be lost. On an inadequate or low protein diet, sweat losses can amount of 0.5 g N/dl. Hair, nail, and menstrual losses can also contribute error to the nitrogen balance technique. Usually sweat, hair, skin, and nail losses are ignored since they are minor in comparison to the urine and fecal losses. Other errors in the method include the possibility of daily cumulative errors in the collection and analysis of the food, urine, and feces and the effects of poor nutritional status on the responses of the subject to this procedure. Good subject cooperation is essential to insure quantitative ingestion of the food and the quantitative collection of the urine and feces.

The main disadvantage of this method is theoretical in character. The basic assumption of "replaceability" of body protein by a food protein is valid only when comparing good quality proteins. When poor proteins such as zein, gelatin, or gluten are evaluated, unrealistically high values result. This overestimation results from the failure of the method to account for the mobilization of body protein to meet particular amino acid needs. If there is a deficiency of one or more of the essential amino acids in the test protein, the animal will catabolize body proteins in an effort to provide the missing amino acid so as to support the synthesis of vital or needed proteins. There appears to be a hierarchy of body proteins — those which are most essential to the survival of the animal are synthesized in preference to those, such as muscle protein, which are not as essential. In any event, when the body proteins are mobilized, the needed amino acids they contain are utilized and the remaining ones are deaminated and used for energy. The amino group is then converted to urea and excreted, contributing to the urinary nitrogen level. The nitrogen balance technique does not differentiate the source of the nitrogen in the excreta and, because of this, is not as valid as a technique to evaluate incomplete proteins.

The nitrogen balance index (NBI) relates the absorbed nitrogen to the nitrogen excretion of a separate but concurrent group of individuals fed a nitrogen-free diet. This technique requires less time than the Thomas-Mitchell method but is subject to many of the same kind of errors. Both methods suffer from the inaccuracies contributed by the methodological measure of the so-called endogenous nitrogen loss. Both methods assume that this loss is represented by the nitrogen excreted by the animal during the nitrogen-free period.

One must consider the dynamic state of the body proteins, that is, the constant need to synthesize proteins having a short half-life. This synthesis must be accommodated by the catabolism of tissue protein; a catabolic process unlikely to occur extensively if good quality proteins are consumed. Because this overestimation of endogenous loss is more serious with proteins of poor quality, inconsistent biological values are obtained. This is particularly true when unrefined proteins or food mixtures are evaluated. The relationship of the nitrogen balance technique to the nitrogen balance index can best be seen in Figure 42.

A more accurate method for the evaluation of protein quality is one which actually measures the retention of nitrogen in the carcass from the ingested protein nitrogen. This is called the NPU-BV or NPU method. Using these methods which calculate biological value from the change in carcass protein, groups of animals, usually rats, are fed diets containing graded amounts of the test protein or a nitrogen-free diet. After a period of 7–10 days, the animals are killed and the nitrogen content of the carcasses determined. Obviously, proteins of high quality will evoke a greater retention of nitrogen in the carcass than proteins of poor quality. Using this technique, biological value can be calculated as follows:

$$\text{NPU BV} = \frac{B_f - B_k + I_k}{I_f} \times 100$$

Where B_f = carcass nitrogen of animals fed test protein diet
        B_k = carcass nitrogen of animals fed nitrogen-free diet
        I_k = absorbed nitrogen of animals fed nitrogen-free diet
        I_f = absorbed nitrogen of animals fed test-protein diet

While this method has the obvious advantage of actually measuring nitrogen retention, its disadvantages are also obvious. This method is inappropriate for large animals because of the technical difficulties associated with the determination of body composition and because of the excessive cost. Obviously, too, human studies would not be possible. However, conceptually, the method has merit and several investigators have devised variations which are useful in a variety of species.

One variation that is useful in man is to measure the changes in body composition indirectly. Using a stable isotope of nitrogen, ^{15}N, the rates of total body protein synthesis and breakdown as a response to variation in amounts of dietary protein can be determined. Constant infusions of ^{15}N-glycine allowed these investigators to assess the value of given proteins in the homeostatic situation where there is constant protein synthesis and breakdown. While a very useful technique, it is also very expensive and requires sophisticated techniques and equipment to make the appropriate measurements.

Another variation of the carcass retention method, which uses a radioactive isotope, measures the change in ^{40}K concentration in the body as a result of consuming a given protein for a period of 7–10 days. This method is based on the constancy of potassium as an intracellular ion. The concentration of potassium in the body can be directly related to the number of cells in the body and indirectly related to the protein in the body. Since a set percentage of this potassium exists as the naturally occurring radioactive isotope ^{40}K, measuring ^{40}K levels is a direct measure of body cell number and an indirect measure of body protein. Again, while this method has the advantage of its applicability to the human, its disadvantage is one of cost and availability of the whole body counters needed to determine the presence of the isotope.

By far, the easiest variation of the carcass retention method is the protein efficiency ratio (PER). In this method, carcass composition is not determined. It makes the assumption that the gain in body weight of a given animal is related to the quality of the protein fed. Thus, young growing animals are fed test protein-containing diets for a period of 28 days. The weight gain is computed and divided by the total protein intake.

The formula, $PER = \dfrac{\text{Weight gain in grams}}{\text{Protein intake in grams}}$ is easy to use and the method requires no

specialized expensive equipment. This is the method used for protein quality evaluation by most food companies and has been adopted by the regulatory agencies of the United States and Canada as their method of choice in evaluating the nutritional quality of foods. The ease and simplicity of the method, however, should not lull the reader into thinking that it is a "choice" method. PER can vary from species to species and within a given species, from strain to strain. Examples of within species variation in the PER of a given protein is given in Table 41. Variation can be introduced if levels of protein intake higher or lower than 10% by weight are used. In addition, the methods make no allowance for the maintenance requirement of the animal. Values obtained from a variety of food proteins are nonlinear. That is, a protein having a PER of 2 may not have twice the nutritional value of a protein having a PER of 1. Examples of the PER for a variety of food proteins is shown in Table 42.

A modification of the PER is the net protein ratio. This method attempts to account for the maintenance needs of the animals. In this method, two groups of animals are used. One is fed a nitrogen-free diet, the other the test diet. This modification is accompanied by all the pitfalls of using the nitrogen-free diets that have been discussed.

A variety of methods employing the assay of enzymes concerned with protein metabolism have also been devised. The determination of the activity of transaminase, xanthine dehydrogenase, renal arginase, and others have been reported as indicators of protein quality. Unfortunately, these methods have not been rigorously tested and compared to the presently available whole body methods.

The holistic approach, while valuable and useful, is nonetheless time consuming and expensive. The approaches discussed above do have the advantage that digestibility and amino acid availability are given due consideration.

TABLE 41
The PER of a Test Protein as Calculated Using the Weight Gain of Rats from Seven Different Strains

Rat Strain	Per			
	Week 1	Week 2	Week 3	Week 4
Holtzman	4.14	3.94	3.61	3.50
Charles River	4.29	3.64	3.54	3.60
ARS-Sprague Dawley	4.31	3.76	3.32	3.36
Osborne-Mendel	4.20	3.52	3.24	3.39
Wistar	4.47	3.59	3.33	3.37
Wistar Lewis	3.69	3.64	3.37	3.28
SSB/PL (NIH)	3.80	3.37	2.96	2.47

TABLE 42
PER of Various Foods

Eggs	3.9–4.0
Fish	3.5
Milk	3.0–3.1
Beef	2.3
Soybeans	2.3
Beans	1.4 –1.9
Nuts	1.8
Peanuts	1.7
Gluten	1.0
Rice	2.0
Corn	1.2

Attempts to circumvent the time and expense of whole animal work have resulted in a number of useful techniques. One method, the amino acid score or chemical score is a nonbiological method and requires the amino acid analysis of the test protein. The amount of the most limiting amino acid (only the essential amino acids are considered) is related to the content of that same amino acid in a reference protein. In most cases, this reference is egg protein, however, a theoretical protein based on the amino acid requirements of the species in question could also be used.

Thus,

$$\text{Chemical Score} = \frac{\text{mg of limiting amino acid/g test protein}}{\text{mg of amino acid/g ideal protein}} \times 100$$

While this method is quick and does not use animals, it does not make any allowance for digestibility or availability of the constituent amino acids. This is a rather important aspect of protein nutrition. Some amino acids form sugar-amino acid complexes which render the amino acids less available to the body. This occurs with the browning of baked goods such as bread; while bread is not considered a prime protein source, evaluation of its protein quality using the amino acid score would be in error due to the browning reaction.

A variation on this chemical method tries to account for digestibility. In this method, test proteins are first digested *in vitro* using conditions resembling those in the gastrointestinal tract. The amino acid score is then determined on the products of this digestion. This is a relatively new but promising approach to evaluating protein quality. It will require considerably more work to validate it, but at present, it represents an innovative approach to the problems associated with assessing protein quality.

Protein structure

Proteins are complex molecules having characteristic primary, secondary, tertiary, and quaternary structures. The primary structure is determined genetically as the particular sequence of amino acids in a given protein.

Under normal pH and temperature conditions, a protein is characterized not only by its amino acid sequence but also its three-dimensional structure; that is, how the chain of amino acids twists and turns and what shape this long chain of amino acids assumes. This three-dimensional shape, unique to each protein's particular amino acid sequence, is known as the native conformation of the protein. This assumption of shape may be spontaneous or may be catalyzed by enzymes and reflects the lowest energy state of the protein in its native environment. Protein conformation is usually divided into two categories — secondary and tertiary. The secondary and tertiary structures of a protein result from interactions between the reactive groups on the amino acids in the protein.

Secondary structure is the local conformation of the protein molecule. It is due to the formation of hydrogen bonds, disulfide bridges, and ionic bonds (in the case of the polar amino acids) between adjacent or nearby amino acids in an amino acid chain. As a result of these bonds, there is a regular recurring arrangement in space of the amino acids within the chain which can extend over the entire chain or only in small segments of it. Two kinds of periodic structures are found in proteins — the helix and the pleated sheet. In the helix, the amino acid chain can be viewed as wrapping itself around a long cylinder. The most common helical arrays are the α-helix and triple helix. The other periodic shape is the pleated sheet. It is essentially a linear array of the amino acid chain. All of these structures are stabilized by hydrogen bonding and sulfide bridges.

Tertiary structure is the regional conformation a protein molecule possesses; it develops after the secondary structure is established. Tertiary structure refers to how the amino acid chain bends or folds in three dimensions to form a compact or tightly folded protein. Tertiary structure results from hydrogen bonding, disulfide cross-linkages, ionic bonds between polar amino acids, and interactions between hydrophobic R groups. This last feature tends to locate the hydrophobic R groups internally in the protein structure, away from the aqueous environment. A protein which clearly demonstrates tertiary structure is hemoglobin. Some parts of the amino acid chains in this molecule can form helices; others cannot. This gives the molecule the fluidity to assume different three-dimensional shapes along the chain — it will bend back upon itself to accomplish the maximum number of hydrogen bonds and disulfide bridges.

As a result of the various bonds that can form within a protein molecule, essentially two kinds of proteins exist — fibrous protein and globular protein. Fibrous proteins resemble long ribbons or hairs. They tend to be insoluble in most solvents and include such tough, resilient protein structures as collagen and elastin. Fibrous protein can have either the helical or pleated sheet structure. Collagen is an example of the triple helix; silk, a pleated sheet structure. Where the fibrous proteins appear to have a long "stringy" shape, globular proteins are roughly spherical or elliptical. Many enzymes and antibodies have a globular structure.

The quaternary structure refers to how groups of individual amino acid chains are arranged in relation to each other within a given protein. It is the structure which results when two or more polypeptide chains combine. The chains (subunits) may be different or identical, yet each subunit still possesses its own primary, secondary, and tertiary structure. The number of subunits in a protein may vary; some proteins have only two subunits while others have as many as 2130 subunits. The protein, hemoglobin, for example, consists of four subunits and is one of the few proteins whose primary, secondary, tertiary, and quaternary structures are known. It contains four separate peptide chains: two α chains which contain 141 amino acid residues and two β chains which contain 146 amino acid residues. To each of these is bound a heme (iron) residue in a noncovalent linkage.

Protein synthesis

Two amino acids joined together form a dipeptide; three form a tripeptide and so on. Each amino acid in a chain is referred to as an amino acid residue. A chain of up to 100 amino acids joined together is called a polypeptide. If more than 100 amino acids are involved, then the compound is called a protein. Proteins have been identified which have as many as 300,000 amino acids residues and molecular weights in excess of 4×10^7.

The sequence of the amino acids which comprise a given protein is represented by a sequential arrangement of abbreviations for each. For example, the polypeptide bradykinin is represented in the following manner: Arg-Pro-Pro-Gly-Phe-Ser-Pro-Phe-Arg. The right hand side of the chain represents the carboxyl terminal while the left hand side represents the amino terminal. The systematic name for bradykinin is arginyldiprolylglyclyphenylalanyl-serylprolylphenylalanylarginine. This systematic name is seldom used except when one wishes to give the amino acid sequence of a given protein. The amino acid sequence of a given protein can vary and its variation is controlled genetically. Some of the proteins of importance in nutrition have been sequenced but these are few in number compared to the vast array of proteins in nature. Even if the proteins were sequenced, their systematic names would not be used because such a name would be very cumbersome.

The number of possible combinations of the 20 amino acids commonly found in proteins to make different protein molecules is almost limitless. In a dipeptide which contains two different amino acids (A and B), two combinations are available: A-B and B-A. In a tripeptide with three different amino acids, six combinations are available if all three amino acids are used and each used only one time: A-B-C, B-A-C, A-C-B, B-C-A, C-A-B, and C-B-A. The number of possible combinations of the sequential arrangement of different amino acids is determined by the expression **n!** (n factorial), when **n** is the number of different amino acids. If 20 amino acids are present in a protein, the number of possible combinations would be $20 \times 19 \times 18 \times 17 \ldots \times 1 = 2 \times 10^{18}$. The molecular weight of this molecule is about 2400 (average molecular weight of an amino acid $\times$ number of amino acids = 120×20), a relatively small protein. If the molecule were larger, and if the amino acids were used more than once, the number of possible combinations is increased even more. That nature can consistently reproduce the same protein when there are so many choices of amino acids and sequences, is due to its dependence on the codes for each of these proteins in the genetic material, DNA. Most of the DNA is in the nucleus, however, a small amount is found in the mitochondria. DNA is composed of four bases — adenine, guanine, thymine, and cytosine. These bases are condensed to form the DNA chain in a process analogous to the condensation of amino acids which comprise the primary structure of a protein. Species vary in the percent distribution of these bases in their DNA. In mammals the adenine-thymidine content varies from 45–53%. Small amounts of the base 5 methyl cytosine as well as methylated derivatives of the other bases can be found.

The sequence of amino acids in each protein synthesized by the body is determined from a subunit of the DNA molecule known as the gene. The gene, through the sequence of bases that are found in its constituent nucleotides, codes for a polypeptide. The DNA in the nucleus is very stable with respect to the base sequence and content. It can be damaged by certain chemicals, free radicals, x-rays, and other agents. However, it also can repair this damage to some extent. If a change in the base sequence does occur and is not repaired, a mutation is said to have occurred. This mutation will then become part of the genetic information transmitted to the next generation.

The chain of nucleotides which comprise DNA is formed by joining these bases through phosphodiester bonds. A typical segment of the chain is illustrated in Figure 48. The hydrophobic properties of the bases plus the strong charges of the polar groups within each of the component units are responsible for the helical conformation of the DNA chain. The bases themselves interact such that two chains are intertwined. Hence, the term double helix applies to the nuclear DNA. Hydrogen bonding between the bases stabilize this conformation as shown in Figure 48. Other factors as well serve to stabilize the structure of the DNA. Unwinding of the DNA, a necessary step in the initiation of protein synthesis, occurs when these stabilizing factors are perturbed. Unwinding exposes a small segment of the DNA allowing its base sequence to be available for complementary base pairing as happens when messenger RNA is synthesized under the influence of RNA polymerase II. The coding segments of most genes contain from 600 to 1800 nucleotides; these nucleotides can code for 200 to 600 amino acids in a polypeptide chain. The nucleotides which code for a specific protein may not be adjacent to each other on the DNA strand but may be located nearby as the DNA exists in a doubly coiled chain of bases, the double helix.

The DNA base sequence is unique for every protein that is synthesized in the body. While only a few bases are used for the DNA, the combinations and sequences of the combinations provide a specific code for each and every protein and peptide. The human genome project sponsored by the National Institutes of Health has as its goal the determination of the complete sequence and the mapping of subsequences. By mapping we mean the identification, within the double helix, of each segment and the protein it encodes. Thus, the function of DNA is to determine the properties of the cell through the provision of a code that directs protein synthesis. It also functions to transmit genetic information from one generation to the next in a given species. Thus, DNA has a broad spectrum of function. It ensures the identity of both specific cell types and specific species. Not all DNA is located in the nucleus. Some is found in the mitochondria. In this organelle, it exists in a circular form rather than as a double stranded coil (helix) as is found in the nucleus. In the nucleus, the DNA is found in the chromosomal chromatin. Chromatin contains very long double strands of DNA and a nearly equal mass of histone and nonhistone proteins. Histones are highly basic proteins varying in molecular weight from ~ 11,000 to ~ 21,000. As a result of their high content of basic amino acids, histones serve to interact with the poly anionic phosphate backbone of the DNA so as to produce uncharged nucleoproteins. The histones also serve to keep the DNA in a very compact form. The nuclear DNA, as soon as its replication is completed, becomes highly condensed into distinct chromosomes of characteristic shapes. These chromosomes exist as pairs and are numbered. There are 46 chromosomes in the human. Included in this number are the sex chromosomes, the X and Y chromosomes. If the individual has one X and one Y he is a male; if two X's are present, she is a female. The chromosomes are the result of a mixing of the nuclear DNA of the egg and sperm. Approximately half of each pair comes from each parent. If identical codes for a given protein are inherited from each parent, the resultant progeny will be a homozygote for that protein. If nonidentical codes are inherited, the progeny will be a heterozygote. Within the heterozygote population, there may be certain codes which are dominant, eye color or hair color for example. These are dominant traits and are expressed despite the fact that the individual has inherited two different codes for this trait. A mutation in a code that is not expressed is a recessive trait. If, by chance, two identical mutated genes are present that encode a certain protein, the expression of this

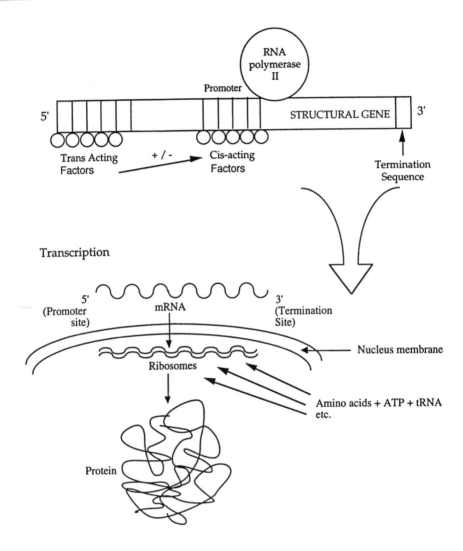

FIGURE 48 Protein synthesis. Signals are transmitted to the nucleus that stimulate the exposure of a gene for a specific protein. A specific messenger RNA is synthesized. The mRNA moves out into the cytosol and attaches to the ribosome whereupon tRNAs attached to amino acids dock at appropriate complementary bases and the amino acids are joined together to make protein.

mutated code will be observed. This is the basis for genetic diseases of the autosomal recessive or dominant type. Autosomal means a mutation in any of the chromosomal DNA except that which is in the X or Y chromosome. A mutation of the DNA in this chromosome is called a sex-linked mutation. If it results in a disease, it is called sex-linked genetic disease.

Having the codes in the nucleus for the synthesis of protein in the cytoplasm implies a communication between the cytoplasm and the nucleus and between the nucleus and the cytoplasm. Signals are sent to the nucleus which "informs" this organelle of the need to synthesize certain proteins. We do not know what all these signals are. Some are substrates for the needed proteins, some are hormones, and some are signalling compounds that have yet to be identified. The communication between the nucleus and the cytoplasm is carried out by messenger RNA (mRNA).

Messenger RNA is used to carry genetic information from the DNA of the chromosomes to the surface of the ribosomes. It is synthesized in the nucleus by a process known as transcription. Chemically, RNA is similar to DNA. It is an unbranched linear polymer in which the monomeric subunits are the ribonucleoside 5' monophosphates. The bases are the purines, adenine and guanine, and the prymidines, uracil and cytosine. Note that thymine is not used in RNA and that uracil is not present in DNA. RNA is single-stranded rather than double-stranded. It is held together by molecular base pairing and will contract if in a solution of high ionic strength. RNA, particularly the mRNA, is a much smaller molecule than DNA and is far less stable.

The synthesis of mRNA, transcription, has been elucidated for many of the important proteins. All known transcription reactions follow the same pattern in that the RNA is made through the use of a DNA template. The synthesis makes use of the RNA polymerase II enzyme. Actually transcription is divided into three parts. The first part is initiation. Initiation refers to the recognition of an active gene starting point by RNA polymerase II and the beginning of the bond formation process. The second part is elongation. This is the synthesis or joining together of the nucleotides. The third and last part is the termination of the chain. This is illustrated in Figure 48. The RNA polymerase synthesizes the mRNA in the 5' to 3' direction using the DNA template. Following transcription is translation. This refers to the synthesis of the protein using the order of the assemblage of constituent amino acids as dictated by the mRNA. As described, this mRNA code is dictated by DNA. There are a number of instances in the nutritional biochemistry literature where a specific nutrient serves to stimulate the transcription of a specific mRNA. Glucose, for example, binds at a specific site on the nuclear DNA which codes for the enzyme glucokinase and has a putative effect on glucokinase mRNA transcription. As the individual consumes a high glucose diet, the glucose in the diet serves as one of the signals which activate the de novo synthesis of glucokinase by the pancreatic β cell and the liver cell. The DNA in these cell types has a glucose sensitive promoter region just preceding the sequence which codes for the glucokinase. Other cell types may not have this promoter region exposed for glucose activation, and glucokinase may not be found in these cells. Similar instances of nutrients acting on promoter regions and stimulating mRNA transcription have been described (see Berdanier, C.D., and Hargrove, J.L., Eds., *Nutrition and Gene Expression*, CRC Press, Boca Raton, FL, 1992).

Ribosomal RNA makes up a large fraction of total cellular RNA. It serves as the "docking" point for the activated amino acids bound to the transfer RNA and the mRNA which dictates the amino acid polymerization sequence. Transfer RNA (tRNA) is used to bring an amino acid to the polysome (ribosome), the site of protein synthesis. Each amino acid has a specific tRNA. Each tRNA molecule is thought to have a cloverleaf arrangement of nucleotides. With this arrangement of nucleotides, there is the opportunity for the maximum number of hydrogen bonds to form between base pairs. A molecule which has many hydrogen bonds is very stable. Transfer RNA also contains a triplet of bases known, in this instance, as the anticodon. The amino acid carried by tRNA is identified by the codon of mRNA through its anticodon; the amino acid itself is not involved in this identification.

The actual site of protein assembly is on the ribosomes; some ribosomes are located on the membrane of the endoplasmic reticulum, and some are free in the cell matrix. Ribosomes consist almost entirely of ribosomal RNA and ribosomal protein. RNA is synthesized in the cell nucleus as a large molecule; there, this molecule is cleaved and leaves the nucleus as two subunits, a large one and a small one. The ribosome is reformed in the cytoplasm by the reassociation of the two subunits; the subunits, however, are not necessarily derived from the same precursor.

A few general statements can be made about the distribution of ribosomes in cells which have different capacities for the synthesis of protein:

1. Cells which synthesize large numbers of protein have numerous ribosomes; conversely, cells which synthesize small numbers of proteins contain few.
2. Of the proteins synthesized by a cell to be secreted from that cell for use elsewhere, most of the ribosomes are attached to the endoplasmic reticulum.
3. Those cells which synthesize protein primarily for intracellular use have relatively few ribosomes attached to the membrane.

Small groups of ribosomes called polysomes are involved in protein synthesis; under physiologic conditions, polysomes are bound to the endoplasmic reticulum. The ribosome is bound to the membrane through its large subunit; the small subunit is involved in the binding of mRNA to the ribosome. The ribosomes have two binding sites used in protein synthesis — the amino-acyl site and the peptidyl site. These two sites have specific functions in protein synthesis.

The synthesis of a protein takes place in four stages. Each stage requires specific cofactors and enzymes. In the first stage, which occurs in the cytosol, the amino acids are activated by esterifying each one to its specific tRNA. This requires a molecule of ATP. In addition to a specific tRNA, each amino acid requires a specific enzyme for this reaction.

During the second stage, the initiation of the synthesis of the polypeptide chain occurs. An initiation complex is formed by the binding of mRNA and the first activated amino acid-tRNA complex to the small ribosomal subunit. The large ribosomal unit then attaches, thus forming a functional ribosome. Three specific protein initiation factors are involved in this initiation step.

In the third stage of protein synthesis, the peptide chain is elongated by the sequential addition of amino acids from the tRNA complexes. The amino acid is recognized by base pairing of the codon of mRNA to the bases found in the anticodon of tRNA, and a peptide bond is formed between the peptide chain and the newly arrived amino acid. The ribosome then moves along the mRNA; this brings the next codon in the proper position for attachment of the next activated amino acyl-tRNA complex. The mRNA and nascent polypeptide appear to "track" through a groove in the ribosomal subunits. This protects them from attack by enzymes in the surrounding environment.

The final stage of protein synthesis is the termination of the chain. The termination is signaled by one of three special codons (stop codons) in the mRNA. After the carboxy terminal amino acid is attached to the peptide chain, it is still covalently attached to tRNA, which is, in turn, bonded to the ribosome. A protein release factor promotes the hydrolysis of the ester link between the tRNA and the amino acid. Once the polypeptide chain is generated and free of the ribosome, it assumes its characteristic three-dimensional structure.

If, during the course of synthesis, there is any interference in the continuity of assembly for lack of a supply of the proper amino acid, synthesis is stopped. Here lies the basis for the time factor of protein synthesis, a feature that nutritionists have recognized for several decades. It was established on the basis of animal feeding experiments that protein synthesis would not occur if all the amino acids were not provided at the proper time. In addition, since protein biosynthesis is very costly in terms of its energy requirement, synthesis is severely inhibited by starvation or caloric restriction. In experimental animals, it has been shown that starvation inhibits the polymerization of mRNA units, thus significantly reducing the activity of the transcription process. Other studies have shown that animals starved and then refed "overcompensate" for this period of reduced mRNA synthesis by markedly increasing mRNA synthesis above normal during the period of realimentation after the starvation period. This starved/refed-induced increase in mRNA is manifested as an increase in the synthesis of enzymes necessary for the metabolism of the various ingredients in the diet used for realimentation. The signal(s) for the release of the starvation induced inhibition of mRNA and enzyme synthesis include the macronutrients in the diet as well as the hormones gluco-corticoid, thyroxine, insulin, and others.

If there is a mutation in the sequence of bases that comprise the genetic code for a given protein, the amino acid sequence in the protein will be incorrect. Whether this substitution of one amino acid for another in the protein being generated affects the functionality of the protein being generated depends entirely on the amino acid in question and its location. Some amino acids can be replaced without affecting the secondary, tertiary, or quaternary structures of the protein (and hence, its chemical and physical properties) whereas others cannot. In addition, genetic errors in amino acid sequence may pose no threat to the individual if the protein in question is of little importance in the maintenance of health and well being, or it can have large effects on health if the protein is a critical one. In the synthesis of the important protein, hemoglobin, if the genetic code calls for the use of valine instead of the usual glutamic acid in the synthesis of the β chain in the hemoglobin molecule, the resulting protein is less able to carry oxygen. This amino acid substitution not only affects the oxygen carrying capacity of the red blood cell but also affects the solubility of the hemoglobin in the red blood cell sap. This, in turn, affects the shape of the red blood cell, changing it from a "dumbbell" shaped donut to a shape resembling a sickle, hence the name, sickle cell anemia. The decreased solubility of the hemoglobin can be understood if one remembers the relative polarity of the glutamic acid and valine molecules. The glutamic acid side chain is more ionic and thus contributes more to the solubility of the protein than the nonpolar side chain of the valine. This change in pH decreases its solubility in water and, of course, a change in solubility leads to an increased viscosity of the blood as the red cells rupture spilling their contents into the blood stream.

The amino acid sequence within a given species for a given protein is usually similar. However, some individual variation does occur. Because of these differences, individuals are able to "recognize" foreign proteins and, through the immune system, reject them. Again, this recognition depends wholly on the amino acid substitutions made and whether the amino acids in question contribute reactive groups that participate in the functional characteristics of the protein or are exposed sufficiently to be "recognized" as a foreign protein. An example of an "acceptable" amino acid substitution would be some of the ones that account for the species differences in the hormone insulin. As a hormone, it serves a variety of important functions in the regulation of carbohydrate, lipid, and protein metabolism. Yet, even though there are species differences in the amino acid sequence of this protein, insulin from one species can be given to another species and be functionally active. Obviously, the species differences in the amino acid sequence of this protein are not at locations in the chains which determine its biological function in promoting glucose use.

Protein turnover

Protein turnover consists of two processes — synthesis and degradation. Synthesis is described in the preceding section. The proteins synthesized by the body have a finite existence. They are subject to a variety of insults and modifications. Some of these modifications have been touched upon as metabolic control processes have been discussed — a prohormone is converted to an active hormone; an enzyme is activated or inactivated with the addition or removal of a substituent and so forth. Thus, it is that a dynamic state within the body exists with respect to its full complement of peptides and proteins. Some proteins have very short lifetimes and very rapid turnover times; other proteins are quite stable and long lived. Their turnover time is quite long. The estimate of the life of a protein, that is, how long it will exist in the body, is its half–life. A half–life is that time interval that occurs when half of the amount of a compound synthesized at time X will have been degraded.

PROTEINURIA
Protein in the urine.

PROTEOLYSIS
Breakdown of protein or peptides.

PROTHROMBIN
Precursor of thrombin. The conversion of thrombin is an essential step in the clotting process.

PROTHROMBIN TIME
A laboratory test performed to identify the time that is needed for clotting after thromboplastin and calcium are added to decalcified plasma.

PROTON
A particle in the nucleus of an atom that has a positive charge.

PROTOPORPHYRIN
A compound found in hemoglobin, myoglobin, and the cytochromes.

PROXIMAL
Toward the center of the body.

PROXIMATE COMPOSITION
The composition of a diet or of an animal in crude (not exact) percentage figures.

P/S RATIO
The ratio of polyunsaturated fatty acids to saturated fatty acids.

PSYLLIUM
An herb that has laxative qualities.

PTH
Parathyroid hormone. Essential to the regulation of blood calcium levels.

PTOMAINES
Very poisonous organic compounds produced by microorganisms in spoiled foods.

PUBERTY
The period of life when the individual undergoes a physical change from childhood to adulthood. The process is orchestrated by the sex hormones.

PUFA
Polyunsaturated fatty acids.

PUFFERFISH POISONING

Intoxication by tetrodotoxin, which is formed by bacteria (*Schewanella putrefaciens*) in the intestines of the pufferfish. The symptoms include tingling of the lips, vomiting, paralysis of the chest muscles, and death. Consumption of this extremely toxic tetrodotoxin results in a mortality of about 60%.

PULMONARY EDEMA

Accumulation of fluids in the lung.

PULMONARY EMBOLISM

Occlusion of one or more of the pulmonary arteries by a thrombus which almost always originates in the leg veins from blood stasis, vessel injury, or changes in clotting factors.

PULMONARY FUNCTION TESTS

Tests used to assess the status of individuals with chronic obstructive pulmonary disease that include vital capacity, residual volume, and total lung capacity.

PULSES

1. Throbbing of blood in response to the heart beat; 2. a family of foods primarily beans, peas, and lentils that are the seeds of their respective plants.

PURINE

A nitrogenous base that is an essential structural unit of DNA and RNA. Includes adenine and guanine.

PURINE RESTRICTED DIET

Therapeutic diet used as an adjunctive therapy to medication for the treatment and control of gout in which foods highest in purines are limited and total protein intake is moderate.

PUTRESCINE

A polyamine derived from arginine.

PVN

Paraventricular nucleus in the hypothalamus. Releases hormones that affect food intake.

PYELONEPHRITIS

Inflammation of the kidney; a common renal disease from acute bacterial infection.

PYLORUS

The connection between the stomach and small intestine.

PYRIDOXAL PHOSPHATE

Coenzyme form of the vitamin pyridoxal.

PYRIDOXINE, PYRIDOXAMINE, PYRIDOXIC ACID

Vitamin B$_6$. An essential nutrient that serves as a coenzyme involved in transamination reactions (see Vitamins, Table 49).

PYRIMIDINE GLYCOSIDES

Nonnutritive natural food components of important toxicological relevance. Favism, a disease caused by the ingestion of fava beans, is characterized by acute hemolysis, in serious cases accompanied by jaundice and hemoglobinuria. It is mainly found in Mediterranean populations with a congenital deficiency of NADPH-dependent glucose-6-phosphate dehydrogenase (G6PD). Fava beans contain two pyrimidine glycosides that have been shown to induce hemolysis — vicine and convicine. The aglycons are divicine and isouramil, respectively. Divicine and isouramil are powerful reducing agents. In red cells, they are readily oxidized by oxyhemoglobin to form methemoglobin, H$_2$O$_2$, and Heinz bodies (thought to consist of denatured hemoglobin). The oxidation products undergo reduction by glutathione, and H$_2$O$_2$ is reduced by glutathione peroxidase. The oxidized glutathione produced by these reactions is reduced by NADPH, generated from glucose-6-phosphate and G6PD. The defect leading to hemolysis lies in the red cells which have insufficient G6PD, i.e., diminished levels of reduced glutathione, to protect them against oxidative attack.

PYRIMIDINES

A group of nitrogenous bases needed for DNA and RNA structures. Includes cytosine, thymine, and uracil.

PYROLYSIS

Decomposition of a compound into smaller, more reactive structures by the action of heat alone. The fragmentation is usually followed by combination of the smaller structures to more stable compounds, provided the conditions do not allow the conversion to CO and CO$_2$. Pyrolysis products may occur in all three of the macronutrient categories. The formation of pyrolysis products depends on the type of parent compound and the temperature. In the case of food, hazardous compounds are formed from about 300°C. Well-known types of pyrolysis products in foods include: (1) polycyclic aromatic hydrocarbons (PAHs) and (2) heterocyclic pyrolysis products from amino acids. PAHs are likely to be formed from degradation products consisting of two- or four-carbon units, such as ethylene and butadiene radicals. The most potent carcinogenic PAH is benz[a]pyrene, which has been identified in the charred crusts of biscuits and bread, in broiled and barbecued meat, in broiled mackerel, and in industrially roasted coffees. Fat is an important precursor for the formation of PAHs (in meat and fish). Furthermore, PAHs are abundantly found in smoked food, originating from the combustion of wood and other fuels. Heterocyclic pyrolysis products from amino acids include 3-amino-1,4-dimethyl-5H-pyrido(4-b)indole (precursor — tryptophan), 3-amino-1-methyl-5H-pyrido (4,3-b)indole (precursor — tryptophan), and 2-amino-5-phenylpyridine (precursor — phenylalanine). These mutagens and several structurally related substances have been isolated from the surface of protein-containing food cooking at 250°C and higher. Other mutagens, such as 2-amino-3-methylimidazo(4,5-f)quinoline and 2-amino-3,8-dimethylimidazole(4,5-f) quinoxaline, have also been isolated from different types of protein-rich foods heated at about 200°C.

PYRUVATE

The end product of glycolysis.

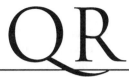

QR

QUADRIPLEGIA

Paralysis of both arms and legs due to damage to the spinal cord in the cervical region.

QUANTITATIVE COMPUTED TOMOGRAPHY

An imaging technique consisting of an array of x-ray sources and radiation detectors aligned opposite each other. As x-ray beams pass through the subject they are weakened or attenuated by the tissues and picked up by the detectors. The signals are then compared using a computer which can construct a cross section of the body using sophisticated modeling techniques.

QUICK BREADS

Baked flour products made without yeast.

QUININE

A compound useful in malaria treatment.

RABBIT FEVER

Tularemia. Caused by microorganism *Fracisella tularensis*. Symptoms include ulcerous lesions of skin, headache, chills, and fever. Organism frequently is carried by wild game.

RADIOACTIVE ISOTOPES

An unstable atom with particles which when released by the atom also results in the release of energy as α, β, or γ rays.

RAFFINOSE

A trisaccharide which is difficult to digest but can be digested by gut flora to result in gas (flatulence) and short chain fatty acids.

RANCIDITY

Deterioration of fats and oils in foods. It is characterized by an unpleasant odor and taste. Two types of rancidity can be defined: (1) hydrolytic rancidity and (2) oxidative rancidity.

RANDOM MISCLASSIFICATION

Errors in the necessary information (e.g., in exposure measurement) which are not related to the state of disease. This is the case if equal proportions of subjects in the groups which are compared are classified incorrectly with respect to exposure or disease. Also known as nondifferential misclassification. This type of misclassification dilutes the true difference and therefore always changes the observed effect toward the null hypothesis (i.e., no relationship between exposure and disease).

RAPESEED

A seed oil plant. A subspecies of rapeseed is the canola seed having no erucid acid in its oil.

RAPID FREEZING

A processing technique affecting the oxidation of dietary fats and oils. Rapid freezing of raw plant material may be accompanied by lipoxygenase-mediated oxidation, depending on the extent of tissue damage and on storage temperature and time.

RATE DIFFERENCE

The difference in incidence rate between exposed and unexposed populations, expressed in absolute terms. It is calculated by subtracting the incidence rate in the unexposed group (I_0) from the incidence rate in the exposed group (I_1). I_0 can be interpreted as the baseline incidence rate, and only the incidence rate exceeding this figure is due to the exposure. Therefore, the rate difference is also known as attributable rate. A difference in incidence rate of 0 means that the disease is not related to exposure $(I_1 = I_0)$.

RBC

Red blood cell. Erythrocyte.

RBP

Retinol binding protein. A protein synthesized in the liver and used to transport retinol in the blood or in the cell.

REACTIVE HYPOGLYCEMIA

Blood levels which fall below 80 mg/dl after a glucose challenge. Can be life threatening. May also be due to an overdose of insulin.

RECALL BIAS

A type of information bias that is of importance in case-control studies. It means that cases differ from controls in the recollection of exposure.

24-HOUR RECALL METHOD

A method used to estimate the food intake of subjects by asking them to recall what they ate over the last 24 hours.

RECEPTOR

This is a general term applied to any protein in any part of the cell that binds to a specific compound and allows that compound to do its job in the cell. Most hormones and many nutrients have specific receptors without which these hormones or nutrients would be ineffective.

RECOMBINANT DNA

DNA isolated and/or synthesized in the laboratory.

RECOMMENDED DIETARY ALLOWANCES (RDA) (U.S.)

Recommended daily **allowance**, not to be confused with requirement. Shown in Table 43.

RECOMMENDED NUTRIENT INTAKES (RDI) FOR CANADIANS

Similar to the U.S. RDA with differences in the recommended intakes for ascorbic acid.

RECORD METHOD

A method for estimating food intake. It is used to obtain detailed information on food intake during a limited number of days, usually 1–7. During that period the subjects write down everything they eat and estimate the quantities. A problem with this method is that people tend to forget to write things down or change their eating habits due to the fact that they have to write down everything they eat. A record method for 2 days cannot be used to obtain information on the usual diet of the study subjects. Due to the large day-to-day variability in the intake of foods, a 2-day period is too short to obtain a valid estimate of the usual food intake. If information on food consumption at an individual level is needed, the record method has to be repeated several times during a certain period of time. However, the 2-day record method can give a good estimate of food consumption at group level, because then a large number of 2-day records is averaged to estimate the mean intake by the group.

RECUMBENT

Lying down.

REDOX STATE

Ratio of oxidized to reduced forms of coenzymes that have two forms — NAD/NADH, FAD/FADH, NADP/NADPH.

REDUCING EQUIVALENTS

Hydrogen ions.

REGISTERED DIETITIAN

See Dietitian.

REGRESSION EQUATION

A statistical method for calculating the relationships between an independent variable such as age with a dependent variable.

RELAPSE

Return of disease symptoms.

RELATIVE RISK (RR)

The difference in incidence rate between exposed and unexposed populations, expressed in relative terms. It can be calculated as the incidence rate in the exposed group (I_1) divided by the incidence rate in the unexposed group (I_0). Also known as rate ratio. A relative risk of 1 indicates that the disease is not related to exposure ($I_1 = I_0$).

REMODELING

Reshaping or degrading and rebuilding a body structure.

RENAL FAILURE

See Chronic renal failure.

RENAL SOLUTE LOAD

Amount of solute that must be excreted by the kidney.

TABLE 43
Recommended Dietary Allowances for Nutrients Needed by Humans of Different Ages (U.S.)

Category	Age	Weight (lbs)	Height (in)	Protein (g)	A (µg/RE)[a]	D (µg)	E (mgαTE)[b]	K (µg)	C (mg)	Thiamin (mg)	Riboflavin (mg)
Infants	0–6 mo	13	24	13	375	7.5	3	5	30	0.3	0.4
	7–12 mo	20	28	14	375	10.0	4	10	35	0.4	0.5
Children	1–3 yr	29	35	16	400	10.0	6	15	40	0.7	0.8
	4–6	44	44	14	500	10.0	7	20	45	0.9	1.0
	7–10	62	52	28	700	10.0	7	30	45	1.0	1.2
Males	11–14	99	62	45	1000	10.0	10	45	50	1.3	1.5
	15–18	145	69	59	1000	10.0	10	65	60	1.5	1.8
	19–24	160	70	58	1000	10.0	10	70	60	1.5	1.7
	25–50	174	70	63	1000	5.0	10	80	60	1.5	1.7
	51+	170	68	63	1000	5.0	10	80	60	1.2	1.4
Females	11–14	101	62	46	800	10.0	8	45	50	1.1	1.3
	15–18	120	64	44	800	10.0	8	55	60	1.1	1.3
	19–24	128	65	46	800	10.0	8	60	60	1.1	1.3
	25–50	138	64	50	800	5.0	8	65	60	1.1	1.3
	51+	143	63	50	800	5.0	8	65	60	1.0	1.2
Pregnancy				60	800	10.0	10	65	70	1.5	1.6
Lactation	0–6 mo			65	1300	10.0	12	65	95	1.6	1.8
	7–12 mo			62	1200	10.0	11	65	90	1.6	1.8

Category											
Infants	5	0.3	25	0.3	400	300	40	6	5	40	10
	6	0.6	35	0.5	600	400	60	10	5	50	15
Children	0	1.0	50	0.7	800	800	80	10	10	70	20
	12	1.1	75	1.0	800	800	120	10	10	90	20
	13	1.4	100	1.4	800	800	170	12	10	120	30
Males	17	1.7	150	2.0	1200	1200	270	12	15	150	40
	20	2.0	200	2.0	1200	1200	400	10	15	150	50
	19	2.0	200	2.0	1200	1200	350	10	15	150	70
	19	2.0	200	2.0	800	800	350	10	15	150	70
	15	2.0	200	2.0	800	800	350	15	15	150	70
Females	15	1.4	150	2.0	1200	1200	280	15	12	150	45
	15	1.5	180	2.0	1200	1200	300	15	12	150	50
	15	1.6	180	2.0	1200	1200	280	15	12	150	55
	15	1.6	180	2.0	800	800	280	15	12	150	55
	13	1.6	180	2.0	800	800	280	10	12	150	55
Pregnancy	17	2.2	400	2.2	1200	1200	320	30	15	175	65
Lactation	20	2.1	280	2.6	1200	1200	355	15	19	200	75
	20	2.1	260	2.6	1200	1200	340	15	16	200	75

[a] RE = retinol equivalent; 1 μg retinol = 6 μg β carotene.

[b] μTE = 1 mg da tocopherol.

[c] NE = niacin equivalents; 1 mg niacin = 60 mg tryptophan.

Data from Food and Nutrition Board, National Academy of Sciences, National Research Council, 1989. These recommendations are periodically re-examined and some are changed.

RENAL THRESHOLD

Concentration of a substance in plasma at which it is excreted in urine.

RENIN-ANGIOTENSIN-ALDOSTERONE SYSTEM

Hormone system that regulates blood pressure and renal function.

REPLICATION

Duplication of the genetic code.

RER

Rough endoplasmic reticulum. That portion of the cell which appears granular due to the profusion of ribosomes.

RESIDUE

Indigestible content of food.

RESPIRATORY ACIDOSIS

Acid-base imbalance of carbon dioxide retention associated with respiratory failure, sedative overdose, chronic obstructive pulmonary disease, chest wall trauma, acute abdominal distention, and obesity which is characterized by a rapid respiratory rate that usually provides inadequate ventilation, rapid heart rate, pale and dry skin, diaphoresis, headache, and coma.

RESPIRATORY ALKALOSIS

Acid-base imbalance of decreased carbon dioxide associated with hyperventilation, anxiety, fever, pain, and mechanical over ventilation which is characterized by increased heart rate, increased rate and depth of respirations, paresthesia, anxiety, irritability, dizziness, and agitation.

RESPIRATORY CHAIN

See oxidative phosphorylation.

RESPIRATORY FAILURE

Inability of the lungs to perform their ventilary function.

RESPIRATORY QUOTIENT (RQ)

The ratio of carbon dioxide exhaled to oxygen consumed.

RESTING ENERGY EXPENDITURE

See basal energy.

RESTENOSIS

Recurrent narrowing of an opening.

RETICULOCYTE

An immature red blood cell with a network of precipitated basophilic substance and occurring during the process of active blood regeneration.

RETINA

The inner neural bilayer of the eye consisting of an outer pigment layer attached to the inner surface of the chorioid ciliary body and iris and an inner layer formed by the expansion of the optic nerve.

RETINOIDS

A group of compounds having Vitamin A activity.

RETINOL-BINDING PROTEIN

A protein required for the transport of Vitamin A in the blood. A separate but similar carrier protein is located within the cells.

RETINOL EQUIVALENT

The activity of one mole of all trans retinol. Not all retinoids have the same biological activity.

RETINYL PALMITATE

A palmitoyl ester of retinol.

RETROSPECTIVE COHORT STUDIES

See follow-up studies.

RHODOPSIN

The visual pigment in the red cells of the eye. Consists of the protein opsin and 11-cis retinal. When light enters the eye, the 11-cis retinal changes to 11-trans retinal which then separates from opsin. Recombination is then needed to restore the rhodopsin. This combination requires more retinol (which is changed to retinal) and the niacin containing coenzyme NAD.

RIA

Radioimmunoassay. Technique useful for determining small quantities of biologically important substances such as hormones.

RIBOFLAVIN

An essential vitamin of the B family. Serves as a coenzyme (FAD, FMN) in reactions where hydrogen ions are transferred (see vitamins, Table 48).

RIBONUCLEASE

An enzyme which catalyzes the destruction of RNA.

RIBONUCLEIC ACID (RNA)

A single strand of nucleosides having ribose instead of deoxyribose and uracil in place of thymine. There are 3 types of RNA — messenger RNA, transfer RNA, and ribosomal RNA. Messenger RNA serves as the template for the order of amino acids of the particular protein being synthesized. Transfer RNA carries these amino acids, and ribosomal RNA serves as the docking place on the ribosome for the messenger RNA.

RIBOSE

A five carbon sugar produced by the hexose monophosphate shunt. When a single oxygen is removed it is deoxyribose and is part of DNA. RNA contains ribose.

RIBOSOME

The organelle of the cell where protein synthesis occurs.

RICKETS

Bone malformation usually due to inadequate intake of vitamins and minerals; some forms of this disease are due to renal disease while other forms may be due to certain toxins.

RIGOR MORTIS

Stiff rigid muscles characteristic of death.

RNA

Ribonucleic acid. A polynucleotide; synthesis of RNA is directed by DNA.

RQ

Respiratory quotient. Ratio of CO_2 to O_2.

RUMINANTS

Animals with a four chambered stomach, one of which is called the rumen. It is a large fermentation vat populated by bacteria that can digest the complex carbohydrates of grasses and grains.

S

SACCHARIN

Non-nutritive sweetener that has 300 times the sweetness of sucrose. Studies with rats fed very high levels developed urinary bladder tumors. The formation of tumors is not identical to the initiation and promotion of a cancer cell. Growth rates differ as do cellular characteristics. Saccharin thus remained on the market while sodium cyclamate was withdrawn.

SAFROLE

A methylenedioxyphenyl substance. Safrole is one of the natural and synthetic flavoring agents. Sassafras, containing high levels of safrole, used to be added to sarsaparilla root beer. Safrole is still present in the diet as a (minor) component of various herbs and spices, e.g., cloves. Safrole and related substances have been shown to be carcinogenic. Biotransformation data suggest that the 1'-hydroxy sulfate ester of safrole is the ultimate carcinogenic species capable of binding to DNA.

SALICYLATES

Salts of salicylic acid; anti-inflammatory agent in the amide form. Salicylic acid has been used as a food preservative.

SALIVA

A clear tasteless secretion of the salivary gland containing a lipase, amylase, and mucin. Its function is to lubricate the food making it easier to swallow.

SALIVARY AMYLASE

An enzyme which initiates starch digestion in the mouth.

SALMONELLA

A genus of bacteria which causes one of the most common foodborne illnesses.

SALT

An inorganic compound having a negative and a positve ion which dissociate in solution. Table salt is sodium chloride.

SAM

S-adenosylmethionine. A principle methyl donor.

SARCOIDOSIS

Disease of unknown etiology characterized by tumor-like lesions that affect any tissue or organ of the body.

SATIETY

Feeling of fullness from consuming food.

SATURATED FATTY ACIDS (SFAs)

Fatty acids with 4 to 18 C atoms. Well-known examples occurring in large quantities in the diet are palmitic acid (C16:0) and stearic acid (C18:0).

SAUERKRAUT

A cabbage product made of thinly sliced cabbage and salt and allowed to ferment.

SCLERODERMA

A disease of the skin characterized by increased thickness.

SCRAPPLE

A pork product using corn meal and meat scraps.

SCURVY

Ascorbic acid deficiency disease.

SECRETIN

A 27 amino acid peptide hormone secreted by duodenal cells in response to the low pH of the chyme entering the small intestine from the stomach. Its function is to inhibit hydrochloric acid secretion while stimulating the release of a watery alkaline juice from the pancreatic exocrine cells.

SECRETOGOGE

A compound such as glucose that stimulates the β cell to release insulin. This term refers to any compound that stimulates a secreting cell to release its product.

SELECTION BIAS

The fact that the effect measured is perverted due to the selection of the study subjects. This means that the association between exposure and disease in the study population differs from the association in the total population. Case-control studies are especially sensitive to selection bias. If subjects are systematically excluded from or included in the case or control group, the comparison of these groups can give biased results. Since cases are often recruited from hospitals, controls are sometimes also selected from the same hospitals. Since hospitalized persons are likely to differ from the general population, this may influence the study results. Therefore, in the study design, special attention should be paid to the selection of controls. Often, several control groups are used, to estimate the consequences of the choice of the source population of controls. Other source populations of controls that are used in addition to hospital controls are neighborhood controls (to control for socio-economic differences between cases and controls) or a random population sample, in order to compare the exposure in the cases with that in the general population.

SELENIUM

An essential mineral needed for the antioxidant enzyme, glutathione peroxidase (see minerals, Table 30).

SEPSIS

Infection due to identifiable microorganisms or their products in the blood or tissues.

SEPTIC SHOCK

The end result of a process initiated by pathogenic organisms, altered mental status, inadequate tissue perfusion, decreased urine output, and refractory hypotension.

SEPTICEMIA

Bloodborne pathogens and their associated toxins.

SER

Smooth endoplasmic reticulum. That portion of the endoplasmic reticulum where certain lipids are synthesized and drugs are detoxified.

SERINE

A three carbon nonessential amino acid containing a hydroxyl group on its terminal carbon (see amino acids, Table 5).

SEROTONIN

A neurotransmitter synthesized in the CNS from tryptophan.

SERUM

The cell-free fluid that surrounds the red blood cells and the white blood cells.

SET POINT WEIGHT

Weight that an individual maintains for extended periods of time without conscious effort.

SEX-LINKED TRAIT

A genetic characteristic carried on either the X or the Y chromosome.

SGOT

Serum glutamate-oxaloacetate transaminase. A Vitamin B_6-dependent enzyme whose level in the serum rises after muscle damage, particularly after a heart attack.

SGPT

Serum glutamate-pyruvate transaminase. Another Vitamin B_6-dependent enzyme. A rise in activity also indicates muscle damage.

SHELLFISH POISONING

A disease resulting from the consumption of shellfish that have ingested toxic algae. Shellfish poisoning manifests itself in two forms — paralytic shellfish poisoning and diarrheic shellfish poisoning.

SHIGELLOSIS

Dysentery caused by food and/or water contaminated by the organism shigella.

SHOCK

Condition in which the peripheral blood flow is inadequate to return blood to the heart; decreased cardiac output (see above) causing poor tissue perfusion.

SI UNITS

Standard units for expressing biological values. Shown in Table 44.

SICKLE CELL ANEMIA

A genetic disease caused by a mutation in the code for one of the subunits of hemoglobin. Because of this mutation, the amino acid sequence of the protein is aberrant which in turn affects its quartenary structure and its ability to carry oxygen. The name comes from the change in shape of the red blood cell. Instead of being round it is sickle shaped.

SIDEROSIS (HEMOSIDEROSIS)

Also called hemochromatosis. A nutritional disorder due to a low protein intake together with a high iron intake. The iron is absorbed and accumulates in the liver causing damage.

SIMPLE SIMILAR ACTION

Combination of substances with common sites of main action and no interaction between the components. The action can be additive. An example is the combined toxic action of mixtures of polychlorinated dibenzodioxins, polychlorinated dibenzofurans, and polychlorinated biphenyls (particularly congeners with planar structures) occurring in, for example, mother's milk. The effects of these substances have been shown to be additive. Usually, the toxicity of such mixtures is expressed in terms of the concentration of 2,3,7,8-tetrachlorodibenzo-p-dioxin (TCDD) by adding the so-called TCDD toxicity equivalent concentrations of the individual components — concentration addition.

SIMPLESSE

A fat substitute derived from egg or milk proteins. It cannot be used in cooked or baked products because it breaks down easily.

SKINFOLD THICKNESS

A double fold of skin and underlying tissue which can be used as a measure of the subcutaneous fat store. The general formulas for calculating body fatness from these measurements are shown in Table 45.

SMALL FOR GESTATIONAL AGE BABY

A baby whose birth weight is small even though the baby has not been born prematurely.

SOAP NOTE

Acronym for a method of organizing information to be written in a medical record given as Subjective data, Objective information, Assessment, and Plan. Subjective data provides pertinent information obtained from the client; objective information includes relevant verifiable facts; assessment is the interpretation of the problems and related facts, and the plan indicates what actions are to be taken to resolve the identified problems.

SOD

Superoxide dismutase. An enzyme important to the suppression of free radicals. See oxidation-autoxidation.

TABLE 44
Conversion Factors for Values in Clinical Chemistry (SI Units)

Component	Present Reference Intervals (examples)	Present Unit	Conversion Factor	SI Reference Intervals	SI Unit Symbol	Significant Digits	Suggested Minimum Increment
acetaminophen (P) - toxic	>5.0	mg/dl	66.16	>330	μmol/l	XXO	10 μmol/l
acetoacetate (S)	0.3–3.0	mg/dl	97.95	30–300	μmol/l	XXO	10 μmol/l
acetone (B,S)	0	mg/dl	172.2	0	μmol/l	XXO	10 μmol/l
acid phosphatase (S)	0–5.5	U/l	16.67	0–90	nkat/l	XX	2 nkat/l
adrenocorticotropin [ACTH] (P)	20–100	pg/ml	0.2202	4–22	pmol/l	XX	1 pmol/l
alanine aminotransferase [ALT] (S)	0–35	U/l	0.01667	0–0.58	μkat/l	X.XX	0.02 μkat/l
albumin (S)	4.0–6.0	g/dl	10.0	40–60	g/l	XX	1 g/l
aldolase (S)	0–6	U/l	16.67	0–100	nkat/l	XXO	20 nkat/l
aldosterone (S)							
normal salt diet	8.1–15.5	ng/dl	27.74	220–430	pmol/l	XXO	10 pmol/l
restricted salt diet	20.8–44.4	ng/dl	27.74	580–1240	pmol/l	XXO	10 pmol/l
aldosterone (U) - sodium excretion							
=25 mmol/d	18–85	μg/24 h	2.774	50–235	nmol/d	XXX	5 nmol/d
=75–125 mmol/d	5–26	μg/24 h	2.774	15–70	nmol/d	XXX	5 nmol/d
=200 mmol/d	1.5–12.5	μg/24 h	2.774	5–35	nmol/d	XXX	5 nmol/d
alkaline phosphatase (S)	0–120	U/l	0.01667	0.5–2.0	μkat/l	X.X	0.1 μkat/l
alpha₁-antitrypsin (S)	150–350	mg/dl	0.01	1.5–3.5	g/l	X.X	0.1 g/l
alpha-fetoprotein (S)	0–20	ng/ml	1.00	0–20	μg/l	XX	1 μg/l
alpha-fetoprotein (Amf)	Depends on gestation	mg/dl	10.0	Depends on gestation	mg/l	XX	1 mg/l
alpha₂-macroglobulin (S)	145–410	mg/dl	0.01	1.5–4.1	g/l	X.X	1 mg/l
aluminum (S)	0–15	μg/l	37.06	0–560	nmol/l	XXO	10 nmol/l
amino acid fractionation (P)							
alanine	2.2–4.5	mg/dl	112.2	245–500	μmol/l	XXX	5 μmol/l

TABLE 44 (CONTINUED)
Conversion Factors for Values in Clinical Chemistry (SI Units)

Component	Present Reference Intervals (examples)	Present Unit	Conversion Factor	SI Reference Intervals	SI Unit Symbol	Significant Digits	Suggested Minimum Increment
alpha aminobutyric acid	0.1–0.2	mg/dl	96.97	10–20	µmol/l	XXX	5 µmol/l
arginine	0.5–2.5	mg/dl	57.40	30–145	µmol/l	XXX	5 µmol/l
asparagine	0.5–0.6	mg/dl	75.69	35–45	µmol/l	XXX	5 µmol/l
citrulline	0.2–1.0	mg/dl	75.13	0–20	µmol/l	XXX	5 µmol/l
cystine	0.2–2.2	mg/dl	57.08	15–55	µmol/l	XXX	5 µmol/l
glutamic acid	0.2–2.8	mg/dl	67.97	15–190	µmol/l	XXX	5 µmol/l
glutamine	6.1–10.2	mg/dl	68.42	420–700	µmol/l	XXX	5 µmol/l
glycine	0.9–4.2	mg/dl	133.2	120–560	µmol/l	XXX	5 µmol/l
histidine	0.5–1.7	mg/dl	64.45	30–110	µmol/l	XXX	5 µmol/l
hydroxyproline	0–trace	mg/dl	76.26	0–trace	µmol/l	XXX	5 µmol/l
isoleucine	0.5–1.3	mg/dl	76.24	40–100	µmol/l	XXX	5 µmol/l
leucine	1.2–3.5	mg/dl	76.24	75–175	µmol/l	XXX	5 µmol/l
lysine	1.2–3.5	mg/dl	68.40	80–240	µmol/l	XXX	5 µmol/l
methionine	0.1–0.6	mg/dl	67.02	5–40	µmol/l	XXX	5 µmol/l
ornithine	0.4–1.4	mg/dl	75.67	30–400	µmol/l	XXX	5 µmol/l
phenylalanine	0.6–1.5	mg/dl	60.54	35–90	µmol/l	XXX	5 µmol/l
proline	1.2–3.9	mg/dl	86.86	105–340	µmol/l	XXX	5 µmol/l
serine	0.8–1.8	mg/dl	95.16	75–170	µmol/l	XXX	5 µmol/l
taurine	0.9–2.5	mg/dl	79.91	25–170	µmol/l	XXX	5 µmol/l
threonine	0.9–2.5	mg/dl	83.95	75–210	µmol/l	XXX	5 µmol/l
tryptophan	0.5–2.5	mg/dl	48.97	25–125	µmol/l	XXX	5 µmol/l
tyrosine	0.4–1.6	mg/dl	55.19	20–90	µmol/l	XXX	5 µmol/l
valine	1.7–3.7	mg/dl	85.36	145–315	µmol/l	XXX	5 µmol/l
amino acid nitrogen (P)	4.0–6.0	mg/dl	0.7139	2.9–4.3	mmol/l	X.X	0.1 mmol/l
amino acid nitrogen (U)	50–200	mg/24 h	0.07139	3.6–14.3	mmol/d	X.X	0.1 mmol/d

delta-aminolevulinate [as levulinic acid] (U)	1.0–7.0	mg/24 h	7.626	8–53	μmol/d	XX	1 μmol/d
amitriptyline (P,S) therapeutic	50–200	ng/ml	3.605	180–270	μmol/l	XO	10 nmol/l
ammonia (vP)							
as ammonia [NH₃]	10–80	μg/dl	0.5872	5–50	μmol/l	XXX	5 μmol/l
as ammonium ion [NH₄⁺]	10–85	μg/dl	0.5543	5–50	μmol/l	XXX	5 μmol/l
as nitrogen [N]	10–65	μg/dl	0.7139	5–50	μmol/l	XXX	5 μmol/l
amylase (S)	0–130	U/l	0.01667	0–2.17	μkat/l	XXX	0.01 μkat/l
androstenedione (S)							
male > 18 years	0.2–3.0	mg/l	3.492	0.5–10.5	nmol/l	XX.X	0.5 nmol/l
female > 18 years	0.8–3.0	mg/l	3.492	3.0–10.5	nmol/l	XX.X	0.5 nmol/l
angiotensin converting enzyme (S)	<40	nmol/ml/min	16.67	<670	nkat/l	XXO	10 nkat/l
arsenic (H) [as As]	<1	μg/g (ppm)	13.35	<13	nmol/g	XX.X	0.5 nmol/g
arsenic (U) [as As]	0–5	μg/24 h	13.35	0–67	nmol/d	XX	1 nmol/d
[as As₂O₃]	<25	μg/dl	0.05055	<1.3	μmol/l	XX.X	0.1 μmol/l
ascorbate (P) [as ascorbic acid]	0.6–2.0	μg/dl	56.78	30–110	μmol/l	XO	10 μmol/l
aspartate amino-transferase [AST] (S)	0–35	U/l	0.0167	0–0.58	μkat/l	O.XX	0.01 μkat/l
barbiturate (S) overdose total expressed as:	Depends on composition of mixture. Usually not known.	...	...	...	...	...	...
phenobarbital		mg/dl	43.06		μmol/l	XX	5 μmol/l
sodim phenobarbital		mg/dl	39.34		μmol/l	XX	5 μmol/l
barbitone		mg/dl	54.29		μmol/l	XX	5 μmol/l
barbiturate (S) therapeutic	...	...	...	...	...	...	...
see phenobarbital							
see pentobarbital							
see thiopental							
bile acids, total (S)							
[as chenodeoxycholic acid]	Trace–3.3	μg/ml	2.547	Trace–8.4	μmol/l	X.X	0.2 μmol/l
cholic acid	Trace–1.0	μg/ml	2.448	Trace–2.4	μmol/l	X.X	0.2 μmol/l
chenodeoxycholic acid	Trace–1.3	μg/ml	2.547	Trace–3.4	μmol/l	X.X	0.2 μmol/l
deoxycholic acid	Trace–1.0	μg/ml	2.547	Trace–2.6	μmol/l	X.X	0.2 μmol/l
lithocholic acid	Trace	μg/ml	2.656	Trace	μmol/l	X.X	0.2 μmol/l

TABLE 44 (CONTINUED)
Conversion Factors for Values in Clinical Chemistry (SI Units)

Component	Present Reference Intervals (examples)	Present Unit	Conversion Factor	SI Reference Intervals	SI Unit Symbol	Significant Digits	Suggested Minimum Increment
bile acids (Df) [after cholcystokinin stimulation] total as							
chenodeoxycholic acid	14.0–58.0	mg/ml	2.547	35–148	mmol/l	XX.X	0.2 mmol/l
cholic acid	2.4–33.0	mg/ml	2.448	6.8–81.0	mmol/l	XX.X	0.2 mmol/l
chenodeoxycholic acid	4.0–24.0	mg/ml	2.547	10.0–61.4	mmol/l1	XX.X	0.2 mmol/l
deoxycholic acid	0.8–6.9	mg/ml	2.547	2–18	mmol/l	XX.X	0.2 mmol/l
lithocholic acid	0.3–0.8	mg/ml	2.656	0.8–2.0	mmol/l	XX.X	0.2 mmol/l
bilirubin, total (S)	0.1–1.0	mg/dl	17.10	2–18	μmol/l	XX	2 μmol/l
bilirubin, conjugated (S)	0–0.2	mg/dl	17.10	0–4	μmol/l	XX	2 μmol/l
bromide (S), toxic							
as bromide ion	>120	mg/dl	0.1252	>15	mmol/l	XX	1 mmol/l
as sodium bromide	>150	mg/dl	0.09719	>15	mmol/l	XX	1 mmol/l
	>15	mEq/l	1.00	>15	mmol/l	XX	1 mmol/l
cadmium (S)	<3	mg/dl	0.08897	<0.3	μmol/l	X.X	0.1 μmol/l
calcitonin (S)	<100	pg/ml	1.00	<100	ng/l	XXX	10 ng/l
calcium (S)							
male	8.8–10.3	mg/dl	0.2495	2.20–2.58	mmol/l	X.XX	0.02 mmol/l
female <50 y	8.8–10.0	mg/dl	0.2495	2.20–2.50	mmol/l	X.XX	0.02 mmol/l
female >50 y	8.8–10.2	mg/dl	0.2495	2.20–2.56	mmol/l	X.XX	0.02 mmol/l
calcium ion (S)	4.4–5.1	mEq/l	0.500	2.20–2.56	mmol/l	X.XX	0.02 mmol/l
	2.00–2.30	mEq/l	0.500	1.00–1.15	mmol/l	X.XX	0.01 mmol/l
calcium (U), normal diet	<250	mg/24 h	0.02495	<6.2	mmol/d	X.X	0.1 mmol/d
carbamazepine (P) - therapeutic	4.0–10.0	mg/l	4.233	17–42	μmol/l	XX	1 μmol/l
carbon dioxide content (B, P, S) [bicarbonate + CO_2]	22–28	mEq/l	1.00	22–28	mmol/l	X	1 mmol/l

Analyte	Conventional	Unit	Factor	SI	SI unit	Round	Sig
carbon monoxide (B) [proportion of Hb which is COHb]	<15	%	0.01	<0.15	1	0.XX	0.01
beta carotenes (S)	50–250	mg/dl	0.01863	0.9–4.6	μmol/l	X.X	0.1 μmol/l
catecholamines, total (U) [as norepinephrine]	<120	mg/24 h	5.911	<675	nmol/d	XXO	10 mg/d
ceruloplasmin (S)	20–35	mg/dl	10.0	200–350	mg/l	XXO	10 mg/l
Chlordiazepoxide (P)							
- therapeutic	0.5–5.0	mg/l	3.336	2–17	μmol/l	XX	1 μmol/l
- toxic	>10.0	mg/l	3.336	>33	μmol/l	XX	1 μmol/l
chloride (S)	95–105	mEq/l	1.00	95–105	mmol/l	XXX	1 mmol/l
chlorimipramine (P) [includes desmethyl metabolite]	50–400	ng/ml	3.176	150–1270	nmol/l	XXO	10 nmol/l
chlorpromazine (P)	50–300	ng/ml	3.136	150–950	nmol/l	XXO	10 nmol/l
chlorpropamide (P) -therapeutic	75–250	mg/l	3.613	270–900	mmol/l	XXO	10 mmol/l
cholestanol (P) [as a fraction of total cholesterol]	1–3	%	0.01	0.01–0.03	1	0.XX	0.01
cholesterol (P)							
- <29 years	<200	mg/dl	0.02586	<5.20	mol/l	X.XX	0.05 mmol/l
- 30–39 years	<225	mg/dl	0.02586	<5.85	mmol/l	X.XX	0.05 mmol/l
- 40–49 years	<245	mg/dl	0.02586	<6.35	mmol/l	X.XX	0.05 mmol/l
- >50 years	<265	mg/dl	0.02586	<6.85	mmol/l	X.XX	0.05 mmol/l
cholesterol esters (P) [as a fraction of total cholesterol]	60–75	%	0.01	0.60–0.75	1	0.XX	0.01
cholinesterase (S)	620–1370	U/l	0.01667	10.3–22.8	mkat/l	XX.X	0.1 mkat/l
chorionic gonadotropin (P) [beta HCG]	0 if not pregnant	mIU/ml	1.00	0 if not pregnant	IU/l	XX	1 IU/l
citrate (B) [as citric acid]	1.2–3.0	mg/dl	52.05	60–160	μmol/l	XXX	5 μmol/l
complement, C3 (S)	70–160	mg/dl	0.01	0.7–1.6	g/l	X.X	0.1 g/l
complement, C4 (S)	20–40	mg/dl	0.01	0.2–0.4	g/l	X.X	0.1 g/l
copper (S)	70–140	μg/dl	0.1574	11.0–22.0	μmol/l	XX.X	0.2 μmol/l
copper (U)	<40	μg/24 h	0.01574	<0.6	μmol/d	X.X	0.2 μmol/l
coproporphyrins (U)	<200	μg/24 h	1.527	<300	nmol/d	XXO	10 nmol/d
cortisol (S)							
-800 h	4–19	μg/dl	27.59	110–520	nmol/l	XXO	10 nmol/l

TABLE 44 (CONTINUED)
Conversion Factors for Values in Clinical Chemistry (SI Units)

Component	Present Reference Intervals (examples)	Present Unit	Conversion Factor	SI Reference Intervals	SI Unit Symbol	Significant Digits	Suggested Minimum Increment
-1600 h	2–15	µg/dl	27.59	50–410	nmol/l	XXO	10 nmol/l
-2400 h	5	µg/dl	7.59	140	nmol/l	XXO	10 nmol/l
cortisol, free (U)	10–110	µg/24 h	2.759	30–300	nmol/d	XXO	10 nmol/d
creatine (S)							
-male	0.17–0.50	µg/dl	76.25	10–40	mmol/l	XO	10 mmol/l
-female	0.35–0.93	µg/dl	76.25	30–70	mmol/l	XO	10 mmol/l
creatine (U)							
-male	0–40	mg/24 h	7.625	0–300	µmol/d	XXO	10 µmol/d
-female	0–80	mg/24 h	7.625	0–600	µmol/d	XXO	10 µmol/d
creatine kinase[CK](S)							
creatine kinase isoenzymes (S)	0–130	U/l	0.01667	0–2.16	µkat/l	X.XX	0.01 µkat/l
-MB fraction	>5 in myocardial infarction	%	0.01	>0.05	1	O.XX	0.01
creatinine (S)	0.6–1.2	mg/dl	88.40	50–110	µmol/l	XXO	10 µmol/l
creatinine (U)	Variable	g/24 h	8.840	Variable	mmol/d	XX.X	0.1 mmol/d
creatinine clearance (S,U)	75–125	ml/min	0.01667	1.24–2.08	ml/s	X.XX	0.02 ml/s

$$\text{creatinine clearance} = \frac{\text{mmol/l (urine creatinine)}}{\text{mmol/l (serum creatinine)}} \times \text{ml/s} \times \frac{1.73}{A} \quad \text{(where A is the body surface area in square meters [m2])}$$

Component	Present Reference Intervals (examples)	Present Unit	Conversion Factor	SI Reference Intervals	SI Unit Symbol	Significant Digits	Suggested Minimum Increment
cyanide (B) - lethal	>0.10	mg/dl	384.3	>40	µmol/l	XXX	5 µmol/l
cyanocobalamin (S) [Vitamin B$_{12}$]	100–200	pg/ml	0.7378	150–750	pmol/l	XXO	10 pmol/l
cyclic AMP (S)	2.6–6.6	µg/l	3.038	8–20	nmol/L	XXX	1 nmol/L
cyclic AMP (U)							

-total urinary	2.9–5.6	µmol/g creatinine	113.1	330–630	nmol/mmol creatinine	XXO	10 nmol/mmol creatinine
-renal tubular	<2.5	µmol/g creatinine	113.1	<280	nmol/mmol creatinine	XXO	10 nmol/mmol creatinine
cyclic GMP (S)	0.6–3.5	µg/l	2.897	1.7–10.1	nmol/l	XX.X	0.1 nmol/l
cyclic GMP (U)	0.3–1.8	µmol/g creatinine	113.1	30–200	nmol/mmol creatinine	XXO	10 nmol/mmol creatinine
cystine (U)	10–100	mg/24 h	4.161	40–420	mmol/d	XXO	10 mmol/d
dehydroepiandrosterone (P,S) [DHEA] - 1–4 years	0.2–0.4	µg/l	3.467	0.6–1.4	nmol/l	XX.X	0.2 nmol/l
4–8 years	0.1–1.9	µg/l	3.467	0.4–6.6	nmol/l	XX.X	0.2 nmol/l
8–10 years	0.2–2.9	µg/l	3.467	0.6–10.0	nmol/l	XX.X	0.2 nmol/l
10–12 years	0.5–9.2	µg/l	3.467	1.8–31.8	nmol/l	XX.X	0.2 nmol/l
12–14 years	0.9–20.0	µg/l	3.467	3.2–69.4	nmol/l	XX.X	0.2 nmol/l
14–16 years	2.5–20.0	µg/l	3.467	8.6–69.4	nmol/l	XX.X	0.2 nmol/l
premenopausal female	2.0–15.0	µg/l	3.467	7.0–52.0	nmol/l	XX.X	0.2 nmol/l
male	0.8–10.0	µg/l	3.467	2.8–34.6	nmol/l	XX.X	0.2 nmol/l
dehydroepiandrosterone (U)	See Steroids						
dehydroepiandrosterone sulphate [DHEA-S] (P, S)		Fractionation	…	…	…	…	…
newborn	1670–3640	ng/ml	0.002714	4.5–9.9	µmol/l	XX.X	µmol/l
pre-pubertal children	100–600	ng/ml	0.002714	0.3–1.6	µmol/l	XX.X	µmol/l
male	2000–3500	ng/ml	0.002714	5.4–9.1	µmol/l	XX.X	µmol/l
female (premenopausal)	820–3380	ng/ml	0.002714	2.2–9.2	µmol/l	XX.X	µmol/l
female (post-menopausal)	110–610	ng/ml	0.002714	0.3–1.7	µmol/l	XX.X	µmol/l
pregnancy [term]	0–1170	ng/ml	0.002714	0.6–3.2	µmol/l	XX.X	µmol/l
11-deoxycortisol (S)	0–2	µg/dl	28.86	0–60	nmol/l	XXO	10 nmol/l
desipramine (P) -therapeutic	50–200	ng/ml	3.754	170–700	nmol/l	XXO	10 nmol/l
diazepam (P) -therapeutic	0.10–0.25	mg/l	3512	350–900	nmol/l	XXO	10 nmol/l
-toxic	>1.0	mg/l	3512	>3510	nmol/l	XXO	10 nmol/l
dicoumarol (P) -therapeutic	8–30	mg/l	2.974	25–90	µmol/l	XX	5 µmol/l
digoxin (P) -therapeutic	0.5–2.2	ng/ml	1.281	0.6–2.8	nmol/l	X.X	0.1 nmol/l

TABLE 44 (CONTINUED)
Conversion Factors for Values in Clinical Chemistry (SI Units)

Component	Present Reference Intervals (examples)	Present Unit	Conversion Factor	SI Reference Intervals	SI Unit Symbol	Significant Digits	Suggested Minimum Increment
digoxin (P) -therapeutic	0.5–2.2	µg/l	1.281	0.6–2.8	nmol/l	X.X	0.1 nmol/l
-toxic	>2.5	ng/ml	1.281	>3.2	nmol/l	X.X	0.1 nmol/l
dimethadione (P) -therapeutic	<1.00	g/l	7.745	<7.7	mmol/l	X.X	0.1 mmol/l
disopyramide (P) -therapeutic	2.0–6.0	mg/l	2.946	6–18	µmol/l	XX	1 µmol/l
doxepin (P) -therapeutic	50–200	n/ml	3.579	180–720	nmol/l	XO	10 nmol/l
electrophoresis, protein (S)							
albumin	60–65	%	0.01	0.60–0.65	1	O.XX	0.01
alpha$_1$-globulin	1.7–5.0	%	0.01	0.02–0.05	1	O.XX	0.01
alpha$_2$-globulin	6.7–12.5	%	0.01	0.07–0.13	1	O.XX	0.01
beta-globulin	8.3–16.3	%	0.01	0.08–0.16	1	O.XX	0.01
gamma-globulin	10.7–20.0	%	0.01	0.11–0.20	1	O.XX	0.01
albumin	3.6–5.2	g/dl	10.0	36–52	g/l	XX	1 g/l
alpha$_1$-globulin	0.1–0.4	g/dl	10.0	1–4	g/l	XX	1 g/l
alpha$_2$-globulin	0.4–1.0	g/dl	10.0	4–10	g/l	XX	1 g/l
beta-globulin	0.5–1.2	g/dl	10.0	5–12	g/l	XX	1 g/l
gamma-globulin	0.6–1.6	g/dl	10.0	6–16	g/l	XX	1 g/l
epinephrine (P)	31–95 (at rest for 15 min)	pg/ml	5.458	170–520	pmol/l	XXO	10 pmol/l
epinephrine (U)	<10	µg/24 h	5.458	<55	nmol/d	XX	5 nmol/d
estradiol (S) male >18 yrs	15–40	pg/ml	3.671	55–150	pmol/l	XX	1 pmol/l
estriol (U) [non pregnant]							
onset of menstruation	4–25	µg/24 h	3.468	15–85	nmol/d	XXX	5 nmol/d
ovulation peak	28–99	µg/24 h	3.468	95–345	nmol/d	XXX	5 nmol/d
luteal peak	22–105	µg/24 h	3.468	75–365	nmol/d	XXX	5 nmol/d
menopausal woman	1.4–19.6	µg/24 h	3.468	5–70	nmol/d	XXX	5 nmol/d
male	5–18	µg/24 h	3.468	15–60	nmol/d	XXX	5 nmol/d

estrogens (S) [as estradiol]							
female	20–300	pg/ml	3.671	70–1100	pmol/l	XXXO	10 pmol/l
peak production	200–800	pg/ml	3.671	750–2900	pmol/l	XXXO	10 pmol/l
male	<50	pg/ml	3.671	<180	pmol/l	XXO	10 pmol/l
estrogens, placental (U) [as estriol]	Depends on period of gestation	mg/24 h	3.468	Depends on period of gestation	µmol/d	XXX	1 µmol/d
estrogen receptors (T)							
negative	0–3	fmol estradiol bound/mg cytosol protein	1.00	0–3	fmol estradiol/mg cytosol protein	XXX	1 fmol/mg protein
doubtful	4–10	fmol estradiol bound/mg cytosol protein	1.00	4–10	fmol estradiol/mg cytosol protein	XXX	1 fmol/mg protein
positive	>10	fmol estradiol bound/mg cytosol protein	1.00	>10	fmol estradiol/mg cytosol protein	XXX	1 fmol/mg protein
estrone (P, S)							
-female 1–10 days of cycle	43–180	pg/ml	3.699	160–665	pmol/l	XXX	5 pmol/l
-female 11–20 days of cycle	75–196	pg/ml	3.699	275–725	pmol/l	XXX	5 pmol/l
-female 20–39 days of cycle	131–201	pg/ml	3.699	485–745	pmol/l	XXX	5 pmol/l
-male	29–75	pg/ml	3.699	105–275	pmol/l	XXX	5 pmol/l
estrone (U) female	2–25	µg/24 h	3.699	5–90	nmol/d	XXX	5 nmol/d
ethanol (P)							
legal limit [driving]	<80	mg/dl	0.2171	<17	mmol/l	XX	1 nmol/l
-toxic	>100	mg/dl	0.2171	>22	mmol/l	XX	1 mmol/l
ethchlorvynol (P) toxic	>40	mg/l	6.915	>280	µmol/l	XXO	10 µmol/l
ethosuximide (P) therapeutic	40–110	mg/l	7.084	280–780	µmol/l	XXO	10 µmol/l
ethylene glycol (P) toxic	>30	mg/dl	0.1611	>5	mmol/l	XX	1 mmol/l
fat (F) [as stearic acid]	2.0–6.0	g/24 h	3.515	7–21	mmol/d	XXX	1 mmol/d
fatty acids, nonesterified (P)	8–20	mg/dl	10.00	80–200	mg/l	XXO	10 mg/l
ferritin (S)	18–300	ng/ml	1.00	18–300	µg/l	XXO	10 µg/l

TABLE 44 (CONTINUED)
Conversion Factors for Values in Clinical Chemistry (SI Units)

Component	Present Reference Intervals (examples)	Present Unit	Conversion Factor	SI Reference Intervals	SI Unit Symbol	Significant Digits	Suggested Minimum Increment
fibrinogen (P)	200–400	mg/dl	0.01	2.0–4.0	g/l	X.X	0.1 g/l
fluoride (U)	<1.0	mg/24 h	52.63	<50	μmol/d	XXO	10 μmol/d
folate (S) [as pteroylglutamic acid]	2–10	ng/ml	2.266	4–22	nmol/l	XX	2 nmol/l
		μg/dl	22.66		nmol/l		2 nmol/l
folate (Erc)	140–960	ng/ml	2.266	550–2200	nmol/l	XXO	10 nmol/l
follicle stimulating hormone [FSH] (P)							
female	2.0–15.0	mIU/ml	1.00	2–15	IU/l	XX	1 IU/l
peak production	20–50	mIU/ml	1.00	20–50	IU/l	XX	1 IU/l
male	1.0–10.0	mIU/ml	1.00	1–10	IU/l	XX	1 IU/l
follicle stimulating hormone [FSH] (U)							
follicular phase	2–15	IU/24 h	1.00	2–15	IU/d	XXX	1 IU/d
midcycle	8–40	IU/24 h	1.00	8–40	IU/d	XXX	1 IU/d
luteal phase	2–10	IU/24 h	1.00	2–10	IU/d	XXX	1 IU/d
menopausal women	35–100	IU/24 h	1.00	35–100	IU/d	XXX	1 IU/d
male	2–15	IU/24 h	1.00	2–15	IU/d	XXX	1 IU/d
fructose (P)	<10	mg/dl	0.05551	<0.6	mmol/l	X.XX	0.1 mmol/l
galactose (P) [children]	<20	mg/dl	0.05551	<1.1	mmol/l	X.XX	0.1 mmol/l
gases (aB)							
pO_2	75–105	mm Hg (= Torr)	0.1333	10.0–14.0	kPa	XX.X	0.1 kPa
pCO_2	33–44	mm Hg (= Torr)	0.1333	4.4–5.9	kPa	X.X	0.1 kPa
gamma-glutamyltransferase [GGT] (S)	0–30	U/l	0.01667	0–0.50	μkat/l	X.XX	0.01 μkat/l
gastrin (S)	0–180	pg/ml	1.00	0–180	ng/l	XXO	10 ng/l

globulins (S) [see immunoglobulins]	...	...	...	...	...	...	...
glucagon (S)	50–100	pg/ml	1.00	50–100	ng/l	XXO	10 ng/l
glucose (P) fasting	70–110	mg/dl	0.05551	3.9–6.1	mmol/l	XX.X	0.1 mmol/l
glucose (Sf)	50–80	mg/dl	0.05551	2.8–4.4	mmol/l	XX.X	0.1 mmol/l
glutethimide (P)							
-therapeutic	<10	mg/l	4.603	<46	µmol/l	XX	1 µmol/l
-toxic	>20	mg/l	4.603	>92	µmol/l	XX	1 µmol/l
glycerol, free (S)	<1.5	mg/dl	0.1086	<0.16	mmol/l	X.XX	0.01 mmol/l
gold (S) therapeutic	300–800	µg/dl	0.05077	15.0–40.0	µmol/l	XX.X	0.1 µmol/l
gold (U)	<500	µg/24 h	0.005077	<2.5	µmol/d	X.X	0.1 µmol/d
palmitic acid (Amf)	Depends on gestation	mmol/l	1000	Depends on gestation	µmol/l	XXX	5 µmol/l
pentobarbital (P)	20–40	mg/l	4.419	90–170	µmol/l	XX	5 µmol/l
phenobarbital (P) -therapeutic	2–5	mg/l	43.06	85–215	µmol/l	XXX	5 µmol/l
phensuximide (P)	4–8	mg/l	5.285	20–40	µmol/l	XX	5 µmol/l
phenylbutazone (P) -therapeutic	<100	mg/l	3.243	<320	µmol/l	XXO	10 µmol/l
phenytoin (P)							
-therapeutic	10–20	mg/l	3.964	40–80	µmol/l	XX	5 µmol/l
-toxic	>30	mg/l	3.964	>12	µmol/l	XX	5 µmol/l
phosphate (S) [as phosphorus, inorganic]	2.5–5.0	mg/dl	0.3229	0.80–1.60	mmol/l	X.XX	0.05 mmol/l
phosphate (U) [as phosphorus, inorganic]	Diet dependent	g/24 h	32.29	Diet dependent	mmol/d	XXX	1 mmol/d
phospholipid phosphorus, total (P)	5–12	mg/dl	0.3229	1.60–3.90	mmol/l	X.XX	0.05 mmol/l
phospholipid phosphorus, total (Erc)	1.2–12.0	mg/dl	0.3229	0.40–3.90	mmol/l	X.XX	0.05 mmol/l
phospholipids (P) substance fraction of total phospholipid							
phosphatidyl choline	65–70	%/total	0.01	0.65–0.70	1	O.XX	0.01
phosphatidyl ethanolamine	4–5	%/total	0.01	0.04–0.05	1	O.XX	0.01
sphingomyelin	15–20	%/total	0.01	0.15–0.20	1	O.XX	0.01

TABLE 44 (CONTINUED)
Conversion Factors for Values in Clinical Chemistry (SI Units)

Component	Present Reference Intervals (examples)	Present Unit	Conversion Factor	SI Reference Intervals	SI Unit Symbol	Significant Digits	Suggested Minimum Increment
lysophosphatidyl choline	3–5	%total	0.01	0.03–0.05	1	O.XX	0.01
phospholipids (Erc) substance fraction of total phospholipid							
phosphatidyl choline	28–33	%total	0.01	0.28–0.33	1	O.XX	0.01
phosphatidyl ethanolamine	24–31	%total	0.01	0.24–0.31	1	O.XX	0.01
sphingomyelin	22–29	%total	0.01	0.22–0.29	1	O.XX	0.01
phosphatidyl serine + phosphatidyl inositol	12–20	%total	0.01	0.12–0.20	1	O.XX	0.01
lysophosphatidyl choline	1–2	%total	0.01	0.01–0.02	1	O.XX	0.01
phytanic acid (P)	Trace–0.3	mg/dl	32.00	<10	µmol/l	XX	5 µmol/l
[human] placental lactogen (SO [HPL]	>4.0 after 30 wk gestation	µg/ml	46.30	>180	nmol/l	XXO	10 nmol/l
porphobilinogen (U)	0–2	mg/24 h	4.420	0–9	µmol/d	X.X	0.5 µmol/d
porphyrins							
coproporphyrin (U)	45–180	µg/24 h	1.527	68–276	nmol/d	XXX	2 nmol/d
protoporphyrin (Erc)	15–50	µg/dl	0.0177	0.28–0.90	µmol/l	X.XX	0.02 µmol/l
uroporphyrin (U)	5–20	µg/24 h	1.204	6–24	nmol/d	XX	2 nmol/d
uroporphyrinogen synthetase (Erc)	22–42	mmol/mL/h	0.2778	6.0–11.8	mmol/(l.s)	X.X	0.2 mmol/(l.s)
potassium ion (S)	3.5–5.0	mEq/l	1.00	3.5–5.0	mmol/l	X.X	0.1 mmol/l
		mg/dl	0.2558		mmol/l	X.X	0.1 mmol/l
potassium ion (U) [diet dependent]	25–100	mEq/24 h	1.00	25–100	mmol/d	XX	1 mmol/d
pregnaediol (U)							
-normal	1–6	mg/24 h	3.120	3.0–18.5	µmol/d	XX.X	0.5 µmol/d
-pregnancy	Depends on gestation						
pregnanetriol (U)	0.5–2.0	mg/24 h	2.972	1.5–6.0	µmol/d	XX.X	0.5 µmol/d

primidone (P)						
-therapeutic	6–10	mg/l	4.582	25–46	μmol/l	XX	1 μmol/l
-toxic	>10	mg/l	4.582	>46	μmol/l	XX	1 μmol/l
procainamide (P)						
-therapeutic	4–8	mg/l	4.249	17–34	μmol/l	XX	1 μmol/l
-toxic	>12.0	mg/l	4.249	>50	μmol/l	XX	1 μmol/l
N-acetyl procainamide (P) -therapeutic	4–8	mg/l	3.606	14–29	μmol/l	XX	1 μmol/l
progesterone (P)						
follicular phase	<2	ng/ml	3.180	<6	nmol/l	XX	2 nmol/l
luteal phase	2–20	ng/ml	3.180	6–64	nmol/l	XX	2 nmol/l
progesterone receptors (T)						
negative	0–3	fmol progesterone bound/mg cytosol protein	1.00	0–3	fmol progesterone bound/mg cytosol protein	XX	1 fmol/mg protein
doubtful	4–10	fmol progesterone bound/mg cytosol protein	1.00	4–10	fmol progesterone bound/mg cytosol protein	XX	1 fmol/mg protein
positive	>10	fmol progesterone bound/mg cytosol protein	1.00	>10	fmol progesterone bound/mg cytosol protein	XX	1 fmol/mg protein
prolactin (P)	<20	ng/ml	1.00	<20	μg/l	XX	1 μg/l
propoxyphene (P) toxic	>2.0	mg/l	2.946	>5.9	μmol/l	X.X	0.1 μmol/l
propranolol (P) [Inderal] therapeutic	50–200	ng/ml	3.856	190–770	nmol/l	XXO	10 nmol/l
protein, total (S)	6.0–8.0	g/dl	10.0	60–80	g/l	XX	1 g/l
protein, total (Sf)	<40	mg/dl	0.01	<0.40	g/l	X.XX	0.1 g/l
protein, total (U)	<150	mg/24 h	0.001	<0.15	g/d	X.XX	0.01 g/d
protrytyline (P)	100–300	ng/ml	3.797	380–1140	nmol/l	XXO	10 nmol/l

TABLE 44 (CONTINUED)
Conversion Factors for Values in Clinical Chemistry (SI Units)

Component	Present Reference Intervals (examples)	Present Unit	Conversion Factor	SI Reference Intervals	SI Unit Symbol	Significant Digits	Suggested Minimum Increment
pyruvate (B) [as pyruvic acid]	0.30–0.90	mg/dl	113.6	35–100	μmol/l	XXX	1 μmol/l
quinidine (P)							
-therapeutic	1.5–3.0	mg/l	3.082	4.6–9.2	μmol/l	X.X	0.1 μmol/l
-toxic	>6.0	mg/l	3.082	>18.5	μmol/l	X.X	0.1 μmol/l
renin (P) normal sodium diet	1.1–4.1	ng/ml/h	0.2778	0.30–1.14	ng/(l.s)	X.XX	0.2 ng/(l.s)
restricted sodium diet	6.2–12.4	ng/ml/h	0.2778	1.72–3.44	ng/(l.s)	X.XX	0.02 ng/(l.s)
salicylate (S) [salicylic acid] toxic	>20	mg/dl	0.07240	>1.45	mmol/l	X.XX	0.05 mmol/l
serotonin (B) [5 hydroxytryptamine]	8–21	μg/dl	0.05675	0.45–1.20	μmol/l/l	X.XX	0.05 μmol/l
sodium ion (S)	135–147	mEq/l	1.00	135–147	mmol/l	XXX	1 mmol/l
sodium ion (U)	Diet dependent	mEq/24 h	1.00	Diet dependent	mmol/d	XXX	2 mmol/d
steroids 17-hydroxy-corticosteroids (U) [as cortisol]							
-female	2.0–8.0	mg/24 h	2.759	5–25	μmol/d	XX	1 μmol/d
-male	3–10	mg/24 h	2.759	10–30	μmol/d	XX	1 μmol/d
17-ketogenic steroids (U) [as dehydroepiandrosterone]							
-female	7–12	mg/24 h	3.467	25–40	μmol/d	XX	1 μmol/d
-male	9–17	mg/24 h	3.467	30–60	μmol/d	XX	1 μmol/d
17-ketosteroids (U) [as dehydroepiandrosterone]							
-female	6–17	mg/24 h	3.467	20–60	μmol/d	XX	1 μmol/d
-male	6–20	mg/24 h	3.467	20–70	μmol/d	XX	1 μmol/d
ketosteroid fractions (U) androsterone							
-female	0.5–2.0	mg/24 h	3.443	1–10	μmol/d	XX	1 μmol/d

-male	2.0–5.0	mg/24 h	3.443	7–17	µmol/d	XX	1 µmol/d
dehydroepiandrosterone							
-female	0.2–1.8	mg/24 h	3.467	1–6	µmol/d	XX	1 µmol/d
-male	0.2–2.0	mg/24 h	3.467	1–7	µmol/d	XX	1 µmol/d
etiocholanolone							
-female	0.8–4.0	mg/24 h	3.443	2–14	µmol/d	XX	1 µmol/d
-male	1.4–5.0	mg/24 h	3.443	4–17	µmol/d	XX	1 µmol/d
sulfonamides (B) [as sulfanilamide] -therapeutic	10–15	mg/dl	58.07	580–870	µmol/l	XXO	10 µmol/l
testosterone (P)							
-female	0.6	ng/ml	3.467	2.0	nmol/l	XX.X	0.5 nmol/l
-male	4.6–8.0	ng/ml	3.467	14–28	nmol/l	XX.X	0.5 nmol/l
theophylline (P) -therapeutic	10–20	mg/l	5.550	55–110	µmol/l	XX	1 µmol/l
thiocyanate (P) (nitroprusside toxicity)	10.0	mg/dl	0.1722	1.7	mmol/l	X.XX	0.1 mmol/l
thiopental (P)	individual	mg/l	4.126	individual	µmol/l	XX	5 µmol/l
thyroid tests:							
thyroid stimulating hormone [TSH] (S)	2–11	µU/ml	1.00	2–11	mU/l	XX	1 mU/l
thyroxine [T$_4$] (S)	4–11	µg/dl	12.87	51–142	nmol/l	XXX	1 nmol/l
thyroxine binding globulin [TGB] (S) [as thyroxine]	12–28	µg/dl	12.87	150–360	nmol/l	XXO	1 nmol/l
thyroxine, free (S)	0.8–2.8	ng/dl	12.87	10–36	pmol/l	XX	1 pmol/l
triiodothyronine [T$_3$] (S)	75–220	ng/dl	0.01536	1.2–3.4	nmol/l	X.X	0.1 nmol/l
T$_3$ uptake (S)	25–35	%	0.01	0.25–0.35	1	O.XX	0.01
tolbuamide (P) -therapeutic	50–120	mg/l	3.699	180–450	mmol/l	XXO	10 mmol/l
transferrin (S)	170–370	mg/dl	0.01	1.70–3.70	g/l	X.XX	0.01 g/l
triglycerides (P) [as triolein]	<160	mg/dl	0.01129	<1.80	mmol/l	X.XX	0.02 mmol/l
trimethadione (P) -therapeutic	<50	mg/l	6.986	<350	µmol/l	XXO	10 µmol/l
trimipramine (P) -therapeutic	50–200	ng/ml	3.397	170–680	nmol/l	XXO	10 nmol/l

TABLE 44 (CONTINUED)
Conversion Factors for Values in Clinical Chemistry (SI Units)

Component	Present Reference Intervals (examples)	Present Unit	Conversion Factor	SI Reference Intervals	SI Unit Symbol	Significant Digits	Suggested Minimum Increment
urate (S) [as uric acid]	2–7	mg/dl	59.48	120–420	µmol/l	XXO	10 µmol/l
urate (U) [as uric acid]	Diet dependent	g/24 h	5.948	Diet dependent	mmol/d	XX	1 mmol/d
urea nitrogen (S)	8–18	mg/dl	0.3570	3.0–6.5	mmol/l UREA	X.X	0.5 mmol/l
urea nitrogen (U)	2–20 diet dependent	g/24 h	35.700	450–700	mmol/d UREA	XXO	10 mol/d
urobilinogen (U)	0–4	mg/24 h	1.693	0.0–6.8	µmol/d	X.X	0.1 µmol/d
valproic acid (P) -therapeutic	50–100	mg/l	6.934	350–700	µmol/l	XO	10 µmol/l
vanillylmandelic acid [VMA], urine	<6.8	mg/24 h	5.046	<35	µmol/d	XX	1 µmol/d
vitamin A [retinol] (P,S)	10–50	µg/dl	0.03491	0.35–1.75	µmol/l	X.XX	0.05 µmol/l
vitamin B₁ [thiamine hydrochloride] (U)	60–500	mg/24 h	0.002965	0.18–1.48	µmol/d	ZX.XX	0.01 µmol/d
vitamin B₂ [riboflavin] (S)	2.6–3.7	µg/dl	26.57	70–100	nmol/l	XXX	5 nmol/l
vitamin B₆ [pyridoxal] (B)	20–90	ng/ml	5.982	120–540	nmol/l	XXX	5 nmol/l
vitamin B₁₂ (P,S) [cyanocobalamin]	200–1000	pg/ml	0.7378	150–750	pmol/l	XO	10 pmol/l
vitamin C [see ascorbate] (B,P,S)	…	…	…	…	…	…	…
vitamin D₃ [cholecalciferol] (P)	24–40	mg/ml	2.599	60–105	nmol/l	XXX	5 nmol/l
25 OH-cholecacliferol	18–36	ng/ml	0.496	45–90	nmol/l	XXX	5 mmol/l
vitamin E [alpha-tocopherol] (P,S)	0.78–1.25	mg/dl	23.22	18–29	µmol/l	XX	1 µmol/l
warfarin (P) -therapeutic	1–3	mg/l	3.243	3.3–9.8	µmol/l	XX.X	0.1 µmol/l

	Conventional reference	Conventional unit	Factor	SI reference	SI unit	Sig.	Minimum increment
xanthine (U) -hypoxanthine	5–30	mg/24	6.574	30–200	µmol/d	XXO	10 µmol/d
D-xylose (B) [25 g dose]	30–40 (30–60 min)	hmg/24 h	7.347	0–2.7 (30–60 min)	µmol/d	XXO	10 µmol/d
		mg/dl	0.06661		mmol/l	X.X	0.1 mmol/l
D-xylose excretion (U) [25 g dose]	21–31	%	0.01	0.21–0.31 (excreted in 5 h)	1	0.XX	0.01
zinc (S)	75–120	µg/dl	0.1530	11.5–18.5	µmol/l	XX.X	0.1 µmol/l
zinc (U)	150–1200	µg/24 h	0.01530	2.3–18.3	µmol/d	XX.X	0.1 µmol/d

From Young, D.S., *Ann. Int. Med.*, 106, 20, 1987.

SODIUM (Na⁺)

An essential cation in the extracellular fluids. This ion is essential for muscle contraction, active transport of solutes, and the maintenance of fluid balance (see minerals, Table 30).

SODIUM BENZOATE

An additive involved in idiosyncratic food intolerance reactions. This preservative is used in foods such as lemonades, margarine, jam, ice cream, fish, sausages, and dressings. Sometimes it is also added to flavorings. Benzoates can elicit asthmatic attacks in asthmatic patients. Furthermore, they may play a role in patients with urticaria.

SODIUM-DEPENDENT ACTIVE TRANSPORT

See active transport.

SODIUM PUMP

The energy requiring process by which a high potassium concentration is maintained inside cells and a high sodium level is maintained outside the cells. The energy is provided by ATP.

SOFT DIET

Therapeutic diet characterized by soft foods and liquids which is typically reduced in fiber and residue.

SOFT TISSUE

Tissues and organs that are not mineralized.

SOLUTE LOAD

The amount of solutes on one side of a membrane. Usually refers to the filtering function of the convoluted tubule in the kidney.

SOMATOSTATIN

Hormone released by D cells of pancreatic islets and other organs (intestine, brain, etc.) (see Table 26).

SOMOGYI EFFECT

Rebound hyperglycemia indicated by change from hypoglycemia to hyperglycemia within one to two hours.

TABLE 45
General Formulas for Calculating Body Fatness from Skinfold Measurements

Males

% Body Fat = 29.288×10^{-2} (X). 5×10^{-4} (X)^2 + 15.845×10^{-2} (Age)

Females

% Body Fat = 29.699×10^{-2} (X) -43×10^{-5} (X)^2 + 29.63×10^{-3} (Age) + 1.4072

  where X = sum of abdomen, suprailiac, triceps and thigh skinfolds and age is in years.

From Committee on Nutritional Anthropometry, Food and Nutrition Board, National Research Council, 1956.

SORBIC ACID

A food additive possessing antimicrobial activity.

SORBITOL

A sugar alcohol derived from the six carbon sugar sorbose. Provides less energy (~2 kcal/g) than glucose.

SORGHUM

A cereal grain; used in both human and animal foods.

SOYBEAN HYDROLYSATE

A protein mixture isolated from soybeans and subjected to hydrolysis to improve its digestibility.

SPECIAL COHORTS

See follow-up studies.

SPECIFIC DYNAMIC ACTION

Heat production resulting from the metabolism of food. It is is estimated to be about 10% of energy value of the food consumed. Also known as thermic effect of food or diet-induced thermogenesis.

SPECIFIC GRAVITY

Ratio of the weight of the body to the weight of an equal volume of water.

SPECIFIC HEAT

The heat absorbing capacity of a substance compared to water.

SPHINCTER

A muscle, surrounding a body opening or vessel, that can contract and close that opening.

SPHINGOMYELIN

A group of phospholipids found in the myelin sheath covering the nerves.

SPHINGOSINE

An alcohol that forms the backbone of Sphingomyelin.

SPINA BIFIDA

Congenital defect in the structure of the spinal column characterized by an open area around the nerve trunk leaving it unprotected and subject to infection or injury.

SPORTS ANEMIA

A decrease in red cell volume due to excessive red cell breakdown due to excessive physical activity.

SPRUE

Malabsorption syndrome caused either by sensitivity to gluten or fat intolerance.

STABLE ISOTOPE

An isotope that is nonradioactive. K^{40} is a stable isotope.

STACHYOSE

A nondigestible carbohydrate found in dried beans and peas.

STANDARD OF IDENTITY

A term used by the U.S. Food and Drug Agency to indicate that standard ingredients in standard amounts are used to make a food product. Deviations from these standards must be so labelled.

STARCH

A glucose polymer having α 1,4 and α 1,6 linkages.

STARVATION

Involuntary absence of feeding.

STASIS

A slowing or stoppage of normal fluid flow.

STEATORRHEA

Excess fat in feces.

STENOSIS

Narrowing of an opening.

STEREOISOMER

Isomers having the same atoms but whose structure has one or two slight differences in the position of these atoms. See carbohydrate structure, protein structure.

STERIGMATOCYSTIN

A carcinogenic mycotoxin, which is primarily produced by *Aspergillus versicolor* and *Aspergillus nidulans*, although other moulds (e.g., *Aspergillus flavus*, *Aspergillus rugulosus*, *Bipolaris* spp., *Penicillium luteum*) are also capable of producing sterigmatocystin. Sterigmatocystin is structurally related to the aflatoxins and is equally stable. It is a potent hepatotoxin causing bile duct hyperplasia in ducklings and hyperplasia of the hepatocytes with little bile duct proliferation and liver necrosis in rats. Factors involved in fungal growth and toxin production include lactose, fat, and some fat hydrolysis products. Occurrence of sterigmatocystin has been reported in grains and the outer layer of hard cheeses, when these have been colonized by *Aspergillus versicolor*.

STEROL

A four ring structure typical of all steroid molecules.

STOMATITIS

Inflammation of the mouth mucous membrane.

STOOL

Feces.

STREPTOCOCCUS MUTANS

A food borne pathogen.

STRESS RESPONSE

Whole body response to physiological or psychological trauma. The response is mediated by hormones listed in Table 46.

STROKE

Blockage or rupture of blood vessel(s) supplying the brain with resulting loss of consciousness, paralysis, and other symptoms. Apoplexy is a common term for stroke.

SUB-UNIT BACTERIAL TOXINS

Compounds produced by foodborne microorganisms.

To this group belong the toxins produced by *Clostridium botulinum*. *Clostridium botulinum* are a group of motile, gram-positive, rod-shaped, spore-forming, anaerobic bacteria, which are capable of producing neurotoxins. According to the toxin they produce, there are seven types and three subtypes of *Clostridium botulinum* — type A, subtype A_f (A toxin); type B (B toxin); type C, subtype $C\alpha$ (C1, C2, and D toxins), subtype $C\beta$ (C2 toxin); type D (C1 and D toxins); type E (E toxin); type F (F toxin); and type G (G toxin). Based on their ability to digest proteins and break down sugars, *Clostridium botulinum* can be divided into four groups — group I, strains which are strongly proteolytic and saccharolytic (all strains of type A, several strains of types B and F); group II, strains which are nonproteolytic but strongly saccharolytic (all strains of type E, several strains of types B and F); group III, strains which are nonproteolytic except that they can digest gelatin (all strains of types C and D); and group IV, strains which are proteolytic but nonsaccharolytic (a single strain of type G). All types can deaminate and decarboxylate amino acids and desulfurize cystine to produce H_2S. Thus, all types can produce NH_3, H_2S, CO_2, and volatile amines from amino acids.

Clostridium botulinum produces an intracellular protoxin consisting of a nontoxic progenitor toxin (a hemagglutinin with a molecular weight of 500,000) and a highly toxic neurotoxin (molecular weight 150,000). The protoxin is released upon lysis of the vegetative bacterial cell. The neurotoxin is formed by proteolytic degradation of the protoxin. This proteolysis is caused by *Clostridium botulinum* proteolytic enzymes or by exogenous proteases (e.g., trypsin) when nonproteolytic strains of *Clostridium botulinum* are involved. Botulinum toxin is heat-sensitive (inactivated at 80°C for 10 minutes or 100°C for a few minutes). It is acid-resistant and survives the gastric passage. Botulinum toxin is an exotoxin; it is excreted by the cell, but most of it is released upon lysis of the cell after sporulation.

Botulism, caused by the ingestion of food containing the neurotoxin, is the most severe bacterial food-borne intoxication known. Humans are susceptible to types A, B, E, and F neurotoxins, whereas type A is toxic to chickens, types $C\alpha$ and E to birds, types $C\beta$ and D to cattle, type $C\beta$ to sheep, types $C\beta$ and E to mink, and types A, B, $C\beta$, and D to horses. Dogs, cats, and pigs are quite resistant to ingested toxin. The minimum lethal oral dose for man based on estimates in lethal poisoning is of the order of 1.4×10^{-2} µg/kg, and doses that have caused nonfatal botulism, as judged from accidental cases, range from 0.1 to 1.0 µg. The toxin appears to be transported by way of the lymph as well as the blood. It has a direct action on the nerves, particularly the peripheral nerves, resulting in neuromuscular paralysis. Clinical symptoms of botulinum poisoning usually occur in 12–36 hours, starting with

TABLE 46
Hormones Directly Involved in the Stress Response

Hormone	Origin	Physiological Functions
Adrenocorticotropic hormone (ACTH)	Anterior pituitary	Synthesis and release of hormones from the adrenal cortex, mainly the glucocorticoids. ACTH acts directly on fatty tissue to liberate free fatty acids into the blood.
Aldosterone (mineralocorticoid)	Adrenal gland (cortex)	Stimulates kidney to excrete potassium into the urine and to conserve sodium.
Epinephrine (adrenaline) norepinephrine (noradrenaline)	Adrenal gland (medulla)	Both hormones alter heart output; dilate or constrict blood vessels; elevate blood pressure; release free fatty acids into the blood; stimulate the brain to increase alertness; increase metabolic rate; cause rapid release of glucose from the liver.
Glucagon	Pancreas (alpha cells of islets of langerhans)	Mobilizes glucose from liver glycogen; increase the formation of glucose from proteins — gluconeogenesis.
Glucocorticoids (cortisone, corticosterone, and cortisol)	Adrenal gland (cortex)	Increase protein catabolism; cause glucose production from protein and fats; elevate blood glucose; make amino acids available for use wherever needed; stimulate protein synthesis in the liver; mobilize fats for energy; antagonistic to action of the hormone insulin.
Growth hormone (GA; somatotropin, STH)	Anterior pituitary	Growth of all tissues; protein synthesis; mobilization of fats for energy while conserving glucose by preventing glucose uptake by some tissues.
Prolactin	Anterior pituitary	Growth of all tissues; protein synthesis; mobilization of fats for energy while conserving glucose by preventing glucose uptake by some tissues.
Triiodothyronine (T_3), Thyroxine (T_4)	Thyroid	Both hormones have similar actions; however, triiodothyronine is more potent and its actions are faster. Steps up metabolic rate; increases heart performance; increases nervous system activity, stimulates protein synthesis, increases motility and secretion of gastrointestinal tract; increases absorption of glucose from the intestine.
Vasopressin (antidiuretic hormone ADH)	Posterior pituitary	Acts on the kidneys to reduce urine volume and conserve body water, thus preventing body fluids from becoming too concentrated, urine becomes concentrated and urine volume decreases.

Adapted from Ensminger et al., *Foods and Nutrition Encyclopedia*, 2nd ed., CRC Press, Boca Raton, FL, 1994, 2057.

vomiting and dizziness, accompanied or followed by weakness, dryness of the mouth with difficulty in swallowing, paralysis, double vision, and respiratory distress. Death, resulting from respiratory paralysis and/or obstruction of the airways, pulmonary infection, and cardiac arrest, may occur as early as 10 hours after symptoms appear.

Factors affecting growth and toxin production by *Clostridium botulinum* include:

1. type and nutrient composition of substrate (in general, complex organic media provide better support for more efficient toxin production than synthetically defined ones);
2. temperature of growth (optimum temperature — 36–37°C at pH 7.0–7.2 [types A, B and D], 33°C at pH 7.6 [type C], 30°C at pH 7.0–7.2 [types E and F]);
3. acidity and salt concentration of substrate (in general, the required inhibitory salt concentration and pH increases and decreases, respectively, as the number of viable spores contaminating a product increases);
4. moisture activity (sufficient water activity is required);
5. oxygen concentration (*Clostridium botulinum*, being an obligate anaerobe, is inhibited by oxygen or may be directly poisoned by it);
6. presence of other microorganisms (effects: (a) lowering of redox potential or production of growth factors; (b) lowering or increasing of pH of medium by production or consumption of acids or acid-forming substances; (c) production of proteolytic enzymes which destroy or activate the toxin; and (d) production of antibiotic or antimicrobial substances);
7. other inhibitors (inhibitors of spore germination, e.g., various metals, rancidified unsaturated fatty acids, some flavonoids and spices, and inhibitors of vegetative growth, e.g., antibiotics).

Sources of *Clostridium botulinum* causing botulism include soil, mud, water, and intestinal tract of animals. At particular risk are low acid foods which are insufficiently heated. Examples are home-canned vegetables contaminated with soil-borne *Clostridium botulinum*, meat and fish contaminated during slaughtering with *Clostridium botulinum* originating from the intestinal tract, and chilled vacuum-packed foods, which usually have had minimal heat treatment, contain no preservatives other than any naturally occurring antimicrobial substances, and are not reheated or only mildly heated prior to consumption. Preventive measures against botulism include the heating and cooking of all foods with high water activity ($a_w > 0.90$) and low acidity (pH > 4) and storage above 3°C. Additionally, sanitary and proper food preservation procedures can minimize botulism.

SUBCUTANEOUS FAT

The fat cell layer just beneath the skin.

SUBSTRATE

The substance upon which an enzyme works.

SUCCINATE

A metabolic intermediate in the citric acid cycle. See citric acid cycle.

SUCCINYL CoA

A metabolic intermediate in the citric acid cycle. See citric acid cycle.

SUCRASE

Enzyme which catalyzes the cleavage of sucrose to glucose and fructose.

SUCROSE

A disaccharide consisting of one molecule of glucose and one molecule of fructose linked together.

SUCROSE DIGESTION/ABSORPTION

See carbohydrate absorption.

SUCROSE-INDUCED FATTY LIVER

Due to the fructose-induced increase in fatty acid synthesis. Adaptation can and does occur and the liver returns to its normal fat level.

SUCROSE-INDUCED LIPEMIA

When rats and some humans are fed sucrose-rich, low-fat diets, blood lipids, particularly triacylglycerols, rise. This is due to the fact that the fructose of the sucrose is metabolized primarily by the liver and the product of this metabolism is triacylglyceride which is then exported to the periphery for storage. In normal individuals, there is adaptation to this diet and the lipemia subsides.

SUCROSE POLYESTER (OLESTRA)

A polymer of sucrose and fatty acids which can be used as a fat substitute.

SULFITES

Additives involved in idiosyncratic food intolerance reactions. Sodium and potassium bisulfite and metabisulfite are used in food products to prevent spoilage by microorganisms as well as oxidative discoloration. They are added, among others, to salads, wine, dehydrated fruits, potatoes, seafood, baked goods, and tea mixtures. Symptoms that may occur in sulfite-intolerant persons are airway constriction, flushing, itching, urticaria, angioedema, nausea, and in extreme cases, hypotension.

SULPHUR

An essential element needed for the formation of disulfide bridges. Also important to hold iron in the centers of heme and the cytochromes and as a structural element in mucopolysaccharides and sulfolipids.

SULPHUR-CONTAINING AMINO ACIDS

Methionine, cysteine, cystine (see Table 5).

SUPINE

Lying on one's back.

SURFACTANT

A compound that reduces the surface tension of a liquid so that another liquid can be mixed with it.

SWEETENING AGENTS

Compounds that elicit a sweet taste. These are listed in Table 47.

SYMPTOMS

Signs or indications of disease.

SYNDROME

A group of signs and symptoms associated with a specific disease.

SYNERGISM

The effect resulting when two substances work together to produce an effect greater than each could produce individually.

TABLE 47
Sweetening Agents, Sugar Substitutes

Name	Sweetness[a]	Classification	Uses	Comments
Acesulfame-K (sold under brand Sunette)	130	Non-nutritive; artificial.	As a tabletop sweetener, chewing gum, dry beverage mixes, and puddings.	This is actually the potassium salt of the 6-methyl derivative of a group of chemicals called oxathiazinone dioxides. Approved by the FDA in 1988.
Aspartame	180	Nutritive; artificial.	It is in most diet sodas. Also used in cold cereals, drink mixes, gelatin, puddings, toppings, dairy products, and at the table by the consumer; not used in cooking due to lack of stability when heated.	Composed of the two naturally occurring amino acids, aspartic acid and phenylalanine; sweeter than sugar, therefore less required, hence fewer calories.
Cyclamate	30	Non-nutritive; artificial.	Used as a tabletop sweetener and in drugs in Canada and 40 other countries.	Discovered in 1937. FDA banned all cyclamate-containing beverages in 1969 and all cyclamate-containing foods in 1970. Cyclamate safety is now being re-evaluated by the FDA.
Dulcin (4-ethoxy-phenyl-urea)	250	Non-nutritive; artificial.	None.	Not approved for food use in the United States; used in some European countries. Also called Sucrol and Valzin.
Fructose (levulose)	1.7	Nutritive; natural.	Beverages, baking, canned goods; anywhere invert sugar or honey may be used.	A carbohydrate; a monosaccharide; naturally occurs in fruits; makes up about 50% of the sugar in honey; commercially found in high-fructose syrups and invert sugars; contributes sweetness and prevents crystallization.
Glucose (dextrose)	0.7	Nutritive; natural.	Primarily in the confection, wine, and canning industries; and in intravenous solutions.	Glucose acts synergistically with other sweeteners.
Glycine	0.8	Nutritive; natural.	Permissible to use to modify taste of some foods.	A sweet-tasting amino acid. Tryptophan is also a sweet-tasting amino acid.

TABLE 47 (CONTINUED)
Sweetening Agents, Sugar Substitutes

Name	Sweetness[a]	Classification	Uses	Comments
Mannitol	0.7	Nutritive; natural.	Candies, chewing gums, confections, and baked goods; dietetic foods.	A sugar alcohol or polyhydric alcohol (polyol); occurs naturally in pineapples, olives, asparagus, and carrots; commercially prepared by the hydrogenation of mannose or glucose; slowly and incompletely absorbed from the intestines; only slightly metabolized, most excreted unchanged in the urine; may cause diarrhea.
Miraculin	—	Nutritive; natural.	None.	Actually a taste-modifying protein rather than a sweetener; after exposing tongue to miraculin sour lemon tastes like sweetened lemon; responsible for the taste changing properties of miracle fruit, red berries of Synsepalum dulcificum, a native plant of West Africa; first described in 1852; one attempt made to commercialize by a U.S. firm but FDA denied approval and marketing was stopped.
Monellin	3000	Nutritive; natural.	None; only a potential low-calorie sweetener.	Extract of the pulp of the light red berries of the tropical plant Dioscoreophyllum cumminsii; also called Serendipity Berry; first protein found to elicit a sweet taste in man; first extracted in 1969; potential use limited by lack of stability; taste sensation is slow and lingering; everything tastes sweet after monellin.
Neohesperidin dihydrochalone (Neo DHC, NDHC)	1250	Non-nutritive; artificial.	None approved; potential for chewing gum, mouthwash, and toothpaste.	Formed from naringen isolated from citrus fruit; slow to elicit the taste sensation; lingering licoricelike aftertaste; animal studies indicate not toxic.

TABLE 47 (CONTINUED)
Sweetening Agents, Sugar Substitutes

Name	Sweetness[a]	Classification	Uses	Comments
P-4,000 (5-nitro-2-propoxyaniline)	4100	Non-nutritive; artificial.	None approved.	Derivative of nitroaniline; used as a sweetener in some European countries but banned in the United States due to toxic effects on rats; no bitter aftertaste; major drawback of p-4000 is powerful local anesthetic effect on the tongue and mouth. Used in the Netherlands during German occupation and during Berlin blockade.
Phyllodulcin	250	Natural.	None approved.	Isolated from Hydrangea macrophylla Seringe in 1916; displays a lagging onset of sweetness with licorice aftertaste; not well studied; possible market for hard candies, chewing gums, and oral hygiene products.
Saccharin (0 benzo-sulfimide)	500	Non-nutritive; artificial.	Used in beverages, as a tabletop sweetener, and in cosmetics, toothpaste, and cough syrup. Used as a sweetener by diabetics.	Both sodium and calcium salts of saccharin used; passes through body unchanged; excreted in urine; originally a generally recognized as safe (GRAS) additive. Subsequently, saccharin was classed as a carcinogen based on experiments with rats. However, recent experiments indicate that saccharin causes cancer in rats, but not in mice and people.
Sorbitol	0.6	Nutritive; natural.	Chewing gum, dairy products, meat products, icing, toppings, and beverages.	A sugar alcohol or polyhydric alcohol (polyol); occurs naturally in many fruits commercially prepared by the hydrogenation of glucose; many unique properties besides sweetness; on the FDA list of generally recognized as safe (GRAS) food additives; the most widely used sugar alcohol; slow intestinal absorption; consumption of large amounts may cause diarrhea.

TABLE 47 (CONTINUED)
Sweetening Agents, Sugar Substitutes

Name	Sweetness[a]	Classification	Uses	Comments
SRI Oxime V (Perilla sugar)	450	Non-nutritive; artificial.	None approved.	Derived from extract of Perilla namkinensis; clean taste; needs research; used as sweetening agent in Japan.
Stevioside	300	Nutritive; natural.	None approved.	Isolated from the leaves of the wild shrub, Stevia rebaudiana Bertoni; used by the people of Paraguay to sweeten drinks; limited evidence suggests nontoxic to humans. Rebaudioside A is isolated from the same plant, and it is said to taste superior to stevioside. Its chemical structure is very similar to stevioside, and it is 190 times sweeter than sugar.
Sucrose (brown sugar, liquid sugar, sugar, table sugar, white sugar) (Also see SUGAR.)	1.0	Nutritive; natural.	Many beverages and processed foods; home use in a wide variety of foods.	The chemical combination of the sugars fructose and glucose; one of the oldest sweetening agents; most popular and most available sweetening agent; occurs naturally in many fruits; commercially extracted from sugarcane and sugar beets.
Thaumatins	1600	Nutritive; natural	None.	Source of sweetness of the tropical fruit from the plant Thaumatococcus daniellii; enjoyed by inhabitants of western Africa; doubtful commercial applications.
Xylitol (Also see XYLITOL.)	0.8	Nutritive; natural	Chewing gums and dietetic foods.	A sugar alcohol or polyhydric alcohol (polyol); occurs naturally in some fruits and vegetables; produced in the body; commercial production from plant parts (oat hulls, corncobs, and birch wood chips) containing xylans — long chains of the sugar xylose; possible diarrhea; one British study suggests xylitol causes cancer in animals.

[a] Sweetness relative to sucrose.

Adapted from Ensminger et al., *Foods and Nutrition Encyclopedia*, 2nd ed., CRC Press, Boca Raton, FL, 1994, pp. 2082–2087.

TU

T₃

Triiodothyronine. The most active of the thyroid hormones.

T₄

Thyroxine. The form of thyroid hormone released by the thyroid gland to the blood.

T-CELLS

Cells of the immune system that originated from the thymus gland. These cells recognize antigens and produce antibodies to them.

TACHYCARDIA

Rapid heart beat.

TALLOW

Beef or sheep fat.

TANGIER DISEASE

Familial HDL deficiency. A genetic disease due to a mutation in the gene for the HDL protein. Characterized by very low plasma HDL and cholesterol levels, an accumulation of cholesterol esters in the tissues, and a peculiar yellow orange color to the tonsils.

TANNINS

A heterogeneous group of widely distributed substances in plants. They include all plant polyphenolic substances with a molecular weight higher than 500. Two types of tannins are distinguished on the basis of certain properties, breakdown products, and botanical distribution — hydrolyzable and condensed tannins. Hydrolyzable tannins are gallic, digallic, and ellagic acid esters of glucose or quinic acid. One type of hydrolyzable tannins is tannic acid (also known as gallotannic acid, gallotannin, or simply tannin). In tannic acid all the hydroxyl groups of glucose are esterified with gallic or digallic acid. It has been reported to cause acute liver injury, i.e., liver necrosis and fatty liver. The condensed tannins (also known as flavolans) are polymers of flavonoids which, in most cases, are leukoanthocyanidins. The monomers are linked through carbon-carbon bonds between position 4 and 6, or position 4 and 8. Occurrence of tannins is reported in many tropical fruits such as mango, dates, and persimmons. The tannins diminish in amounts as the fruits ripen. Furthermore, tannins are found in variable amounts in coffee (regular coffee: 1.1% tannins; instant coffee: 4.3% tannins; decaffeinated ground coffee: 1.2% tannins; instant decaffeinated coffee: 5.2% tannins), cocoa (unsweetened cocoa: 2.5% tannins; cocoa made by by treatment with alkali: 4% tannins), and tea (bulk black tea and green tea: 10.5–11.8% tannins; tea bags [black and green tea]: 9.1–13.1% tannins; black instant tea: 14.7% tannins). Green tea may yield more soluble tannins, while black tea contains tannins with a higher molecular mass, as a result of oxidation of phenolic precursors during fermentation. Other important sources of tannins are grapes (condensed tannins, on average 500 mg/kg of grapes), grape juice, wines (red wine: 1.2–4.4 g/l of wine), many varieties of sorghum grains, and in bracken.

TASTE BUDS

Sensory cells on the surface of the tongue, soft palate, cheeks, and throat.

TASTE THRESHOLD

Lowest concentration of a food or beverage at which its taste can be determined. Altered taste thresholds are often noted by individuals undergoing chemotherapy.

TAURI'S DISEASE

Glycogen storage disease type VII due to a mutation in the gene for phosphofructokinase. Characterized by excess glycogen stores in muscles.

TAURINE

2-aminoethyl sulfonic acid; synthesized from methionine and excreted via the kidneys; is involved in neurotransmission; is an end product of taurochloic acid (a bile acid) degradation.

TAUROCHOLATE

A biosalt derived from taurine; a bile acid produced by the liver, stored in the gall bladder, and released into the duodenum to serve as an emulsifier of lipid in the ingesta.

TAY-SACHS DISEASE

A genetic disease due to a mutation in the gene for the enzyme, hexo-amidase A that is involved in the normal degradation of brain gangliosides. When these accumulate, the brain disintegrates, the child loses mental function, and dies.

TBF

Total body fat.

TBG

Thyroxine binding globulin. The protein which carries the thyroxine from the thyroid gland to its target tissue.

TBW

Total body water.

TCA CYCLE

See citric acid cycle.

TDP, TPP

Thiamin-containing coenzyme required for decarboxylation reactions.

TERATOGENIC RISK

Risk associated with specific compounds, based on the chance that these compounds will have deleterious effects on the embryo or fetus.

TETANY

A disorder characterized by intermittent tonic muscular contractions accompanied by fibrillary tremors, paresthesias, and muscle pain.

TETRAHYDROFOLATE

A coenzyme form of the vitamin folacin; a carrier of methyl groups.

THALASSEMIA

A genetic disorder characterized by a defect in one of the homoglobin chains which reduce its oxygen carrying capacity.

THEOPHYLLINE

An alkaloid found in tea; acts as a diuretic, vasodilator, and a cardiac stimulant.

THERAPEUTIC DIETS

Diets designed to manage the symptoms of metabolic disorders such as obesity, diabetes, hypertension, etc.

THERMIC EFFECT OF FOOD

Heat producing response of the body to the ingestion of food.

THERMOGENESIS

Heat production.

THERMOPHILES

Bacteria that thrive or tolerate temperatures above 55°C.

THIAMIN

Vitamin that serves as a coenzyme (TPP, thiamin pyrophosphate) and is required for oxidative decarboxylation reactions (see vitamins, Table 49).

THIAMIN DIPHOSPHATE

Coenyzme form of thiamin also called thiamin pyrophosphate.

THIAMINASE

An enzyme found in raw fish that destroys thiamin.

THIOESTER BOND

An energy rich bond of the general formula: R-S-C-R-.

THIRST MECHANISM

Control mechanism in which cells of the anterior hypothalamus of the brain are stimulated and result in drinking behavior.

THREONINE
An essential four carbon amino acid having a hydroxyl group attached to carbon 3 (see amino acids, Table 5).

THRESHOLD DOSE
Dose required to have a measurable or expected effect.

THROMBOPLASTIN
A substance present in tissues, platelets, and leukocytes that in the presence of Ca^{++} brings about the conversion of prothrombin to thrombin and thence the formation of a clot.

THROMBOSIS
Obstruction of blood vessel by a blood clot.

THROMBUS
Blood clot that obstructs a blood vessel or cavity in the heart.

THYMIDINE PHOSPHATE (TMP, TDP, TTP)
A nucleotide consisting of thymine (a pyrimidine base) deoxyribose and 1, 2, or 3 phosphate groups.

THYMINE
A pyrimidine base in DNA.

TSH
Thyroid stimulating hormone. A hormone released by the pituitary which stimulates the thyroid gland to make and release thyroxine.

THYROCALCITONIN — CALCITONIN
A hormone that regulates blood calcium levels.

THYROGLOBULIN
Protein which carries the thyroxine in the blood.

THYROIDECTOMY
Removal of the thyroid gland.

THYROIDITIS
Inflammation of thyroid gland.

THYROTOXICOSIS
Hyperactive thyroid gland; excess levels of thyroid hormone also known as Graves Disease. Characterized by elevated oxygen consumption, elevated energy need, increased irritability and nervousness, bulging eyes, and weight loss.

THYROXINE
See T_4.

TOCOPHEROLS

A family of fat soluble compounds having Vitamin E activity.

TOLBUTAMIDE

A hypoglycemic oral agent; a derivative of sulfonylurea that works by stimulating insulin release by the β cells of the pancreas.

TONUS

Tonicity.

TOTAL IRON BINDING CAPACITY

The relative saturation of the iron binding protein, transferrin.

TOTAL LUNG CAPACITY

Total amount of gas that the lungs can hold.

TOTAL PARENTERAL NUTRITION (TPN)

See parenteral nutrition.

TOXEMIA OF PREGNANCY

See eclampsia, pre-eclampsia. Condition associated with pregnancy characterized by hypertension and inadequate renal function.

TOXIC REACTION

A food-intolerance reaction caused by toxic food components. Also known as food poisoning.

TOXICITY

The potential of a chemical to induce an adverse effect in a living organism. Each chemical, and thus also each food component, has its own specific toxicity. In general, information on the toxicity of food components is obtained from studies in experimental animals, *in vitro* studies, studies in volunteers, or epidemiological studies. The aims of these studies are to determine: (1) the type of adverse effect; (2) dose-effect relationships including the no-observed-adverse-effect level; and 3) the mechanism underlying the adverse effect.

TOXICITY OF NUTRIENTS.

Some nutrients (fat soluble Vitamins A and D, some minerals) if consumed in excess can elicit undesirable effects. These effects can be life threatening.

TOXINS

Chemicals which elicit symptoms of poisoning. Table 48 lists some of these.

TPN

Total parenteral nutrition. A method of providing all nutrient needs through a solution infused into a large blood vessel.

TABLE 48
Some Potentially Poisonous (Toxic) Agents

Aflatoxins (See Mycotoxins in this table).

Poison (Toxin)	Source	Symptoms and Signs	Distribution; Magnitude	Prevention; Treatment	Remarks
Aluminum (Al) (Also see Mineral(s).)	Food additives, mainly presented in such items as baking powder, pickles, and processed cheeses. Aluminum-containing antacids. Utensils.	Abnormally large intakes of aluminum irritate the digestive tract. Also, unusual conditions have sometimes resulted in the absorption of sufficient aluminum from antacids to cause brain damage. Aluminum may form nonabsorbable complexes with essential trace elements, thereby creating deficiencies of these elements.	Distribution — Aluminum is widely used throughout the world. Magnitude — The United States uses more aluminum than any other product except iron and steel. However, known cases of aluminum toxicity are rare.	Prevention — Based on the evidence presented herein, no preventative measures are recommended.	Aluminum toxicity has been reported in patients receiving renal dialysis.
Arsenic (As)	Consuming foods and beverages contaminated with excessive amounts of arsenic-containing sprays used as insecticides and weed killers. Arsenical insecticides used in vineyards exposing the workers (1) when spraying or (2) by inhaling contaminated dusts and plant debris. Arsenic in the air from three major sources — smelting of metals, burning of coal, and use of arsenical pesticides.	Burning pains in the throat or stomach, cardiac abnormalities, and the odor of garlic on the breath. Other symptoms may be diarrhea and extreme thirst along with a choking sensation. Small doses of arsenic taken into the body over a long period of time may produce hyperkeratosis (irregularities in pigmentation, especially on the trunk), arterial insufficiency, and cancer. There is strong evidence that inorganic arsenic is a skin and lung carcinogen in man.	Distribution — Arsenic is widely distributed, but the amount of the element consumed by man in food and water, or breathed, is very small and not harmful. Magnitude — Causes of arsenic toxicity in man are infrequent. Two note-worthy episodes occurred in Japan in 1955. One involved tainted powdered milk; the other contaminated soy sauce. The toxic milk caused 12,131 cases of infant poisoning, with 130 deaths. The soy sauce poisoned 220 people.	Treatment — Induce vomiting, followed by an antidote of egg whites in water or milk. Afterward, give strong coffee or tea, followed by Epsom salts in water or castor oil.	Arsenic is known to partially protect against selenium poisoning. The highest residues of arsenic are generally in the hair and nails. Arsenic in soils may sharply decrease crop growth and yields, but it is not a hazard to people or livestock that eat plants grown in these fields.

Chromium (Cr)	Food, water, and air contaminated by chromium compounds in industrialized areas.	Inorganic chromium salt reduces the absorption of zinc; hence, zinc deficiency symptoms may become evident in chronic chromium toxicity.	Distribution — Chromium toxicity is not common. Magnitude — Chromium toxicity is not very common.	Prevention — It is unlikely that people will get too much chromium because; (1) only minute amounts of the element are present in most foods, (2) the body utilizes chromium poorly, and (3) the toxic dose is about 10,000 times the lowest effective medical dose.	
Copper (Cu)	Diets with excess copper, but low in other minerals that counteract its effects. Acid foods or beverages (vinegar, carbonated beverages, or citrus juices) that have been in prolonged contact with copper metal may cause acute gastrointestinal disturbances.	Acute copper toxicity — Characterized by headache, dizziness, metallic taste, excessive salivation, nausea, vomiting, stomachache, diarrhea, and weakness. If the disease is allowed to get worse, there may also be racing of the heart, high blood pressure, jaundice, hemolytic anemia, dark-pigmented urine, kidney disorders, and even death. Chronic copper toxicity — May be contributory to iron-deficiency anemia, mental illness following childbirth (postpartum psychosis), certain types of schizophrenia, and perhaps heart attacks.	Distribution — Copper toxicity may occur wherever there is excess copper intake, especially when accompanied by low iron, molybdenum, sulfur, zinc, and vitamin C. Magnitude — The incidence of copper toxicity is extremely rare in man. Its occurrence in significant form is almost always limited to (1) suicide attempted by ingesting large quantities of copper salt or (2) a genetic defect in copper metabolism inherited as an autosomal recessive, known as Wilson's disease.	Prevention — Avoid foods and beverages that have been in prolonged contact with copper metal. Administration of copper chelating agents to remove excess copper.	Copper is essential to human life and health, but like all heavy metals, it is potentially toxic, also.

TABLE 48 (CONTINUED)
Some Potentially Poisonous (Toxic) Agents

Poison (Toxin)	Source	Symptoms and Signs	Distribution; Magnitude	Prevention; Treatment	Remarks
Ergot	Rye, wheat, barley, oats and triticale carry this mycotoxin. Ergot replaces the seed in the heads of cereal grains, in which it appears as a purplish-black, hard, banana-shaped, dense mass from 1/4 to 3/4 in. (6–9 mm) long.	When a large amount of ergot is consumed in a short period, convulsive ergotism is observed. The symptoms include itching, numbness, severe muscle cramps, sustained spasms and convulsions, and extreme pain. When smaller amounts of ergot are consumed over an extended period, ergotism characterized by gangrene of the finger-tips and toes, caused by blood vessel and muscle contraction stopping blood circulation in the extremities. These symptoms include cramps, swelling, inflammation, alternating burning and freezing sensations ("St. Anthony's fire"), and numbness; eventually the hands and feet may turn black, shrink, and fall off. Ergotism is a cumulative poison, depending on the amount of ergot eaten and the length of time over which it is eaten.	Distribution — Ergot is found throughout the world, wherever rye, wheat, barley, oats, or triticale are grown. Magnitude — There is considerable ergot, especially in rye. But, normally, screening grains before processing alleviates ergotism in people.	Prevention — Consists of an ergot-free diet. Ergot in food and feed grains may be removed by screening the grains before processing. In the United States, wheat and rye containing more than 0.3% ergot are classed as "ergoty." In Canada, government regulations prohibit more than 0.1% ergot in feeds. Treatment — An ergot-free diet; good nursing; treatment by a doctor.	Six different alkaloids are involved in ergot poisoning. Ergot is used to aid the uterus to contract after childbirth, to prevent loss of blood. Also, another ergot drug (ergotamine) is widely used in the treatment of migraine headaches.

| Fluorine (F) (fluorosis) | Ingesting excessive quantities of fluorine through either the food or water, or a combination of these. Except in certain industrial exposures, the intake of fluoride inhaled from the air is only a small fraction of the total fluoride intake in man. Pesticides containing fluorides, including those used to control insects, weeds, and rodents. Although water is the principal source of fluoride in an average human diet in the United States, fluoride is frequently contained in toothpaste, toothpowder, chewing gums, mouthwashes, vitamin supplements, and mineral supplements. | Acute fluoride poisoning — Abdominal pain, diarrhea, vomiting, excessive salivation, thirst, perspiration, and painful spasms of the limbs. Chronic fluoride poisoning — Abnormal teeth (especially mottled enamel) during the first 8 years of life and brittle bones. Other effects, predicted from animal studies, may include loss of body weight, and altered structure and function of the thyroid gland and kidneys. Water containing 3–10 ppm of fluoride may cause mottling of the teeth. An average daily intake of 20–80 mg of fluoride over a period of 10–20 years will result in crippling fluorosis. | Distribution — The water in parts of Arkansas, California, South Carolina, and Texas contains excess fluorine. Occasionally, throughout the United States, high-fluorine phosphates are used in mineral mixtures. Magnitude — Generally speaking, fluorosis is limited to high-fluorine areas. Only a few instances of health effects in man have been attributed to airborne fluoride, and they occurred in persons living in the vicinity of fluoride-emitting industries. | Prevention — Avoid the use of food and water containing excessive fluorine. Treatment — Any damage may be permanent, but people who have not developed severe symptoms may be helped to some extent if the source of excess fluorine is eliminated. Calcium and magnesium may reduce the absorption and utilization of fluoride. | Fluorine is a cumulative poison. The total fluoride in the human body averages 2.57 g. Susceptibility to fluoride toxicity is increased by deficiencies of calcium, Vitamin C, and protein. Virtually all foods contain trace amounts of fluoride. |

TABLE 48 (CONTINUED)
Some Potentially Poisonous (Toxic) Agents

Poison (Toxin)	Source	Symptoms and Signs	Distribution; Magnitude	Prevention; Treatment	Remarks
Lead (Pb)	Consuming food or medicinal products (including health food products) contaminated with lead. Inhaling the poison as a dust by workers in such industries as painting, lead mining, and refining. Inhaling airborne lead discharged into the air from auto exhaust fumes. Consuming food crops contaminated by lead being deposited on the leaves and other edible portions of the plant by direct fallout. Consuming food or water contaminated by contact with lead pipes or utensils. Old houses in which the interiors were painted with leaded paints prior to 1945, with the chipped wall paint eaten by children. Such miscellaneous sources as illicitly distilled whiskey, improperly lead-glazed earthenware, old battery casings used as fuel, and toys containing lead.	Symptoms develop rapidly in young children, but slowly in mature people. Symptoms of acute lead poisoning — Colic, cramps, diarrhea or constipation, leg cramps, and drowsiness. The most severe form of lead poisoning, encountered in infants and in heavy drinkers of illicitly distilled whiskey, is characterized by profound disturbances of the central nervous system, and permanent damage to the brain; damage to the kidneys; and shortened life span of the erthrocytes. Symptoms of chronic lead poisoning — Colic, constipation, lead palsy especially in the forearm and fingers, the symptoms of chronic nephritis, and sometimes mental depression, convulsions, and a blue line at the edge of the gums.	Distribution — Predominantly among children who may eat chips of lead-containing paints, peeled off form painted wood. Magnitude — The Center for Disease Control, Atlanta, Georgia, estimates that (1) lead poisoning claims the lives of 200 children each year, and (2) 400,000 to 600,000 children have elevated lead levels in the blood. Lead poisoning has been reduced significantly with the use of lead-free paint.	Prevention — Avoid inhaling or consuming lead. Treatment — Acute lead poisoning — An emetic (induce vomiting), followed by drinking plenty of milk and 1/2 oz (14 g) of Epsom salts in half a glass of water. Chronic lead poisoning — Remove the source of lead. Sometimes treated by administration of magnesium or lead sulphate solution as a laxative and antidote on the lead in the digestive system, followed by potassium iodide which cleanses the tracts. Currently, treatment of lead poisoning makes use of chemicals that bind the metal in the body and help in its removal.	Lead is a cumulative poison. When incorporated in the soil, nearly all the lead is converted into forms that are not available to plants. Any lead taken up by plant roots tends to stay in the roots, rather than move up to the top of the plant. Lead poisoning can be diagnosed positively by analyzing the blood tissue for lead content; clinical signs of lead poisoning usually are manifested at blood lead concentrations above 80 µg/100 g.

Mercury (Hg)	Mercury is discharged into air and water from industrial operations and is used in herbicide and fungicide treatments. Mercury poisoning has occurred where mercury from industrial plants has been discharged into water then accumulated as methylmercury in fish and shellfish. Accidental consumption of seed grains treated with fungicides that contain mercury, used for the control of fungus diseases of oats, wheat, barley, and flax.	The toxic effects of organic and inorganic compounds of mercury are dissimilar. The organic compounds of mercury, such as the various fungicides (1) affect the central nervous system and (2) are not corrosive. The inorganic compounds of mercury include mainly mercuric chloride, a disinfectant; mercurous chloride (calomel), a cathartic; and elemental mercury. Commonly the toxic symptoms are: corrosive gastrointestinal effects, such as vomiting, bloody diarrhea, and necrosis of the alimentary mucosa.	Distribution — Wherever mercury is produced in industrial operations or used in herbicide or fungicide treatments. Magnitude — Limited. But about 1200 cases of mercury poisoning identified in Japan in the 1950s were traced to the consumption of fish and shellfish from Japan's Minamata Bay contaminated with methyl-mercury. Some of the offspring of exposed mothers were born with birth defects, and many victims suffered central nervous system damage. Still another outbreak of mercury toxicity occurred in Iraq, where more than 6000 people were hospitalized after eating bread made from wheat that had been treated with methyl-mercury.	Control mercury pollution form industrial operations.	Mercury is a cumulative poison. Food and Drug Administration prohibits use of mercury-treated grain for food or feed. Grain crops produced form mercury-treated seed and crops produced on soils treated with mercury herbicides have not been found to contain harmful concentrations of this element.
Polybrominated biphenls (PBBs), a fire retardant which may cause cancer when taken into the food supply.	All of the 1973 Michigan toxicity problem was traced to livestock feed which became contaminated with PBB when the fire retardant was shipped by mistake to a feed manufacturer.	People exposed to PBB in Michigan reported suffering from neurological symptoms such as loss of memory, muscular weakness, coordination problems, headaches, painful swollen joints, acne, abdominal pain, and diarrhea.	In 1973, the accidental contamination of animal feeds exposed many people in Michigan to PBB in dairy products and other foods. The Michigan incident eventually led to the slaughter and burial of nearly 25,000 cattle, 3500 hogs, and 1.5 million chickens; and the disposal of about 5 million eggs and tons of milk, butter, cheese, and feed.	Treatment — Follow the prescribed treatment of a medical doctor.	PBBs are long-term, low-level contaminants, very stable and resistant to decay.

TABLE 48 (CONTINUED)
Some Potentially Poisonous (Toxic) Agents

Poison (Toxin)	Source	Symptoms and Signs	Distribution; Magnitude	Prevention; Treatment	Remarks
Polychlorinated biphenyls (PCBs), industrial chemicals; chlorinated hydrocarbons which may cause cancer when taken into the food supply.	Sources of contamination to man include: 1. Contaminated foods. 2. Mammals or birds that have fed on contaminated foods of fish. 3. Residues on foods that have been wrapped in papers and plastics containing PCBs. 4. Milk from cows that have been fed silage from silos coated with PCB-containing paint; and eggs from layers fed feeds contaminated with PCBs. 5. Absorption by human beings of PCBs through the lungs, the gastrointestinal tract, and the skin.	The clinical effects of people are: an eruption of the skin resembling acne, visual disturbances, jaundice, numbness, and spasms. Newborn infants from mothers who have been poisoned show discoloration of the skin which regresses after 2–5 months.	Distribution — PCBs are widespread packaging materials.	Prevention — Avoid harmfully contaminated food. Treatment — People afflicted with PCB should follow the prescribed treatment of their doctor.	Although the production of PCBs was halted in 1977 and the importing of PCBs was banned January 1, 1979, the chemicals had been widely used for 40 years, and they are exceptionally long-lived. PCBs have been widely used in dielectric fluids in capacitors and transformers, hydraulic fluids, and heat transfer fluids. Also, they have more than 50 minor uses, including plasticizers and solvents in adhesives, printing ink, sealants, moisture retardants, paints, and pesticide carriers. PCB will cause cancer in laboratory animals (rats, mice, and rhesus monkeys). It is not know if it will cause cancer in humans. More study is needed to gauge its effects on the ecological food chain and on human health. When fed coho salmon from Lake Michigan with 10–15 ppm PCB, mink in Wisconsin stopped reproducing or their kits died. In 1977, polar bears at the very top of the Arctic food chain showed PCB levels of up to 8 ppm in their fatty tissue. This indicates that PCBs are spread throughout the atmosphere.

Salt (NaCl — sodium chloride) poisoning	Consumption of high levels of the salt in food or drinking water.	Salt may be toxic (1) when it is fed to infants or others whose kidneys cannot excrete the excess in the urine, or (2) when the body is adapted to a chronic low-salt diet.	Distribution — Salt is used all over the world. Hence, the potential for salt poisoning exists everywhere. Magnitude — Salt poisoning is relatively rare.	Treatment — Drink large quantities of fresh water.	Even normal salt concentration may be toxic if water intake is low.
Selenium	Consumption of high levels of the element in food or drinking water. Presence of malnutrition, parasitic infestation, or other factors which make people highly susceptible to selenium toxicity.	Abnormalities in the hair, nails, and skin. Children in a high-selenium area of Venezuela showed loss of hair, discolored skin, and chronic digestive disturbances. Normally, people who have consumed large excesses of selenium excrete it as trimethyl selenide in the urine and/or as dimethyl selenide on the breath. The latter substance has an odor resembling garlic.	Distribution — In certain regions of western United States, especially in South Dakota, Montana, Wyoming, Nebraska, Kansas, and perhaps areas in other states in the Great Plains and Rocky Mountains. Also, in Canada. Magnitude — Selenium toxicity in people is relatively rate.	Treatment — Selenium toxicity may be counteracted by arsenic or copper, but such treatment should be carefully monitored.	Confirmed cases of selenium poisoning in people are rare because (1) only traces are present in most foods, (2) foods generally come from a wide area, and (3) the metabolic processes normally convert excess selenium into harmless substances which are excreted in the urine or breath.
Tin (Sn)	From acid fruits and vegetables canned in tin cans. The acids in such foods as citrus fruits and tomato products can leach tin from the inside of the can. Then the tin is ingested with the canned food. In the digestive tract tin goes through a methylation process in which nontoxic tin is converted to methylated tin, which is toxic.	Methylated tin is a neurotoxin — a toxin that attacks the central nervous system, the symptoms of which are numbness of the fingers and lips followed by a loss of speech and hearing. Eventually, the afflicted person becomes spastic, then coma and death follow.	Distribution — Tin cans are widely used throughout the world. Magnitude — The use of tin in advanced industrial societies has increased 14-fold over the last 10 years.	Prevention — Many tin cans are coated on the inside with enamel or other materials.	Currently, not much is known about the amount of tin in the human diet.

Adapted from Ensminger et al., *Foods and Nutrition Encyclopedia*, 2nd ed., CRC Press, Boca Raton, FL, 1994, pp. 1790–1803.

tRNA

Transfer ribonucleic acid. Form of nucleic acid responsible for transferring specific amino acids to specific sites on the mRNA in the process of protein synthesis.

TRACE ELEMENTS

Minerals needed in trace amounts (see minerals, Table 29).

TRANS FATTY ACIDS

Fatty acids that assume the chain form rather than the boat form around a double bond.

TRANSAMINATION

Process or reaction where the amino group ($-NH_3$) is transferred from one compound to another.

TRANSCRIPTION

The synthesis of messenger RNA using the DNA as a template. The process is catalyzed by RNA polymerase II and is illustrated in Figure 48.

TRANSFER RNA (tRNA)

Small stable RNA molecules that dock onto the messenger RNA and ribosomes and which carry amino acids. Each amino acid has its own specific tRNA.

TRANSFERRIN

Iron carrying protein in blood.

TRANSKETOLASE

Enzyme that catalyzes the transfer of a two carbon keto group from a keto sugar to an aldehyde sugar.

TRANSLATION

The synthesis of protein using the message for amino acid sequence carried by messenger RNA. Occurs on the ribosomes.

TRANSLOCASES

Proteins that move smaller molecules through a membrane.

TRAUMA

Injury.

TREE NUT ALLERGY

In several studies, a cross-reactivity has been reported between birch pollen and nuts. This cross-reactivity shows itself in a syndrome that is known as the para-birch-syndrome. The complaints of people suffering from this syndrome result from a birch pollen allergy (sneezing, nasal obstruction and conjunctivitis during the birch pollen season) and also from an allergy to nuts and/or certain fruits. The allergic reactions to these foods mainly cause symptoms such as itching in and around the mouth and pharynx and swelling of the lips. In some cases, however, more severe reactions occur. Related fruits in this context are apple, peach, plum, cherry, and orange. Also, some vegetables such as celery and carrot have been shown to be cross-reactive with the birch allergen. Other known cross-reactivity combinations are grass pollen with carrot, potato, wheat, and celery. A grass pollen-allergic person may become allergic to wheat as well. The exact mechanisms underlying these phenomena are not known.

TRIACYLGLYCEROL (TRIGLYCERIDES)

Lipid consisting of three fatty acids esterified to a glycerol backbone.

TRICHINOSIS

Disease caused by a parasite found in pork.

TRICHOTHECENES

The most important mycotoxins produced by the mold Fusarium. They can be classified as 12,13-epoxytrichothecenes and macrocyclic resorcyclates (naturally occurring derivatives of β-resorcyclic acid). The production of trichothecenes is shared by the species of Trichothecium, Myrothecium, Trichoderma, and Cephalosporium. There are three types of trichothecenes: (1) monoepoxytrichothecenes (8-deoxymonoepoxytrichothecenes (structure I), including diacetoxyscirpenol and T-2 toxin; 8-ketomonoepoxytrichothecenes (structure II), including trichothecin and fusarenone; (2) diepoxytrichothecenes (structure III), including crotocin and crotocol; (3) macrocyclic trichothecenes (macrocyclic diesters [structure IV], including the roroidins; and (4) macrocyclic triesters (structure V), including the verrucarins). Most trichothecenes are phytotoxic and zootoxic. The *in vitro* toxic effects of the trichothecenes include skin necrosis, inflammatory effects, massive hemorrhages, and effects on heart and respiration rates. Furthermore, many of the trichothecenes have been shown to be inhibitors of protein synthesis; the most toxic types inhibiting at the initiation step (e.g., T-2 toxin, diacetoxyscirpenol, many of the verrucarins), the least toxic types at the elongation-termination process (e.g., crotocin, trichothecin, trichodermin). The actual toxicities of some of the trichothecenes were probably demonstrated in the field by both animal and human mycotoxicoses. An example of the latter is Alimentary Toxic Aleukia, a toxic syndrome caused by *Fusarium* spp. This disease was traced to the consumption of grain that was allowed to overwinter in the fields. The grains became invaded by cryophilic molds from which several fungal genera and species were identified. In order to produce toxins, the most important requirement of these molds appeared to be the presence of alternate freezing and thawing cycles. The clinical course of Alimentary Toxic Aleukia occurs in four stages — 1st stage (3–9 days): burning sensation in the mouth and tongue and in the gastrointestinal tract, headache, dizziness, weakness, fatigue; latent 2nd stage (2–8 weeks): progressive leukopenia, granulopenia, lymphocytosis, anemia, bacterial infections, disturbances in the central and autonomic nervous system, such as weakness, headache, palpitation, asthmatic attacks, icterus, hypotension, dilation of the pupils, soft and labile pulse, diarrhea, or constipation; 3rd stage: petechial hemorrhages in the skin, mucous membranes in the mouth, tongue, gastrointestinal tract and nasal area, necrosis in parts of the buccal cavity, enlargement and edema of the cervical lymph nodes, lesions in the esophagus and epiglottis, and edema in the larynx; 4th stage (≥2 months): if death does not intervene, the patient may recover.

TRIIODOTHYRONINE

T$_3$. The active thyroid hormone.

TRIMESTER
Three months.

TRIPEPTIDES
Three amino acids joined together via the peptide bond.

TRISTEARIN
Triacylglyceride having three stearic acids esterified to the glycerol backbone.

TRITIUM
Radioactive hydrogen.

TRYPSIN
A proteolytic enzyme that attacks peptide bonds adjacent to arginine or lysine.

TRYPSINOGEN
Precursor of trypsin; trypsin is available after trypsinogen is acted on by enterokinase.

TRYPTOPHAN
An essential amino acid. See Table 5.

TSH
Thyroid stimulating hormone. A pituitary hormone which stimulates the thyroid gland to produce thyroid hormone.

TUBE FEEDING
See Enteral nutrition.

TULAREMIA
See rabbit fever.

2,3,7,8-TETRACHLORODIBENZO-P-DIOXIN (TCDD)
A well-known environmental pollutant, formed at high temperatures (as in incinerators) from chlorinated hydrocarbons. It is also a contaminant of the herbicide 2,4,5-trichlorophenoxy-acetic acid (2,4,5-T). On acute exposure it is highly toxic. In experimental animals, it has been shown to induce liver damage, teratogenic effects, immune suppression, enzyme induction, and increased tumor incidence. In man, occupational exposures and industrial accidents involving TCDD have been associated with chloracne, liver damage, and polyneuropathy. The principal source of TCDD exposure is food: 1) via spraying of crops with 2,4,5-T, (2) via ingestion of contaminated feed by livestock, (3) via magnification through food chains, and (4) via contamination of fruits and vegetables in the proximity of incinerators. The average daily intake of TCDD is set at 10 pg/kg/day.

TXA2
Thromboxane A2. An eicosanoid involved in stimulating platelet aggregation.

TYPE A ANTINUTRITIVES

Substances primarily interfering with the digestion of proteins or the absorption and utilization of amino acids. Also known as antiproteins. People depending on vegetables for their protein supply, as in less developed countries, are in danger of impairment by this type of antinutritives. The most important type A antinutritives are protease inhibitors and lectins.

Protease inhibitors, occurring in many plant and animal tissues, are proteins which inhibit proteolytic enzymes by binding to the active sites of the enzymes. Proteolytic enzyme inhibitors were first found in avian eggs around the turn of the century. They were later identified as ovomucoid and ovoinhibitor, both of which inactivate trypsin. Chymotrypsin inhibitors also are found in avian egg whites. Other sources of trypsin and/or chymotrypsin inhibitors are: soybeans and other legumes and pulses; vegetables; milk and colostrum; wheat and other cereal grains; guar gum; and white and sweet potatoes. The protease inhibitors of kidney beans, soybeans, and potatoes can additionally inhibit elastase, a pancreatic enzyme acting on elastin, an insoluble protein in meat. Animals given food containing active inhibitors show growth depression. This appears to be due to interference in trypsin and chymotrypsin activities and to excessive stimulation of the secretory exocrine pancreatic cells, which become hypertrophic. Valuable proteins may be lost to the feces in this case. *In vitro* experiments with human proteolytic enzymes have been shown that trypsin inhibitors from bovine colostrum, lima beans, soybeans, kidney beans, and quail ovomucoid were active against human trypsin, whereas trypsin inhibitors originating from bovine and porcine pancrease, potatoes, chicken ovomucoid, and chicken ovoinhibitor were not. The soybean and lima bean trypsin inhibitors are also active against human chymotrypsin. Many protease inhibitors are heat labile, especially with moist heat. Relatively heat resistant protease inhibitors include the antitryptic factor in milk, the alcohol-precipitable and nondialyzable trypsin inhibitor in alfalfa, the chymotrypsin inhibitor in potato, the kidney bean inhibitor, and the trypsin inhibitor in lima beans.

Lectin is the general term for plant proteins that have highly specific binding sites for carbohydrates. They are widely distributed among various sources such as soybeans, peanuts, jack beans, mung beans, lima beans, kidney beans, fava beans, vetch, yellow wax beans, hyacinth beans, lentils, peas, potatoes, bananas, mangoes and wheat germ. Most plant lectins are glycoproteins, except concanavalin A from jack beans, which is carbohydrate-free. The most toxic lectins include ricin in castor bean (oral toxic dose in man: 150–200 mg; intravenous toxic dose: 20 mg) and the lectins of kidney bean and hyacinth bean. The mode of action of lectins may be related to their ability to bind to specific cell receptors in a way comparable to that of antibodies. Because they are able to agglutinate red blood cells, they are also known as hemagglutinins. The binding of bean lectin on rat intestinal mucosal cells has been demonstrated *in vitro*, and it has been suggested that this action is responsible for the oral toxicity of the lectins. Such bindings may disturb the intestines' absorptive capacity for nutrients and other essential compounds. The lectins, being proteins, can easily be inactivated by moist heat. Germination decreases the hemagglutinating activity in varieties of peas and species of beans.

TYPE B ANTINUTRITIVES

Substances interfering with the absorption or metabolic utilization of minerals. Also known as antiminerals. Although they are toxic per se, the amounts present in foods seldom cause acute intoxication under normal food consumption. However, they may harm the organism under suboptimum nutriture. The most important type B antinutritives are phytic acid, oxalates, and glucosinolates.

Phytic acid, or myo-inositol hexaphosphate, is a naturally occurring strong acid which binds to many types of bivalent and trivalent heavy metal ions, forming insoluble salts.

Consequently, phytic acid reduces the availability of many minerals and essential trace elements. The degree of insolubility of these salts appear to depend on the nature of the metal, the pH of the solution, and for certain metals, on the presence of another metal. Synergism between two metallic ions in the formation of phytate complexes has also been observed. For instance, zinc-calcium phytate precipitates maximally at pH 6, which is also the pH of the duodenum, where mainly calcium and trace metals are absorbed. Phytates are occurring in a wide variety of foods, such as cereals (e.g., wheat, rye, maize, rice, and barley); legumes and vegetables (e.g., bean, soybean, lentil, pea, and vetch); nuts and seeds (e.g., walnut, hazelnut, almond, peanut, and cocoa bean); and spices and flavoring agents (e.g., caraway, coriander, cumin, mustard, and nutmeg). From several experiments in animals and man it has been observed that phytates exert negative effects on the availability of calcium, iron, magnesium, zinc, and other trace essential elements. These effects may be minimized considerably, if not eliminated, by increased intake of essential minerals. In the case of calcium, intake of cholecalciferol must also be adequate, since the activity of phytates on calcium absorption is enhanced when this vitamin is inadequate or limiting. In many food-stuffs the phytic acid level can be reduced by phytase, an enzyme occurring in plants, that catalyzes the dephosphorylation of phytic acid.

Oxalic acid is a strong acid which forms water soluble Na^+ and K^+ salts but less soluble salts with alkaline earth and other bivalent metals. Calcium oxalate is particularly insoluble at neutral or alkaline pH, whereas it readily dissolves in acid medium. Oxalates mainly exert effects on the absorption of calcium. These effects must be considered in terms of the oxalate/calcium ratio (in milliequivalent/milliequivalent): foods having a ratio greater than 1 may have negative effects on calcium availability, whereas foods with a ratio of 1 or below do not. Examples of foodstuffs having a ratio greater than 1 are: rhubarb (8.5), spinach (4.3), beet (2.5–5.1), cocoa (2.6), coffee (3.9), tea (1.1), and potato (1.6). Harmful oxalates in food may be removed by soaking in water. Consumption of calcium-rich foods (e.g., dairy products and seafood), as well as augmented cholecalciferol intake, are recommended when large amounts of high oxalate food are consumed.

A variety of plants contain a third group of type B antinutritives, the glucosinolates, also known as thioglucosides. Many glucosinolates are goitrogenic. They have a general structure and yield on hydrolysis the active or actual goitrogens, such as thiocyanates, isothiocyanates, cyclic sulfur compounds, and nitriles. Three types of goiter can be identified: (1) cabbage goiter; (2) brassica seed goiter; and (3) legume goiter. Cabbage goiter, also known as struma, is induced by excessive consumption of cabbage. It seems that cabbage goitrogens inhibit iodine uptake by directly affecting the thyroid gland. Cabbage goiter can be treated by iodine supplementation. Brassica seed goiter can result from the consumption of the seeds of Brassica plants (e.g., rutabaga, turnip, cabbage, and rape) which contain goitrogens that prevent thyroxine synthesis. This type of goiter can only be treated by administration of the thyroid hormone. Legume goiter is induced by goitrogens in legumes like soybeans and peanuts. It differs from cabbage goiter in that the thyroid gland does not lose its activity for iodine. Inhibition of the intestinal absorption of iodine or the reabsorption of thyroxine has been shown in this case. Legume goiter can be treated by iodine therapy. Glucosinolates which have been shown to induce goiter, at least in experimental animals, are found in several foods and feedstuffs: broccoli (buds), brussels sprouts (head), cabbage (head), cauliflower (buds), garden cress (leaves), horseradish (roots), kale (leaves), kohlrabi (head), black and white mustard (seed), radish (root), rape (seed), rutabaga (root), and turnips (root and seed). One of the most potent glucosinolates is progoitrin from the seeds of Brassica plants and the roots of rutabaga. Hydrolysis of this compound yields 1-cyano-2-hydroxy-3-butene, 1-cyano-2-hydroxy-3,4-butylepisulfide, 2-hydroxy-3,4-butenylisothiocyanate, and (S)-5-vinyl-oxazoli-done-2-thione, also known as goitrin. The latter product interferes, together with its

R-enantiomer, in the iodination of thyroxine precursors, so that the resulting goiter cannot be treated by iodine therapy.

TYPE C ANTINUTRITIVES

Naturally occurring substances which can decompose vitamins, form unabsorbable complexes with them, or interfere with their digestive or metabolic utilization. Also known as antivitamins. The most important type C antinutritives are ascorbic acid oxidase, antithiamine factors, and antipyridoxine factors.

Ascorbic acid oxidase is a copper-containing enzyme that catalyzes the oxidation of free ascorbic acid to diketogluconic acid, oxalic acid, and other oxidation products. It has been reported to occur in many fruits (e.g., peaches and bananas) and vegetables (e.g., cucumbers, pumpkins, lettuce, cress, cauliflowers, spinach, green beans, green peas, carrots, potatoes, tomatoes, beets, and kohlrabi). The enzyme is active between pH 4 and 7 (optimum pH 5.6–6.0); its optimum temperature is 38°C. The enzyme is released when plant cells are broken. Therefore, if fruits and vegetables are cut, the Vitamin C content decreases gradually. Ascorbic acid oxidase can be inhibited effectively at pH 2 or by blanching at around 100°C. Ascorbic acid can also be protected against ascorbic acid oxidase by substances of plant origin. Flavonoids, such as the flavonoles quercetin and kempferol, present in fruits and vegetables, strongly inhibit the enzyme.

A second group of type C antinutritives are the antithiamine factors, which interact with thiamine, also known as Vitamin B_1. Antithiamine factors can be grouped as thiaminases, catechols, and tannins. Thiaminases, which are enzymes that split thiamine at the methylene linkage, are found in many freshwater and saltwater fish species and in certain species of crab and clam. They contain a nonprotein coenzyme, structurally related to hemin. This enzyme is the actual antithiamine factor. Thiaminases in fish and other sources can be destroyed by cooking. Antithiamine factors of plant origin include catechols and tannins. The most well-known ortho-catechol is found in bracken fern. In fact, there are two types of heat-stable antithiamine factors in this fern, one of which has been identified as caffeic acid, which can also by hydrolyzed from chlorogenic acid (found in green coffee beans) by intestinal bacteria. Other ortho-catechols, such as methylsinapate occurring in mustard seed and rapeseed, also have antithiamine activity. The mechanism of thiamine inactivation by these compounds requires oxygen and is dependent on temperature and pH. The reaction appears to proceed in two phases: a rapid initial phase, which is reversible by addition of reducing agents (e.g., ascorbic acid), and a slower subsequent phase, which is irreversible. Tannins, occurring in a variety of plants, including tea, similarly possess antithiamine activity. Thiamine is one of the vitamins that are likely to be deficient in the diet. Thus, persistent consumption of antithiamine factors and the possible presence of thiaminase-producing bacteria in the gastrointestinal tract may compromise the already marginal thiamine intake.

A variety of plants and mushrooms contain pyridoxine (a form of Vitamin B_6) antagonists. These antipyridoxine factors have been identified as hydrazine derivatives. Linseed contains the water-soluble and heat-labile antipyridoxine factor linatine (γ-glutamyl-1-amino-D-proline). Hydrolysis of linatine yields the actual antipyridoxine factor 1-amino-proline. Antipyridoxine factors have also been found in wild mushrooms, the common commercial edible mushroom, and the Japanese mushroom shiitake. Commercial and shiitake mushrooms contain agaritine. Hydrolysis of agaritine by γ-glutamyl transferase, which is endogenous to the mushroom, yields the active agent 4-hydroxymethylphenylhydrazine. Disruption of the cells of the mushroom can accelerate hydrolysis; careful handling of the mushrooms and immediate blanching after cleaning and cutting can prevent hydrolysis. The mechanism underlying the antipyridoxine activity is believed to be condensation of the hydrazines with the carbonyl compounds pyridoxal and pyridoxal phosphate (the active form of the vitamin), resulting in the formation of inactive hydrazones.

TYRAMINE

The amine of tyrosine; an amine with vasoactive effects similar to epinephrine. A vasoactive amine, which is found in french cheese, cheddar, yeast, chianti, and canned fish. It can also be produced by microorganisms in the gut. Symptoms like migraine and urticaria can occur in sensitive persons.

TYROSINASE

A copper-containing enzyme which catalyes the conversion of tyrosine to melanin.

TYROSINE

An amino acid that results from the hydroxylation of phenylalanine. See Table 5.

TYROSINOSIS

A genetic disorder due to a lack of parahydroxyphenylpyruvic acid oxidase which catalyzes the conversion of tyrosine to homogentisic acid. Characterized by elevated blood and urine levels of tyrosine, liver damage, mental retardation, and rickets.

UBIQUINONE

Coenzyme Q, an electron carrier that is part of the respiratory chain in the mitochondria.

UDP, UTP

Uridine di- or triphosphate. A high energy compound essential to glycogen synthesis.

ULCERATIVE COLITIS

A type of inflammatory bowel disease that primarily affects the rectum and colon.

ULTRA TRACE ELEMENTS

Minerals required in extremely small amounts.

UMBILICAL CORD

Connection between the developing fetus and the placenta.

UMP

Uridine monophosphate.

URACIL

Pyrimidine base used in DNA.

UREA

Waste product of amino acid degradation.

UREA CYCLE

A cyclic series of reactions shown in Figure 49 that converts carbamyl phosphate to urea.

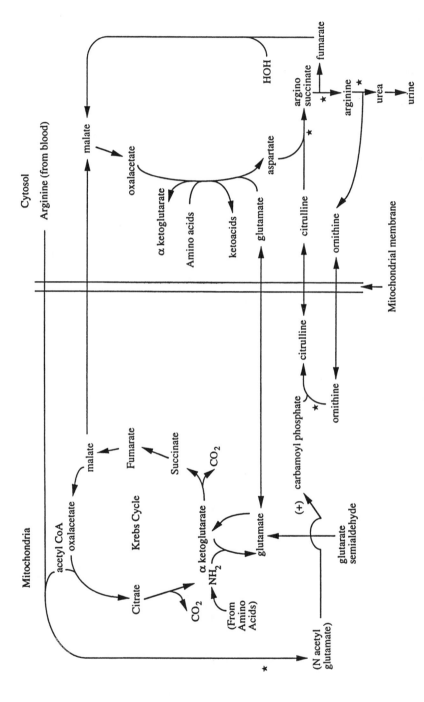

FIGURE 49 The urea cycle. Locations of mutations in the urea cycle enzymes are indicated with a ★. Persons with these mutations have very short lives with evidence of mental retardation, seizures, coma, and early death due to the toxic effects of amomnia accumulation.

UREMIA

Blood urea levels above 25 mg/dl. Retention of nitrogenous substances in the blood.

URIC ACID

Crystalline acid, excreted in urine, from purine metabolism.

URIDINE

Uracil with a ribose group attached.

URIDINE MONOPHOSPHATE

Uridine with a single phosphate group attached.

UROLITHIASIS

Urinary tract stone or calculi.

URTICARIA

A vascular reaction of the skin characterized by severe itching and rash.

UTERUS

Womb. Vessel which houses the embryo and developing fetus.

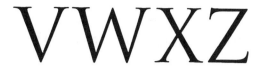

VALIDITY (OF A MEASUREMENT)

The concordance between the value of a measurement and the true value. A high reproducibility is a prerequisite for validity but does not automatically imply validity. With regard to the validity of the results of epidemiological studies a distinction is made between internal and external validity.

VALINE

An essential amino acid. See Table 5.

VASOACTIVE COMPOUNDS

Compounds that elicit either vasoconstriction or vasodilation.

VASOCONSTRICTION

Constriction of the vascular tree with the result of an increase in blood pressure.

VASODILATION

Relaxation of the vascular tree with the result of a fall in blood pressure.

VASOPRESSIN

Antidiuretic hormone (ADH) released by the pituitary. Functions to stimulate water reabsorption by the kidney.

VEAL

Meat from an immature bovine.

VEGAN

An individual who subsists on a meat-milk-egg-cheese-fish-free diet.

VEGETABLE ALLERGY

This kind of allergy may be provoked by beans (soy), peas, and peanuts. Especially, peanut allergy is well-known. Extensive reactions include urticaria, angioedema, nausea, vomiting, rhinitis, and dyspnea. Anaphylactic shock is not uncommon. The peanut allergen is very stable; it is resistant to all kinds of processing. In peanut butter and peanut flour (which is added to quite a few food products), the peanut allergen is still detectable, whereas it is not or seldom present in peanut oil. Similarly, the soy allergen is rarely found in soy oil. Allergy to a particular legume does not invariably imply allergic sensitivity to all members of the legume family.

VERY LOW CALORIE DIET

Diet containing <1000 calories per day.

VILLI

Finger-like projections from the small intestinal wall that function in the absorption of nurients.

VIP

Vasoactive peptide. A neuropeptide originating in the neurons of the gastrointestinal system.

VIRAL HEPATITIS

Inflammation of the liver caused by a viral infection. Five types of viral hepatitis (hepatitis A, B, C, D, and E) have been identified by their unique method of transmission, onset, and laboratory findings.

VISCERAL PROTEIN

Body protein in components other than muscle tissue such as internal organs and blood.

VITAL CAPACITY

Maximal amount of gas that can be exhaled after a maximal inspiration.

VITAMINS

A group of small organic compounds that cannot be synthesized in the body and therefore must be consumed as part of the diet. Table 49 summarizes our knowledge about these compounds.

VLDL

Very low density lipoprotein. A lipid-protein complex involved in the transport of lipids from the liver and gut to storage sites.

VOLATILE FATTY ACIDS

Short chain (carbons less than 8) fatty acids which volitilize at room temperature.

VON GIERKE'S DISEASE

Genetic disorder characterized by excess glycogen stores in liver and muscles; due to a mutation in the gene for the enzyme glucose-6-phosphatase.

WATER BALANCE

The water intake is equal to the water loss.

WATER INTOXICATION

Excess water intake.

WATER MISCIBLE

Substance or liquid that mixes freely with water.

WATER OF METABOLISM

See metabolic water.

WERNICKE-KORSAKOFF SYNDROME

Condition resulting from severe deficiency of thiamin marked by loss of memory and personality changes.

TABLE 49
Vitamins

Functions	Deficiency and Toxicity Symptoms	Sources	Comments
Fat-Soluble Vitamins			
Vitamin A Helps maintain normal vision in dim light — prevents night blindness and xerophthamia. Essential for body growth. Necessary for normal bone growth and normal tooth development. Is an essential component of nuclear transcription factors and, as such, has an important role in cell replication gene expression and embryogenesis.	Deficiency symptoms — Night blindness (nyctalopia), xerosis, and xerophthalmia. Stunted bone growth, abnormal bone shape, and paralysis. Unsound teeth, characterized by abnormal enamel, pits, and decay. Rough, dry, scaly skin — a condition known as follicular hyperkeratosis (it looks like "gooseflesh"); increased sinus, sore throat, and abscesses in ears, mouth, or salivary glands; increased diarrhea and kidney and bladder stones. Reproductive disorders, including poor conception, abnormal embryonic growth, placental injury, and death of the fetus. Toxicity — Toxicity of Vitamin A is characterized by loss of appetite. headache, blurred vision, excessive irritability, loss of hair, dryness and flaking of skin (with itching), swelling over the long bones, drowsiness, diarrhea, nausea, and enlargement of the liver and spleen.	Liver, carrots, dark-green leafy vegetables. Yellow vegetables — pumpkins, sweet potatoes, squash (winter). Yellow fruits — apricots, peaches. Some seafoods (crab, halibut, oysters, salmon, swordfish), milk and milk products, eggs. Supplemental sources — Synthetic Vitamin A, cod and other fish liver oils.	The forms of Vitamin A are: alcohol (retinol), ester (retinyl palmitate), aldehyde (retinal or retinene), and acid (retinoic acid.) Retinol, retinyl palmitate, and retinal are readily converted from one form to other forms. Retinoic acid fulfills some of the functions of Vitamin A, but it does not function in the visual cycle. β carotene found in vegetables serves as a Vitamin A precursor.

TABLE 49 (CONTINUED)
Vitamins

	Functions	Deficiency and Toxicity Symptoms	Sources	Comments
Vitamin D	Increases calcium absorption from the small intestine. Promotes growth and mineralization of bones. Promotes sound teeth. Increases absorption of phosphorus through the intestinal wall, and increases resorption of phosphates from the kidney tubules. Maintains normal level of citrate in the blood. Protects against the loss of amino acids through the kidneys.	Deficiency symptoms — Rickets in infants and children, characterized by enlarged joints, bowed legs, knocked knees, outward projection of the sternum (pigeon breast), a row of beadlike projections on each side of the chest at the juncture of the rib bones and joining (costal) cartilage (called rachitic rosary), bulging forehead, pot belly, and delayed eruption of temporary teeth and unsound permanent teeth. Osteomalacia in adults, in which the bones soften, become distorted, and fracture easily. Tetany, characterized by muscle twitching, convulsions, and low serum calcium. Toxicity — Excessive Vitamin D may cause hypercalcemia (increased intestinal absorption, leading to elevated blood calcium levels), characterized by loss of appetite, excessive thirst, nausea, vomiting, irritability, weakness, constipation alternating with bouts of diarrhea, retarded growth in infants and children, and weight loss in adults.	D-fortified foods — Milk (400 IU/qt) and infant formulas. Other foods to which Vitamin D is often added include: breakfast and infant cereals, breads, margarines, milk flavorings, fruit and chocolate beverages, and cocoa. Supplemental sources — Fish liver oils (from cod, halibut, or swordfish); irradiated ergosterol or 7-dehydro-cholesterol such as viosterol. Exposure to sunlight or sunlamp — Converts the Vitamin D precursor to active Vitamin D.	Vitamin D includes both D_2 (ergocalciferol, calciferol, or viosterol) and D_3 (cholecalciferol). Vitamin D is unique among vitamins because it can be formed in the body and in certain foods by exposure to ultraviolet rays, and the active compound of Vitamin D (1, 25-$(OH)_2$-D_3) functions as a hormone.
Vitamin E (Tocopherols)	As an antioxidant which protects body cells from free radicals formed from the unsaturated fatty acids. Maintains the integrity of red blood cells by its action as a suppressor of free radicals. As an agent essential to cellular respiration, primarily in heart and skeletal muscle tissues.	Deficiency symptoms — Newborn infants (especially the premature). Anemia caused by shortened life span of red blood cells, edema, skin lesions, and blood abnormalities. Patients unable to absorb fat have low blood and tissue tocopherol levels, decreased red blood cell life span, and increased urinary excretion of creatine. Toxicity — Vitamin E is relatively nontoxic. Some persons consuming daily doses of more than 300 IU of Vitamin E have complained of nausea and intestinal distress. Excess intake of Vitamin E appears to be excreted in the feces.	Vegetable oils (except coconut oil), alfalfa seeds, margarine, nuts (almonds, Brazil nuts, filberts, peanuts, pecans), sunflower seed kernels. Good sources — Asparagus, avocados, beef and organ meats, blackberries, butter, eggs, green leafy vegetables, oatmeal, potato chips, rye, seafoods (lobster, salmon, shrimp, tuna), tomatoes. Supplemental sources — Synthetic di-alpha-tocopherol acetate, wheat germ, and intestinal tocopherol acetate, wheat germ, wheat germ oil.	There are 8 tocopherols and tocotrienols, of which α-tocopherol has the greatest Vitamin E activity.

Vitamin K

Vitamin K is essential for the synthesis in the liver of four bloodclotting proteins:
1. Factor II, prothrombin
2. Factor VII, proconvertin
3. Factor IX, Christmas factor
4. Factor X, Stuart-Power.

Its action is on the post-translational carboxylation of glutamic acid residues.

Deficiency symptoms — 1. Delayed blood clotting, 2. Hemorrhagic disease of newborn.
Vitamin K deficiency symptoms are likely in:
1. Newborn infants.
2. Infants born to mothers receiving anticoagulants.
3. Obstructive jaundice (lack of bile).
4. Fat absorption defects (celiac disease, sprue).
5. Anticoagulant therapy or toxicity.

Toxicity — The natural forms of Vitamin K_1 and K_2 have not produced toxicity even when given in large amounts. However, synthetic menadione and its various derivatives have produced toxic symptoms in rats and jaundice in human infants when given in amounts of more than 5 mg daily.

Vitamin K is fairly widely distributed in foods and is available synthetically.

Two forms: K_1 (phylloquinone, or phytylmenaquinone), and K_2 (meanquinones), multiprenyl-menaquinones.
Vitamin K is synthesized by bacteria in the intestinal tracts of human beings and other species.
There are several synthetic compounds, the best known of which is menadione, formerly known as K_3.

Water-Soluble Vitamins

Biotin

Biotin functions as a coenzyme mainly in decarboxylation-carboxylation and in deamination reactions.

Deficiency symptoms — The deficiency symptoms in man include a dry scaly dermatitis, loss of appetite, nausea, vomiting, muscle pains, glossitis (inflammation of the tongue), pallor of skin, mental depression, a decrease in hemoglobin and red blood cells, a high cholesterol level, and a low excretion of biotin; all of which respond to biotin administration.
Toxicity — There are no known toxic effects.

Rich sources — Cheese (processed), kidney, liver, soybean flour.
Good sources — Cauliflower, chocolate, eggs, mushrooms, nuts, peanut butter, sardine and salmon, wheat bran.
Supplemental sources — Synthetic biotin, yeast (brewer's torula), alfalfa leaf meal (dehydrated).
Considerable biotin is synthesized by the microorganisms in the intestinal tract.

Avidin, found in raw egg white, binds biotin making it unavailable. Avidin is destroyed by cooking.

Choline

1. As part of the neurotransmitter acetyl choline, transmits nerve impulses.
2. Is essential for one of the membrane phospholipids (phosphatidylcholine).
3. Serves as a methyl donor.

Deficiency symptoms — Poor growth and fatty livers are the deficiency symptoms in most species except chickens and turkeys. Chickens and turkeys develop slipped tendons (perosis). In young rats, choline deficiency produces hemorrhagic lesions in the kidneys and other organs.
Toxicity — No toxic effects have been observed.

Rich sources — Egg yolk, eggs, liver (beef, pork, lamb).
Good sources — Soybeans, potatoes (dehydrated), cabbage, wheat bran, navy beans, alfalfa leaf meal, dried buttermilk, dried skimmed milk, rice polish, rice bran, whole grains (barley, corn, oats, rice, sorghum, wheat), hominy, turnips, wheat flour, blackstrap molasses.
Supplemental sources — Yeast (brewers', torula), wheat germ, soybean lecithin, egg yolk lecithin, and synthetic choline and choline derivatives.

The classification of choline as a vitamin is debated because it does not meet all the criteria for vitamins, especially those of the B vitamins. The body manufactures choline from methionine, with the aid of folacin and Vitamin B-12.

TABLE 49 (CONTINUED)
Vitamins

Functions	Deficiency and Toxicity Symptoms	Sources	Comments
Folacin/Folate (Folic Acid) Folacin coenzymes are responsible for the following important functions: 1. The formation of purines and pyrimidines which, in turn, are needed for the synthesis of the nucleic acids DNA and RNA. 2. The formation of heme, the iron-containing protein in hemoglobin. 3. The interconversion of the three-carbon amino acid serine from the two-carbon amino acid glycine. 4. The formation of the amino acids tyrosine from phenylalanine and glutamic acid from histidine. 5. The formation of the amino acid methionine from homocysteine. 6. The synthesis of choline from ethanolamine. 7. The conversion of nicotinamide to N-methylnicotinamide, one of the metabolites of niacin that is excreted in the urine.	Deficiency symptoms — Megaloblastic anemia (of infancy), also called macrocyticanemia (of pregnancy), in which the red blood cells are larger and fewer than normal, and also immature. The anemia is due to inadequate formation of nucl-proteins, causing failure of the megaloblasts (young red blood cells) in the one marrow to mature. The hemoglobin level is low because of the reduced number of red blood cells, and the white blood cell, blood platelet, and serum folate levels are low. Other symptoms include a sore, red, smooth red tongue (glossitis), disturbances of the digestive tract (diarrhea), and poor growth. Toxicity — Normally, no toxicity.	Rich sources — Liver and kidney. Good sources — Avocados, beans, beets, celery, chickpeas, eggs, fish, green leafy vegetables (such as asparagus, broccoli, Brussels sprouts, cabbage, cauliflower, endive, lettuce, parsley, spinach, turnip greens), nuts, oranges, orange juice, soybeans, and whole wheat products. Supplemental sources — Yeast, wheat germ, and commercially synthesized folic acid (pteroyl-glutamic acid, or PGA).	There is no single vitamin compound with the name folacin; rather, the term folacin is used to designate folic acid and a group of closely related substances which are essential for all vertebrates, including man. Ascorbic acid, vitamin B-12, and vitamin B-6 are essential for the activity of the folacin coenzymes. Folacin deficiencies are thought to be a health problem in the United States and throughout the world. Infants, adolescents, and pregnant women are particularly vulnerable. The folacin requirement is increased by tropical sprue, certain genetic disturbances, cancer, parasitic infection, alcoholism, and oral contraceptives. Raw vegetables stored at room temperature for 2–3 days lose as much as 50–70% of their folate content. Between 50 and 95% of food folate is destroyed in cooking. Intestinal synthesis provides some folacin.

Niacin (Nicotinic acid; nicotinamide) is a constituent of two important coenzymes in the body nicotinamide adenine dinucleotide (NAD) and nicotinamide adenine dinucleotide phosphate (NADP). These coenzymes function as reducing equivalent (H^+) acceptors or donors.

Deficiency symptoms — A deficiency of niacin results in pellagra, the symptoms of which are: dermatitis, particularly of areas of skin which are exposed to light or injury; inflammation of mucous membranes, including the entire gastrointestinal tract, which results in a red, swollen, sore tongue and mouth, diarrhea, and rectal irritation; and psychic changes, such as irritability, anxiety, depression, and in advanced cases, delirium, hallucinations, confusion, disorientation, and stupor.

Toxicity — Only large doses of niacin, sometimes given to an individual with mental illness, are known to be toxic. However, ingestion of large amounts may result in vascular dilation, or "flushing" of the skin, itching, liver damage, elevated blood glucose, elevated blood enzymes, and/or peptic ulcer.

Generally speaking, niacin is found in animal tissues as nicotinamide and in plant tissues as nicotinic acid. Both forms are of equal niacin activity.

Rich sources — Liver, kidney, lean meats, poultry, fish, rabbit, corn flakes (enriched), nuts, peanut butter, milk, cheese, and eggs, although low in niacin content, are good antipellagra foods, because their niacin is in available form. Enriched cereal flours and products are good sources of niacin.

Supplemental sources — Both synthetic nicotinamide and nicotinic acid are commercially available. For pharmaceutical use, nicotinamide is usually used; for food nutrification, nicotinic acid is usually used. Also, yeast is a rich natural source of niacin.

An average mixed diet in the United States provides about 1% protein as tryptophan. Thus, a diet supplying 60 g of protein contains about 600 mg of tryptophan, which will yield about 10 mg of niacin (on the average, 1 mg of niacin is derived from each 60 mg of dietary tryptophan).

Niacin is the most stable of the B-complex vitamins. Cooking losses of a mixed diet usually do not amount to more than 15–25%.

Pantothenic acid (Vitamin B-3)
Pantothenic acid functions as part of two enzymes — coenzyme A (CoA) and acyl carrier protein (ACP).
CoA functions in the following important reactions:
1. The formation of acetyl-choline, a substance of importance in transmitting nerve impulses.
2. The synthesis of porphyrin, a precursor of heme, of importance in hemoglobin synthesis.
3. The synthesis of cholesterol and other sterols.
4. The steroid hormones formed by the adrenal and sex glands.
5. The maintenance of normal blood sugar, and the formation of antibodies.
6. The excretion of sulfonamide drugs. ACP, along with CoA, required by the cells in the synthesis of fatty acids.

Deficiency symptoms — The symptoms: irritableness and restlessness; loss of appetite, indigestion, abdominal pains, nausea; headache; sullenness, mental depression; fatigue, weakness; numbness and tingling of hands and feet, muscle cramps in the arms and legs; burning sensation in the feet; insomnia; respiratory infections; rapid pulse; and a staggering gait. Also, in these subjects there was increased reaction to stress; increased sensitivity to insulin, resulting in low blood sugar levels; increased sedimentation rate for erythrocytes; decreased gastric secretions; and marked decrease in antibody production.

Toxicity — Pantothenic acid is relatively nontoxic. However, doses of 10–20 g per day may result in occasional diarrhea and water retention.

Organ meat (liver, kidney, and heart), cottonseed flour, wheat bran, rice bran, rice polish, nuts, mushrooms, soybean flour, salmon, blue cheese, eggs, buckwheat flour, brown rice, lobster, sunflower seeds.

Supplemental sources — Synthetic calcium pantothenate is widely used as a vitamin supplementation. Yeast is a rich natural supplement.

Intestinal bacteria synthesize pantothenic acid, but the amount and availability is unknown.

Coenzyme A, of which pantothenic acid is a part, is one of the most important substances in body metabolism. It functions in acetyl group transfer and thus is important to fatty acid synthesis and degradation.

TABLE 49 (CONTINUED)
Vitamins

Functions	Deficiency and Toxicity Symptoms	Sources	Comments
Riboflavin (Vitamin B-2) Riboflavin is an integral part of the coenzymes FAD and FMN. These coenzymes accept or donate reducing equivalents.	Deficiency symptoms — Unlike all the other vitamins, riboflavin deficiency is not the cause of any severe or major disease of man. Rather, riboflavin often contributes to other disorders and disabilities such as beriberi, pellagra, scurvy, keratomalacia, and nutritional megaloblastic anemia. Riboflavin deficiency symptoms are: sores at the angles of the mouth (angular stomatitis); sore, swollen, and chapped lips (cheilosis); swollen, fissured, and painful tongue (glossitis); redness and congestion at the edges of the cornea of the eye; and oily, crusty, scaly skin (seborrheic dermatitis). Toxicity — There is no known toxicity of riboflavin.	Rich sources — Organ meats (liver, kidney, heart). Good sources — Corn flakes (enriched), almonds, cheese, eggs, lean meat (beef, pork, lamb), mushrooms (raw), wheat flour (enriched), turnip greens, wheat bran, soybean flour, bacon, cornmeal (enriched). Supplemental sources — Yeast (brewers', torula). Riboflavin is the only vitamin present in significant amounts in beer.	Riboflavin is destroyed by light; and by heat in an alkaline solution.
Thiamin (Vitamin B-1) As a coenzyme in transketolation (Keto-carrying). In direct functions in the body, including (1) maintenance of normal appetite, (2) the tone of the muscles, and (3) a healthy mental attitude.	Moderate thiamin deficiency symptoms include fatigue; apathy (lack of interest); loss of appetite; nausea; moodiness; irritability; depression; retarded growth; a sensation of numbness in the legs; and abnormalities of the electrocardiogram. Severe thiamin deficiency of long duration culminates in beriberi, the symptoms of which are polyneuritis (inflammation of the nerves), emaciation and/or edema, and disturbances of heart function. Toxicity — None.	Thiamin is found in a large variety of animal and vegetable products but is abundant in few. Rich sources — Lean pork, sunflower seed, corn flakes (enriched), peanuts, safflower flour, soybean flour. Good sources — Wheat bran, kidney, wheat flour (enriched), rye flour, nuts (except peanuts, which are a rich source), whole wheat flour, cornmeal (enriched), rice (enriched), white bread (enriched), soybean sprouts. Supplemental sources — Thiamin hydrochloride, thiamin mononitrate, yeast (brewers', torula), rice bran, wheat germ, and rice polish. Enriched flour (bread) and cereal which was initiated in 1941 has been of special significance in improving the dietary level of thiamin in the United States.	

Vitamin B-6

(Pyridoxine; pyridoxal; pyridoxamine)

Vitamin B-6 functions as a coenzyme (pyridoxal phosphate)

a. Transamination
b. Decarboxylation
c. Transsulfuration
d. Tryptophan conversion to nicotinic acid.
e. Absorption of amino acids.
f. The conversion of glycogen to glucose-1-phosphate.
g. The conversion of linoleic acid to arachidonic acid.

Rice bran, wheat bran, sunflower seeds, avocados, bananas, corn, fish, kidney, lean meat, liver, nuts, poultry, rice (brown), soybeans, whole grain.

Supplemental sources — Pyridoxine hydrochloride is the most commonly available synthetic form, and yeast (torula, brewers'), rice polish, and wheat germ are used as natural source supplements.

Deficiency symptoms — In adults, greasy scaliness (seborrheic dermatitis) in the skin around the eyes, nose, and mouth, which subsequently spread to other parts of the body; a smooth, red tongue; loss of weight; muscular weakness; irritability; mental depression. In infants, the deficiency symptoms are irritability, muscular twitchings, and convulsions.

Toxicity — B-6 is relatively nontoxic. But large doses may result in sleepiness and be habit-forming when taken over an extended period.

In rats, the three forms of Vitamin B-6 have equal activity, and it is assumed that the same applies to man.

Processing or cooking foods may destroy up to 50% of the B-6.

Because Vitamin B-6 is limited in many foods, supplemental B-6 with synthetic pyridoxine hydrochloride may be indicated, especially for infants and during pregnancy and lactation.

Vitamin B-12

(Cobalamins)

1. Synthesis or transfer of single carbon units.
2. Biosynthesis of methyl groups (–CH3), and in reduction reactions such as the conversion of disulfide (S–S) to the sulfhydryl group (–SH).

Liver and other organ meats — kidney, heart, muscle meats, fish, shellfish, eggs, and cheese.

Supplemental sources — Cobalamin, of which there are at least three active forms, produced by microbial growth; available at the corner drugstore.

Some B-12 is synthesized in the intestinal tract of human beings. However, little of it may be absorbed.

Deficiency symptoms — Vitamin B-12 deficiency in man may occur as a result of (1) dietary lack, which sometimes occurs among vegetarians who consume no animal food, or (2) deficiency of intrinsic factor due to pernicious anemia, total or partial removal of the stomach by surgery, or infestation with parasites such as the fish tapeworm.

The common symptoms of a dietary deficiency of Vitamin B-12 are sore tongue, weakness, loss of weight, back pains, tingling of the extremities, apathy, and mental and other nervous abnormalities. Anemia is rarely seen in dietary deficiency of B-12.

In pernicious anemia, the characteristic symptoms are abnormally large red blood cells, lemon-yellow pallor, anorexia, prolonged bleeding time, abdominal discomfort, loss of weight, glossitis, an unsteady gait, and neurological disturbances, including stiffness of the limbs, irritability, and mental depression. Without treatment death follows.

Toxicity — No toxic effects of Vitamin B-12 are known.

Plants cannot manufacture Vitamin B-12.

Vitamin B-12 is the largest and the most complex of all vitamin molecules.

Vitamin B-12 is the only vitamin that requires a specific gastrointestinal factor for its absorption (intrinsic factor), and the absorption of Vitamin B-12 in the small intestine requires about 3 hours.

TABLE 49 (CONTINUED)
Vitamins

Functions	Deficiency and Toxicity Symptoms	Sources	Comments
Vitamin C (Ascorbic acid) Formation and maintenance of collagen, the substance that binds body cells together. Metabolism of the amino acids tyrosine and tryptophan. Absorption and movement of iron. Metabolism of fats and lipids and cholesterol control. Sound teeth and bones. Strong capillary walls and healthy blood vessels. Metabolism of folic acid.	Deficiency symptoms — Early symptoms, called latent scurvy: loss in weight, listlessness, fatigue, fleeting pains in the joints and muscles, irritability, shortness of breath, sore and bleeding gums, small hemorrhages under the skin, bones that fracture easily, and poor wound healing. Scurvy — Swollen, bleeding and ulcerated gums; loose teeth; malformed and weak bones, fragility of the capillaries with resulting hemorrhages throughout the body; large bruises; big joints, such as the knees and hips, due to bleeding into the joint cavity; anemia; degeneration of muscle fibers, including those of the heart; and tendency of old wounds to become red and break open. Sudden death from severe internal hemorrhage and heart failure. Toxicity — Adverse effects reported of intakes in excess of 8 g per day (more than 100 times the recommended allowance) include nausea, abdominal cramps, and diarrhea; absorption of excessive amounts of iron; destruction of red blood cells; increased mobilization of bone minerals; interference with anticoagulant therapy; formation of kidney and bladder stones; inactivation of Vitamin B-12; rise in plasma cholesterol; and possible dependence upon large doses of Vitamin C.	Natural sources of Vitamin C occur primarily in fruits (especially citrus fruits) and leafy vegetables — acerola cherry, *camu-camu*, and rose hips, raw, frozen, or canned citrus fruit or juice, oranges, grapefruit, lemons, and limes. Guavas, peppers (green, hot), black currants, parsley, turnip greens, poke greens, and mustard greens. Good sources — Green leafy vegetables: broccoli, Brussels sprouts, cabbage (red), cauliflower, collards, kale, lamb's-quarter, spinach, Swiss chard, and watercress. Also, cantaloupe, papaya, strawberries, and tomatoes and tomato juice (fresh or canned). Supplemental sources — Vitamin C (ascorbic acid) is available wherever vitamins are sold.	All animal species appear to require Vitamin C, but dietary need is limited to humans, guinea pigs, monkeys, fruit bats, birds, certain fish, and certain reptiles. Of all the vitamins, ascorbic acid is the most unstable. It is easily destroyed during storage, processing, and cooking; it is water-soluble, easily oxidized, and attacked by enzymes.

Note: Some nutritionists include inositol, coenzyme Q (ubiquinone), the bioflavinoids and carnitine as essential nutrients or as vitamins. While these compounds are essential to normal metabolism, the needs for them as essential nutrients can depend on the physiologic state of the consumer. Premature infants require carnitine in the diet because they do not synthesize adequate amounts. Similarly, inositol is synthesized in the body; however, there may be instances where that synthesis is inadequate. Ubiquinone and the bioflavinoids have yet to be shown as essential dietary ingredients for humans. Some drugs interfere with vitamin use. These are listed in Table 50.

TABLE 50
Drugs that Influence Vitamin Use

Drug Class	Nutrient Affected
Diuretics	
Spironolactone	Vitamin A
Thiazide	Potassium
Bile Acid Sequestrant	
Cholestyramine	Vitamin A, Vitamin B_{12}, Folacin
Colestipol	Vitamin A, Vitamin K, Vitamin D
Laxative	
Phenolphthalein	Vitamin A, Vitamin D, Vitamin K, Potassium
Anticonvulsant	
Phenytoin	Vitamin D, Vitamin K, Folacin
Anticoagulant	
Coumarin, decoumarol	Vitamin K
Warafin	
Immunosuppressant	
Cyclosporin	Vitamin K
Antibacterial	
Isoniazid	Niacin, B_6
Sulfasalazine	Folacin
p-aminosalicylic acid	Vitamin B_{12}
Neomycin	Vitamin B_{12}
Tetracycline	Calcium, Magnesium, Iron, Zinc
Antiinflammatant	
Phenylbutazone	Niacin
Chelating agents	
EDTA	Calcium, Magnesium, Lead
Penicillamine	Copper, Vitamin B_6
Thiosemicarbazide	Vitamin B_6
Anticholinergic	
L-DOPA	Vitamin B_6
Antihypertensive	
Hydralazine	Vitamin B_6
Antimalarial	
Pyrimethamine	Folacin
Antineoplastic	
Methotrexate	Folacin
Antihistamine	
Ametidine	Vitamin B_{12}
Theophylline	Protein
Antacids	
Aluminum hydroxide	Folate, phosphate
Magnesium hydroxide	Phosphate
Sodium bicarbonate	Folacin
Other	
Ethanol	Niacin, Folacin, Thiamin
Mineral Oil	Vitamin A, β carotene

WHEAT ALLERGY

A condition where the individual is intolerant to wheat products in the diet.

Wheat contains water, starch, lipids, and the proteins albumin, globulins, and gluten. Gluten consists of gliadin and glutenine. The various proteins in wheat can cause different symptoms. One example is the so-called baker's asthma in bakers allergic to wheat albumin. This reaction shows itself when wheat dust is inhaled. In food allergy, globulins and glutenine are the most important allergens. Allergic reactions can occur following the ingestion of wheat. In celiac disease, an allergy to gliadin plays an important role in the pathogenesis. After exposure to gluten, infiltration of eosinophils and neutrophils, along with edema and an increase in vascular permeability of the mucosa of the small intestine, can be observed. If the allergic reaction is chronic, the infiltration consists mainly of lymphocytes and plasma cells. Furthermore, flattening of the mucosal surface is found. The disorder manifests itself typically 6–12 months after introduction of gluten into the diet. It is characterized initially by intermittent symptoms such as abdominal pain, irritability, and diarrhea. If not treated, anemia, various deficiencies and growth failure may occur as a result of malabsorption. Improvement is seen about 2 weeks after elimination of gluten from the diet. In addition to the immunological reaction to gluten, a direct toxic effect may also play a role in causing the disease.

WHEAT GERM

The fatty portion of the wheat grain; rich source of Vitamin E.

WHEY

Proteins in milk that separate out when milk is coagulated with renin. These are the proteins that comprise cheese.

WHOLE GRAIN CEREALS

Cereals which contain all parts of the grain from which it is made.

WILSON'S DISEASE

Abnormal accumulation of copper in tissues.

XANTHINE

Nitrogenous extract formed during the metabolism of nucleoproteins. Three methylated xanthines include caffeine, theophylline, and theobromine.

XEROPHTHALMIA

Vitamin A deficiency. One of the leading causes of blindness in the world.

ZEARALENONE

A mycotoxin produced by *Fusarium tricinctum*, *Fusarium gibbosum*, *Fusarium roseum*, and three subspecies of the latter, *Fusarium roseum culmorum*, *Fusarium roseum equiseti*, and *Fusarium roseum graminearum*. In animals, it has been shown to possess oestrogenic and anabolic properties. The production of zearalenone by *Fusarium roseum* required alternating high (24–27°C) and low (12–14°C) temperatures. The lower temperature is necessary for the induction of the biosynthetic enzyme for zearalenone, whereas the higher temperature is important in the proceeding of the biosynthesis. Food types involved in the contamination of zearalenone include maize, wheat, flour, and milk.

ZELLWEGER SYNDROME

Rare fatal genetic disease. Victims of this disorder do not make bile acids or plasmalogens nor are they able to shorten the very long fatty acids. These biochemical deficiencies are seemingly unrelated to the structural abnormalities observed in liver, kidney, muscle, and brain.

ZINC

A cofactor of a variety of enzymes mediating metabolic pathways, such as alcohol dehydrogenation, lactic dehydrogenation, superoxide dismutation, and alkaline phosphorylation. It occurs especially in meat, (whole) grains, and legumes. The Recommended Dietary Allowance for zinc is 12–15 mg, depending on the age, while the zinc intake is about 10 mg per day. Acute toxicity, including gastrointestinal irritation and vomiting, has been observed following the ingestion of 2 g or more of zinc in the form of sulfate (see Table 28 on minerals).

ZYMOGENS

An inactive enzyme.

APPENDIX

General Guidelines for Food Selection to Optimize Health. Before one can provide general statements about food choice we must recognize that these choices are not only due to the recognition of the need for food to avoid starvation but also due to a variety of nonfood, nonhealth, considerations. Among these are food availability, ethnic identity, economic status, education, occupation, gender, age, physiological status, religious beliefs, and individual factors of likes, dislikes, tolerances, and intolerances. Advertising of specific food products, peer pressure, and availability of restaurants and take-out food producers also influence food acceptance and food choice. Having acknowledged the above, there are some general guidelines that if followed will result in a healthy diet. In the United States the Department of Agriculture has developed a food guide called the Food Guide Pyramid. This consists of six groups of foods arranged in order of number of servings a day as follows:

Bread, cereal, rice, pasta	6–11 servings/day
Fruits	2–4 servings/day
Vegetables (including potatoes)	3–5 servings/day
Meat, poultry, fish, dry beans, nuts, eggs	2–3 servings/day
Milk, yogurt, cheese	2–3 servings/day
Fats, oils, sweets	use sparingly

What does this food guide mean? A serving can be defined in varying amounts. Is a serving of meat 4 oz or 8 oz? One can use this guide to translate desired energy intakes into a real diet as follows:

Energy Intake (kcal)	1600	2200	2800
Bread	6	9	11
Vegetable	3	4	5
Fruits	2	3	4
Meats	2	2	3
Milk	2	2	3

A serving of bread = 1 slice bread or 1/2 cup pasta, rice, cereal
A serving of vegetable = 1/2 cup cooked vegetable, 1 cup raw
A serving of fruit = 1/2 cup
A serving of meat = 2-3 oz
A serving of milk = 8 fluid oz or cheese equivalent (1.5 oz)

Restricted energy diets

Weight loss will be achieved if energy intake is exceeded by energy expenditure. Energy expenditure = Basal energy need (see Table 12) plus Activity increment (see Table 2).

To reduce energy intake delete as much fat and free sugar from the diet. Substitute reduced fat products for regular products; substitute artifically sweetened products for products containing sucrose or/and fructose; select lean meat; substitute chicken (without skin), turkey, or fish for well marbled meat; avoid fried foods substitute broiling, boiling, or steaming cooking methods for deep fat grilling methods for food preparation; substitute raw unprocessed fruits and vegetables for cooked or prepared fruits and vegetables; substitute skim milk for whole milk. Making these substitutions to the 1600 kcal diet described above will result in a 20–30% reduction in energy intake. If the energy intake is less than 1200 kcal, the individual may not be well-nourished with respect to the micronutrients. A supplement may be needed under these conditions. See Tables 28 and 32 for assessing nutritional status.

Low income diets

Diets for people under economic stress are difficult to prescribe because of local factors which influence food cost. However, using the Food Guide Pyramid some general suggestions can be made:

1. Avoid prepared/processed foods. If a kitchen is available it is generally less expensive to make a given dish than to buy it already prepared.
2. Substitute eggs, cheese, chicken, peanut butter, dried beans, and peas for beef, veal, and pork.
3. Avoid snack foods; they are high cost items with little nutritional value.
4. Use fresh fruits and vegetables in season when their cost is lowest.
5. If good storage is possible, buy large volumes of foods that store well, i.e., potatoes, root vegetables, apples, and oranges in season. These items need cool, well-ventilated storage and will last several months.

Diets for the elderly

Food choices for the elderly are not much different for younger adults providing these elders have good teeth (or well-fitting dentures) and are not constrained by degenerative disease or economic/social factors. The elderly may have more fixed ideas about food choice and may also need to reduce their energy intake, yet may need larger amounts of essential micronutrients (see Table 43). Malnutrition in the elderly can result if one ignores these two factors.

Diets for infants and children

Again the Food Guide Pyramid can be used as a general guide and Table 43 should be consulted. Infants usually consume milk as their main source of nutrients. Solid foods are gradually introduced such that by the age of two a variety of foods are consumed. Because young children are far more sensitive to flavors and textures the foods offered to children should be monitored with these factors in mind. Highly seasoned items may be rejected as well as items that are tough or gritty or rough textured. Older children may develop food "jags" which means that they wish to eat only certain food items over many days. With time these behaviors change.